Threats to Fetal, Placental and Myometrial Oxygenation

Thomas L. Archer

Threats to Fetal, Placental and Myometrial Oxygenation

A Unified Hemodynamic Approach

Springer

Thomas L. Archer
San Antonio, TX, USA

ISBN 978-3-031-60363-1 ISBN 978-3-031-60364-8 (eBook)
https://doi.org/10.1007/978-3-031-60364-8

This Springer imprint is published by the registered company Springer Nature Switzerland AG
The registered company address is: Gewerbestrasse 11, 6330 Cham, Switzerland

Foreword

For the nine months before birth we are totally dependent on the functioning of our placenta, the afterbirth, for our well-being. Although the basic structure of the organ is well known, there are many aspects of placental physiology that are still poorly understood. In this book, the author, a former obstetric anesthetist, sheds new light on a critical issue that affects all pregnant women especially in the later stages, namely how their body position affects blood flow to the placenta and hence the supply of oxygen to their baby. Through the text and copious illustrations, entertainingly embellished with personal experiences and informative clinical anecdotes, Dr. Archer sets out the hemodynamic principles governing the placental circulations. The key message he promotes is that it is now possible to monitor, and hence maximize, the mother's blood flow to the placenta non-invasively rather than relying on what may be inaccurate assumptions. If adopted, his technique could prevent periods when the uterus and baby are starved of oxygen, hypoxia, and so improve obstetric outcomes.

The placenta has two separate circulations, a maternal and a fetal circulation, and the relationship between the two poses unique hemodynamic challenges. The maternal placental circulation is very unusual in that the uterine arteries terminate at the surface of the placenta. The maternal blood flows out from the ends of the vessels into a cavity within the placenta, the intervillous space, where it bathes the fetal component of the organ, a series of highly branched villous trees. After percolating between the villi, exchanging nutrients and respiratory gases as it does so, the maternal blood re-enters the maternal vascular system by draining into the uterine veins. The finger-like fetal villi contain a network of arteries, capillaries, and veins that connect to the baby via the umbilical cord. This maternal–fetal relationship has been likened to the fronds of a sea anemone (fetal) wafting in the water of a rock pool (maternal). Oxygen and many nutrients pass between the two circulations by simple diffusion through the covering of the villi. To aid this process, there are dome-like specializations along the surface of the villi where that covering is very thin, reducing the distance between the maternal and fetal circulations to as little as 2–3 thousandths of a millimeter. And herein lies the problem: how can such delicate areas be maintained when the villi are immersed in maternal arterial blood that is normally at a much higher pressure than that of the baby?

To avoid potential compression of the specializations, the maternal vessels supplying the placenta display another unique feature. Whereas in other circulations arteries reduce in diameter as they run to their target organ, in the case of the uterus and placenta they dilate. This is especially true of the terminal branches of the uterine arteries as they approach the placenta, for they are transformed into funnel-shaped dilations by the actions of placental cells. This remodeling has the opposite effect of placing your finger over the end of a hose pipe, enabling a high volume of flow but at a slow velocity and a low pressure.

While considerable attention has been paid to the dynamics of the inflowing blood over the last few decades, much less has been paid to another key determinant, that maternal venous outflow from the intervillous space must be unimpeded. Dr. Archer rightly champions the importance of this neglected requirement, placing it as the central tenet in this book and updating ideas of how obstruction of placental venous outflow may lead to adverse obstetric outcomes. The pregnant uterus is a large and heavy object, and when a woman lies on her back it rests against the spine. Interposed between the two is the vena cava, the main vein draining the lower half of the body, including the uterus. As Dr. Archer illustrates, compression of the vein can impede uteroplacental blood flow, causing the wall of the uterus and the baby to become hypoxic. Even more seriously, digital compression of the vein at the time of caesarean section has been reported to result in premature separation of the placenta from the uterine wall, placental abruption. Because of these dangers, women in late pregnancy are recommended to lie on their left sides on the assumption that this avoids compression of the vena cava.

As Dr. Archer highlights, this perceived wisdom is an oversimplification of the true situation. Firstly, there are alternative routes by which the venous blood can return to the heart, and the magnitude of the effects of caval compression will depend on the efficacy of those routes. Secondly, from his own clinical experience, he has shown that even when women lie on the left side, compression of the vena cava can still occur. Until now, obstetricians have had no way of assessing how compromised the placental circulation is when the mother adopts different positions. Dr. Archer elegantly demonstrates how the degree can be accurately quantified by measuring the impact on cardiac output. Obstruction of the vena cava results in less venous return to the heart and so a reduction in cardiac output. Hence, monitoring cardiac output can provide a proxy measure of acute uteroplacental hypoxia.

By identifying this easily assessed clinical index, Dr. Archer enables uteroplacental blood flow to be maximized on an individual basis when a heavily pregnant woman lies down. His quantitative data confirm what has long been suspected but never proven and provide a robust scientific foundation to inform clinical practice. Future generations will be grateful for Dr. Archer's insightful intellectual musings while administering anesthetics at the head-end of the delivery couch.

Cambridge, UK Graham J. Burton

Preface

I have been wanting to write this book since 2010 when, one morning at Board Rounds in Labor and Delivery at the University Hospital of the University of California San Diego, I started to try to look at maternal hemodynamics from the point of view of the uterus itself, rather than the mother. The dangers to the mother of "aortocaval compression" in pregnancy have been taught for decades in medical schools and nursing programs, but always with an emphasis on short-term maternal problems with blood pressure or—if the discussion was more sophisticated—with cardiac output. But no one seemed to look at the question from the point of view of the uterus itself and to try to imagine what might happen to the uterus and its precious contents earlier in gestation, long before term. Specifically, no one seemed to try to imagine what extended periods of increased uterine venous pressure from aortocaval compression might do to the fetus, placenta, myometrium, or vagina.

The main theory of this book—that unrecognized and chronic or recurrent obstruction of uterine venous return might harm the fetus, placenta, myometrium, or vagina during the second half of pregnancy—may seem incredibly simple, old-fashioned, and very low-tech. It does not involve genomics, transcriptomics, or proteomics and it probably does not offer many opportunities to develop new medications. The theory—besides appearing difficult to investigate (which it is not)—may seem boring. But this boring theory might be true, and it might be important. But it has not been investigated yet, and that is why I have written this book—to encourage you to investigate it.

But even if this theory is true, preventing or mitigating the impact of obstruction of uterine venous return on maternal and fetal health might still face obstacles. There would be no easy pill to take, and preventing the problem would involve changes in perspective and behavior on the part of pregnant women and their obstetricians, midwives, nurses, and anesthesiologists. Obstetrics and obstetric nursing care have been focused on fetal heart rate since the introduction of electronic fetal monitoring in the 1970s, but it may well be that fetal heart rate changes—as well as preeclampsia, fetal growth restriction, preterm birth, dysfunctional labor, and postpartum uterine atony—are the late-appearing *results* of a fetal environment which has been unfavorable for a long time. Also, fetal heart rate changes may not occur at all when serious injury to the fetus, placenta, or myometrium develops slowly and gradually over time. Preeclampsia and fetal growth restriction are almost certainly the late results of ongoing injury—to which we respond at present only in a reactive manner. It would be far better to prevent that injury in the first place!

Fetal heart rate is easy to understand, but cardiac output—and the technologies used to measure or trend it—represents a whole new world for health care providers outside of critical care medicine. Furthermore, fully understanding this new world would require an exercise of the imagination—looking at gestation and labor from a hemodynamic perspective and trying to understand the individual oxygen requirements of four different entities: the fetus, the placenta, the myometrium, and the vagina.

If the theory turns out to be true, additional good news is that we probably now have an easy way of knowing when obstruction of uterine venous return is really taking place and when it is not, rather than relying on the simplistic assumption that "supine is bad" and "left side down is good" when it comes to maternal positioning. Reproducible, positional reductions in maternal cardiac output can be used as an immediate "early warning" signal that uterine venous return has been obstructed at the inferior vena cava, *and this early warning—if heeded—might enable the patient and her care-givers to rectify an unfavorable hemodynamic situation in the female reproductive system before it can cause serious problems.* It is possible that this ability to *prevent* serious pregnancy-related disease, rather than merely reacting to it, might be a breakthrough in maternal and fetal health. Of course, this may just be a dream, but the possible benefit is so great that this theory cries out for investigation (at least in my highly prejudiced opinion).

You may be wondering, "Why is Dr. Archer bringing this crazy idea up now? Haven't we known about this problem since the 1950s? What's so special now?" The answer—in part—is that certain pregnancy-related problems have not gone away, despite the dramatic advances in obstetrics and general medical care of the last 70 years. The incidences of preeclampsia, fetal growth restriction, preterm birth, and dysfunctional labor have not decreased over the last 70 years, and in fact, some of those conditions appear to be more common than they were a few decades ago. Of course, pregnant women are older and have more pre-existing conditions than in the past—but could it also be that we are missing something very simple in the picture that is fundamental and should be obvious, were it not so simple and well-known? *In other words, there may be a problem hiding in plain sight.*

Could it be that the obesity epidemic or our increasingly sedentary life-style has something to do with some of these pregnancy-related problems? With respect to dysfunctional labor, is it possible that our method of managing epidural labor analgesia has something to do with allowing it to develop? Could it be that the midwives, with their emphasis on mobility and physical activity during labor are promoting optimal uteroplacental perfusion in a way that mainstream obstetrics and anesthesiology are neglecting? Might there be a way of achieving both excellent labor analgesia and optimal perfusion of the placenta and myometrium during labor?

If the ideas presented in this book have any validity, they would best be understood and presented as a means of optimizing the fetal, placental, myometrial, and vaginal environment during pregnancy in order to prevent problems in pregnancy from arising in the first place. Improving the fetal, placental, myometrial, and vaginal environment through optimal placental, myometrial, and pelvic perfusion would best be understood and practiced as a routine part of prenatal care—like taking prenatal vitamins: very simple, routine, and important and with the possible benefit of fewer cesarean deliveries and fewer neonatal intensive care unit admissions.

I will close this Preface by admitting that this book mostly presents ideas and theories, but I also believe that the amount of circumstantial evidence which supports—or at least is compatible with—the ideas presented this book is substantial. There has also been a revolution in non-invasive technology that now makes investigation of these ideas quite easy. I am not asking you to *believe* the theories presented in this book. All I am asking is that you believe that they *might* be true and that they are important enough to be investigated further.

San Antonio, TX, USA
April 4, 2024

Thomas L. Archer

Acknowledgements

I want to begin by thanking Graham J. Burton for his immensely beneficial help. For almost a year now, he has helped me clarify and refine my thinking about multiple issues regarding placental anatomy, function, and oxygenation. I am very grateful to him for his time and patience and his intellectual support has encouraged me greatly while writing this book. I also want to thank Jerasimos ("Jerry") Ballas and Erin Martin, who helped me develop these ideas while we worked together in San Diego over a decade ago.

I also want to thank the following wonderful obstetricians with whom I had the honor and pleasure to work for seven years at the University of California San Diego: Thomas Moore, Steve Hebert, Yvette Lacoursiere, Doug Woelkers, Andy Hull, Sandy Ramos, and Bob Resnik. I also want to thank Karen Perdion and all of the other midwives with whom it was such a pleasure to work at UCSD and from whom I learned so much.

The atmosphere I experienced on Labor and Delivery at UCSD from 2008 until I retired in 2015 was—for me—an unprecedented experience of the highest quality clinical care combined with a remarkable atmosphere of friendly, constructive, and respectful collegiality. I am profoundly grateful for my opportunity to work in that environment, and my years at UCSD as the Director of Obstetric Anesthesia were—for me—the highlight of my career and my happiest time in medical practice. Lastly, I want to express my gratitude to my wife Azucena—for being the wonderful person and wife that she is. Her wisdom, common sense, and loving support have made all the difference.

Contents

Obstruction of Uterine Venous Return

1

Personal Note
In 1978 when I was getting ready to graduate from anesthesiology residency and start private practice at a local hospital, I went to an obstetric anesthesiology conference organized by practitioners in the community to see what I might have missed during my residency. After the conference I was sure that there had been no coordination between the speakers because all their talks delivered the same basic message: avoid aortocaval compression when caring for pregnant patients in order to avoid maternal hypotension and fetal distress. Of course, I had heard about this concept repeatedly during medical school and residency and had become fully aware of the dangers of the "supine hypotensive syndrome of pregnancy." But no one had ever suggested that obstruction of the inferior vena cava and uterine venous return could be more than an acute problem which can occur during the later stages of pregnancy. Specifically, no one suggested that it might cause problems in a less obvious and dramatic manner—and much earlier in gestation. I began to develop that idea in 2009—some 31 years later—when I was Director of Obstetric Anesthesia at the University of California San Diego.

Can Obstruction of Uterine Venous Return Injure the Fetus, Placenta, or Myometrium During the Second Half of Pregnancy?

Obstruction of uterine venous return occurs when the gravid uterus compresses the inferior vena cava against the lower lumbar spine, as shown in panel (a) on the left side of Figs. 1.1 and 1.2. Relief of that obstruction is shown in panel (b) on the right side of Figs. 1.1 and 1.3. The aorta can be compressed by the uterus to some extent as well, but most authors agree that most of the hemodynamic effects of what is called "aortocaval compression" are caused by obstruction of the inferior vena cava.

T. L. Archer, *Threats to Fetal, Placental and Myometrial Oxygenation*,
https://doi.org/10.1007/978-3-031-60364-8_1

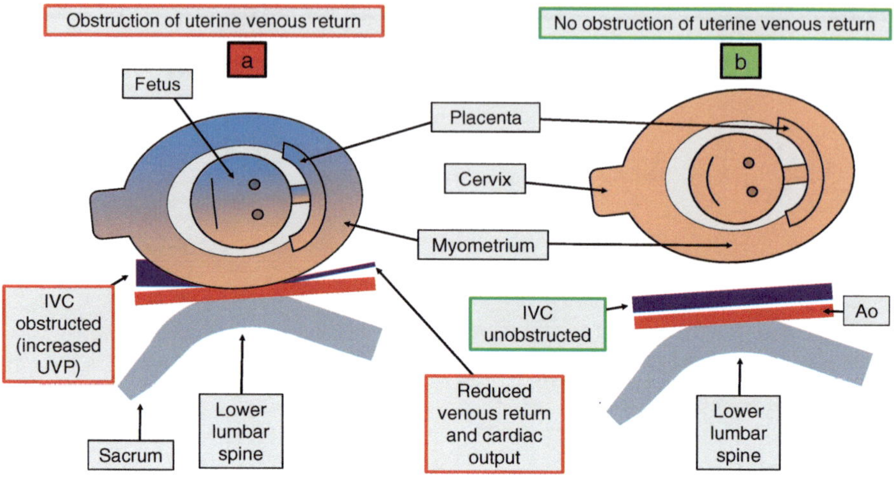

Fig. 1.1 The gravid uterus can compress the inferior vena cava and aorta against the lumbar spine in many different positions—not just the supine position. This figure contains two schematic lateral views of the abdomen of a pregnant woman, centered on the lower lumbar spine and lumbosacral promontory where the gravid uterus often obstructs uterine venous return at the inferior vena cava. The gravid uterus often—but not always—obstructs the inferior vena cava in the lumbar region when a pregnant woman lies supine near term, but the specific anatomy and effects of this obstruction vary widely. Some women are asymptomatic, whereas other women become nauseated, sweaty, light-headed, tachycardic and can even lose consciousness in what is known as the "supine hypotensive syndrome of pregnancy." Also, obstruction of uterine venous return can occur in positions other than supine. *The lesson is that obstruction of uterine venous return is variable, both in terms of the positions which cause it and in terms of the effects that this obstruction has on the mother.* The situation shown in panel (**a**) on the left—obstruction of uterine venous return which is causing fetal, placental, and myometrial hypoxia—*might* occur in the supine position, or it might occur in other positions, *and it might or might not cause maternal symptoms, depending on the mother's cardiovascular response to the decrease in cardiac output.* With respect to panel (**b**) on the right, unobstructed uterine venous return with optimal uteroplacental perfusion and oxygenation *often* occurs in the left lateral position but may also occur in other positions—including the supine position. The figure also indicates that when obstruction of uterine venous return occurs at the inferior vena cava, the maternal cardiac output decreases—and these decreases in cardiac output can be used as an objective and early warning signal for the need to change a pregnant patient's position. *This book argues that some objective method is needed to know when the inferior vena cava is obstructed and when it is not, and this use of positional reductions of maternal cardiac output to identify obstruction of the inferior vena cava has been termed "cardiac output-guided maternal positioning." Ao* aorta, *IVC* inferior vena cava, *UVP* uterine venous pressure

It has been well known for decades that such obstruction—late in gestation and in the short term—can cause severe maternal symptoms and fetal death [1–8]. Much less well considered and investigated is the possibility that unrecognized and prolonged obstruction of uterine venous return might occur much earlier in gestation and might play a role in causing preeclampsia, fetal growth restriction, preterm birth, dysfunctional labor, and postpartum uterine atony [9–15].

In the past, even considering this possibility might have been considered a pointless theoretical exercise, since obstruction of uterine venous return could not be

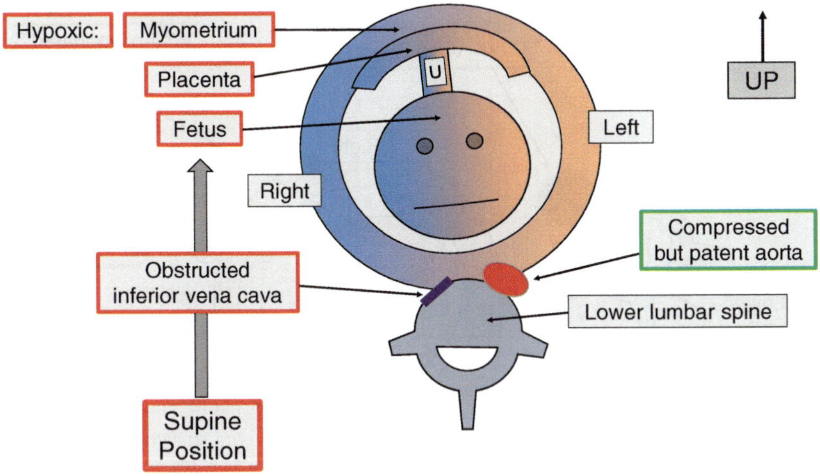

Fig. 1.2 Obstruction of uterine venous return by the gravid uterus may injure the fetus, placenta, or myometrium during the second half of gestation. This figure is a schematic transverse view of the abdomen of a pregnant woman at the level of the lower lumbar spine. In this example, the woman is lying supine and her gravid uterus is obstructing its own venous return. This obstruction causes two things to happen: (1) reduced perfusion of the placental intervillous spaces and myometrium and (2) increased uterine venous and intervillous space pressure. In this example, the obstruction of uterine venous return is caused by the supine position, but this same obstruction could occur in other positions, and the supine position does not invariably cause this unfavorable situation. I am not aware of any technique currently in common use for the *early* detection of suboptimal uteroplacental perfusion during pregnancy—but cardiac output-guided maternal positioning might serve that purpose. *U* umbilical cord

detected easily and objectively, but techniques now appear to be available for detecting hemodynamically significant inferior vena cava obstruction easily, safely, and on a continuous and real-time basis. One technique for detecting this obstruction of venous return at the inferior vena cava depends on the fact that such obstruction decreases maternal cardiac output within less than a minute, and maternal cardiac output can now be trended easily, safely, non-invasively, and on a continuous and hands-free basis. In short, obstruction of uterine venous return at the inferior vena cava can now be detected by detecting the decrease in maternal cardiac output which it causes.

This new capability may now make it possible to prevent injury to mothers and fetuses if obstruction of uterine venous return during the second half of gestation is found to be detrimental to fetal or maternal health. The new non-invasive technology may also enable the early detection of obstruction of uterine venous return during labor, before it results in recognized maternal hypotension or overt "fetal distress" as manifest by changes in fetal heart rate and variability [10, 16, 17]. This new "early-warning" capability might make labor management both safer for the mother and fetus and less crisis-driven for the obstetric care team.

This possibility of preventing or mitigating a large burden of disease using well-known concepts and readily available non-invasive technology may represent

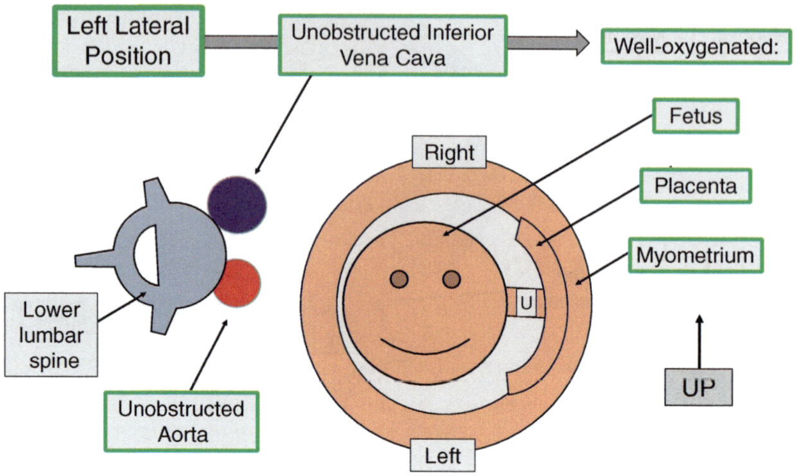

Fig. 1.3 Unobstructed uterine venous return is probably essential for optimal fetal, placental, and myometrial health. This figure represents the same anatomy as shown in the preceding figure—a transverse section through a pregnant abdomen at the level of the lower lumbar spine. The woman is lying on her left side and both the inferior vena cava and the aorta are completely unobstructed, allowing excellent uteroplacental perfusion and fetal oxygenation, since aortic pressure is normal and uterine venous pressure is low. In this example, excellent uterine perfusion is being achieved in the left lateral position, which tends to displace the uterus off the inferior vena cava and aorta, but equally good uteroplacental perfusion might occur in other positions as well. Unfortunately, in the absence of maternal symptoms or fetal heart rate changes suggestive of fetal hypoxia, we currently have no way of knowing in a specific person which maternal positions provide optimal uteroplacental perfusion and which do not—unless we use cardiac output-guided maternal positioning. *U* umbilical cord

"low-hanging fruit" in the effort to improve the health care of pregnant women and their fetuses. Of course, this is just a theory—but it is a biologically plausible one that merits further investigation, and it is a major purpose of this book to stimulate such investigation.

Electrical Cardiometry for Trending Maternal Cardiac Output During Pregnancy

In 2009, my colleagues and I at the University of California San Diego began to use electrical cardiometry (a type of impedance cardiography) to trend cardiac output in pregnant patients. Avoiding aortocaval compression through proper patient positioning was (and still is) a cornerstone of the care of the pregnant patient, and it had always been emphasized in training that obstruction of the inferior vena cava by the gravid uterus causes a reduction in maternal cardiac output. But we had never actually *seen* the cardiac output before now. We only saw the blood pressure that resulted from the product of the cardiac output and the systemic vascular resistance, and both of these latter concepts had always seemed somewhat mysterious—they were frequently discussed but never really *seen*! In 2009, we were hoping to start measuring—or at least trending—maternal cardiac output continuously, and I was hoping to actually *see* cardiac output—and to see it change in real time. At that point, I started to make simple drawings to help me think about the hemodynamics of pregnancy.

The Hemodynamics of Pregnancy

Figure 1.4 shows the normal circulation of a healthy pregnancy. The mother, fetus, placenta, and myometrium are all well oxygenated by maternal blood, which then easily returns to the mother's heart, resulting in a robust cardiac output. Specifically—as shown in the figure—the mother's arterial blood pressure is adequate to perfuse a low-impedance placenta and myometrium. The deoxygenated blood from the uterus then flows easily into a low-pressure system of uterine and iliac veins which then empty into a patent inferior vena cava—which then provides an unobstructed

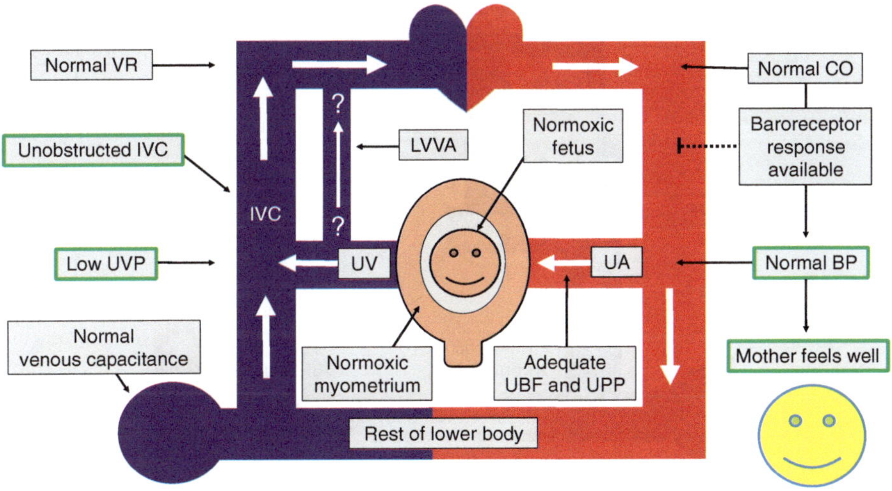

Fig. 1.4 Hemodynamics of healthy pregnancy *without* inferior vena cava obstruction. In a healthy pregnancy, the blood volume and cardiac output increase and the systemic vascular resistance and blood pressure decrease. The uterine veins normally drain into the iliac veins and then into the inferior vena cava, but a collateral lumbar, vertebral venous, and azygos venous system exists in many patients (labeled LVVA in the figure) which carries venous blood back to the heart if the inferior vena cava is obstructed. Venous return becomes cardiac output within less than a minute and therefore any reduction in venous return will cause an immediate reduction of cardiac output. The aortic and carotid sinus baroreceptor system is available to activate the sympathetic nervous system to maintain maternal blood pressure if the cardiac output decreases, but that system varies in its activity and effectiveness from person to person. *BP* arterial blood pressure, *CO* cardiac output, *IVC* inferior vena cava, *LVVA* lumbar, vertebral venous, and azygos collateral venous return pathways to heart, *UA* uterine arteries, *UBF* uterine blood flow, *UPP* uterine perfusion pressure (arterial minus venous), *UV* uterine veins, *UVP* uterine venous pressure, *VR* venous return

route for the venous blood to return to the heart and be immediately converted into cardiac output. The baroreceptors that help maintain normal maternal blood pressure during daily events are not being called upon to work especially hard in the situation shown in Fig. 1.4, since the cardiac output is normal, and therefore strong activation of the sympathetic nervous system is not required to maintain adequate blood pressure.

Another important detail of Fig. 1.4 is that there are two separate ways for the venous blood emerging from the uterus to get back to the heart: (1) via the inferior vena cava, which is the normal route, and (2) via an alternate lumbar, vertebral venous, and azygos collateral pathway labeled LVVA. Figure 1.5 shows how the LVVA pathway can compensate for obstruction of the inferior vena cava by the uterus, *but only if the LVVA pathway is sufficiently well developed* [18–23]. The following is a key point: *unobstructed uterine venous return—either through the inferior vena cava or through a compensatory collateral lumbar, vertebral venous, and azygos system—is important not only because it keeps the maternal cardiac output high but also because it keeps the uterine venous pressure low.*

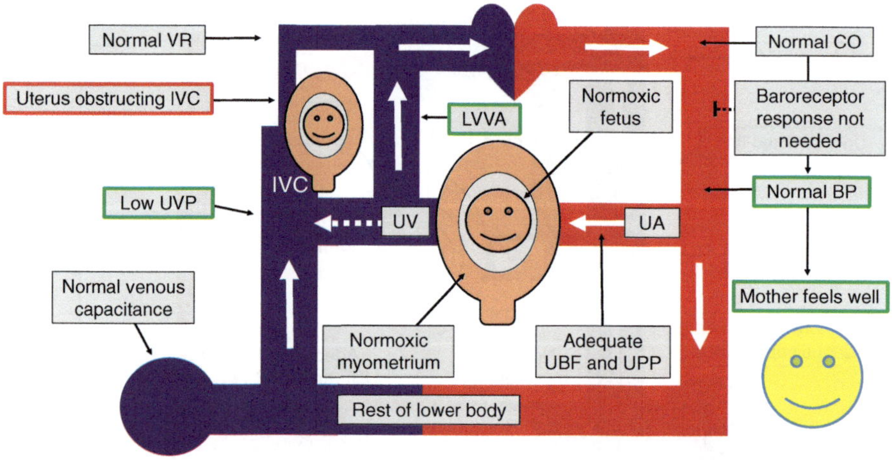

Fig. 1.5 Hemodynamics of healthy pregnancy with inferior vena cava obstruction, but *with* adequate venous collaterals. This figure shows how adequate lumbar, vertebral venous, and azygos (LVVA) collateral venous pathways can compensate for obstruction of the inferior vena cava by the gravid uterus. In this situation, robust baroreflex support of maternal blood pressure may not be required, since venous return and cardiac output are maintained at normal levels by a widely patent LVVA collateral system. An important—but perhaps not widely recognized—additional benefit of having a widely patent collateral venous return system is that the uterine venous pressure remains low in the supine position, despite obstruction of the inferior vena cava. *BP* blood pressure, *CO* cardiac output, *IVC* inferior vena cava, *LVVA* lumbar, vertebral venous, and azygos collateral venous return pathway, *UA* uterine arteries, *UBF* uterine blood flow, *UPP* uterine perfusion pressure (arterial minus venous), *UV* uterine veins, *UVP* uterine venous pressure, *VR* venous return

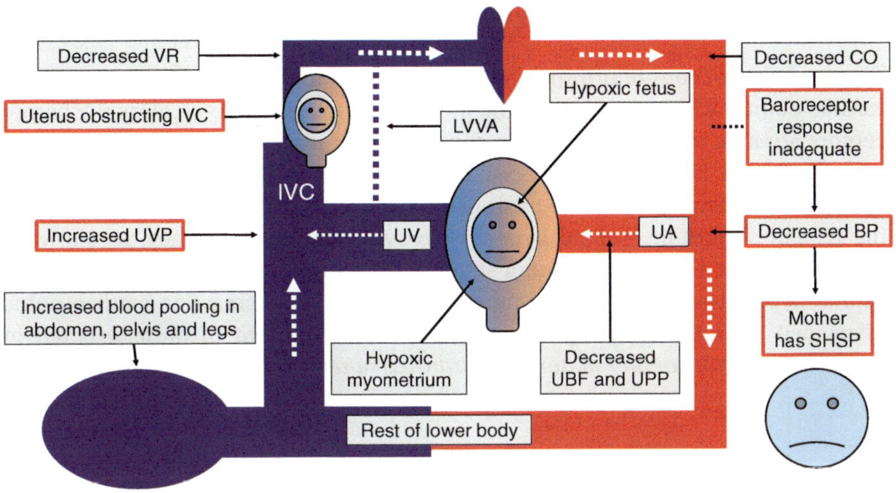

Fig. 1.6 Hemodynamics of obstruction of the inferior vena cava, *without* adequate collateral pathways for venous return. Four interrelated unfavorable events occur in this figure. First of all, the gravid uterus is obstructing the inferior vena cava. Second, there is no adequate collateral venous return system to compensate for the blocked inferior vena cava, so venous return from the uterus and the lower half of the body will decrease, followed within a minute by a decrease in the cardiac output. Third, the baroreceptor and sympathetic nervous systems do not increase systemic vascular resistance sufficiently to maintain an adequate maternal blood pressure, and therefore the mother will experience the supine hypotensive syndrome of pregnancy. Fourth, uteroplacental perfusion will decrease because maternal arterial pressure is lower and uterine venous pressure is higher than before obstruction of the inferior vena cava. In this situation, a conscious mother would almost certainly change her body position because she was not feeling well, and such a position change would probably restore adequate venous return to her heart and adequate blood flow to her brain. The other beneficiaries of the position change would be the fetus, placenta, and myometrium since they—like the mother's brain—would have their perfusion restored to normal. The mother's change of position in response to the supine hypotensive syndrome of pregnancy will not only preserve her well-being but that of the fetus as well. *But what would happen if the fetus is becoming hypoxic due to obstruction of uterine venous return, but the mother feels perfectly well and feels no need to change her body position?* (see Fig. 1.8). *BP* blood pressure, *CO* cardiac output, *IVC* inferior vena cava, *LVVA* lumbar, vertebral venous, and azygos collateral veins, *SHSP* supine hypotensive syndrome of pregnancy, *UA* uterine arteries, *UBF* uterine blood flow, *UPP* uterine perfusion pressure (arterial minus venous), *UV* uterine veins, *UVP* uterine venous pressure, *VR* venous return

Figure 1.6 shows what happens when the uterus obstructs the inferior vena cava and there is no adequate collateral pathway for venous blood from the lower part of the body to easily return to the heart. In this case, the venous return "backs up" in the veins of the uterus, pelvis, and legs, limiting continued uterine perfusion and perhaps causing the lower extremity edema so common in pregnancy. Uterine venous pressure also increases and this increased pressure may have important consequences within the intervillous spaces, as we will discuss later on.

The Supine Hypotensive Syndrome of Pregnancy

The decreased venous return shown in Fig. 1.6 is rapidly converted into a decreased cardiac output, which then lowers the mother's blood pressure—unless the baroreceptors are able to provoke a strong compensatory response from the sympathetic nervous system. If the baroreceptors and sympathetic nervous system fail to increase the systemic vascular resistance sufficiently to maintain adequate blood pressure, the patient suffers the supine hypotensive syndrome of pregnancy, as shown in Fig. 1.6. Figure 1.7 shows that in a study of 10 pregnant women who suffered the supine hypotensive syndrome of pregnancy, the mean decrease in cardiac output associated with the supine position was 20.3% [19], *and in these hypotensive patients the inadequate maternal cardiovascular response obviously did not*

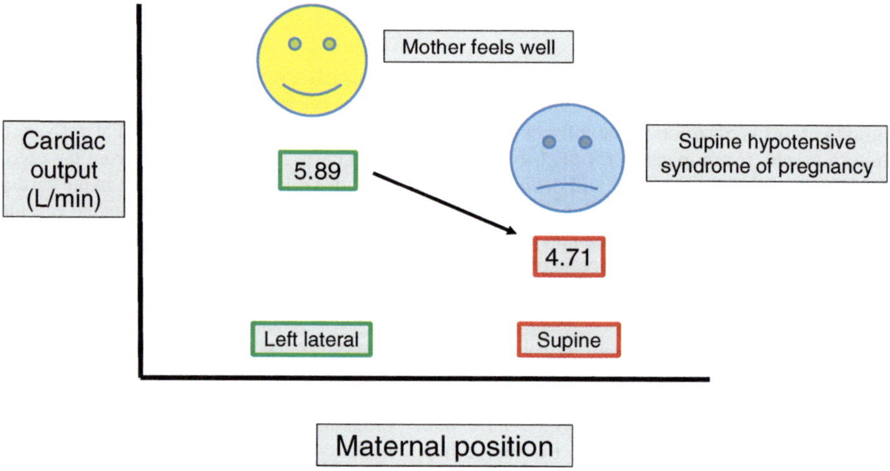

Fig. 1.7 Women who suffer the supine hypotensive syndrome of pregnancy show a 20% reduction in cardiac output. The supine hypotensive syndrome of pregnancy is associated with about a 20% reduction in cardiac output, in a series of ten patients [19]. *But this does not mean that all women who have a positional 20% reduction in cardiac output due to obstruction of uterine venous return will experience the supine hypotensive syndrome of pregnancy!* The baroreceptor systems of many women who experience a 20% reduction in cardiac output may maintain a normal blood pressure and the women may not even know that anything bad is happening with their circulatory system—or with their fetuses! The author created this figure from data from [19]

increase the systemic vascular resistance sufficiently to maintain an adequate maternal blood pressure.

The Supine Position, Cardiac Output, and Maternal Symptoms: Not Always Related!

The relationships between the supine position, cardiac output, and maternal symptoms are complicated. In fact—despite common beliefs—there is no definite relationship between the three factors! There may be relationships between the factors on average, but there appears to be no relationship between the factors as a rule [23–25], and this fact has probably caused a lot of confusion in both clinical care and research. To be explicit: not all women suffer the supine hypotensive syndrome of pregnancy when they adopt the supine position. Not all women have a reduction in cardiac output when they adopt the supine position, and (to consummate the confusion), not all women who *do* adopt the supine position and who *do* have a reduction in cardiac output will go on to suffer symptoms!

These three negative statements appear to contradict all clinical teaching, which is that: *the supine position is bad for pregnant women because it reduces maternal cardiac output and may cause the supine hypotensive syndrome of pregnancy in the mother as well as harm the fetus.* This classical clinical teaching is wise, *because it is true on average*, but it is also confusing—especially for research—*because it is not always true.*

Due to the presence of adequate venous collaterals to the inferior vena cava (the "LVVA system"), not all pregnant women in the supine position have a reduction of venous return and cardiac output. And of those women who do have a reduction of cardiac output in the supine position (with an increase in uterine venous pressure), not all of them suffer symptoms, probably due to the presence of highly active baroreceptor and sympathetic nervous systems which maintain blood pressure by increasing systemic vascular resistance. A remarkable paper by Kerr presented this possibility in 1965 [26], but it appears that the full implications of this possible but imperfect hemodynamic compensation for reduced cardiac output have not been adequately identified and investigated.

Maternal Cardiovascular Compensation for Reduced Cardiac Output in the Short and Long Term: A Suboptimal "Solution" with Harmful Consequences?

Figure 1.8 illustrates this possible scenario, in which the baroreceptors and the sympathetic nervous system increase the systemic vascular resistance in the short term, and the renin–angiotensin–aldosterone and vasopressin systems act over the longer

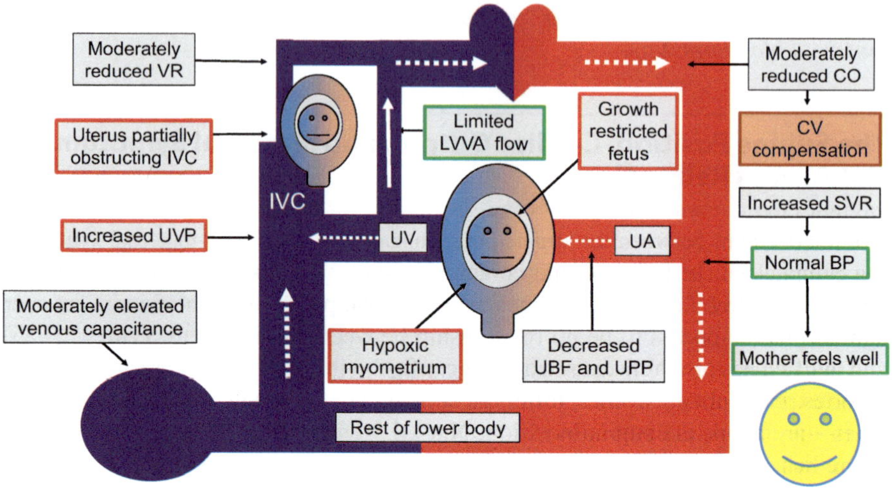

Fig. 1.8 Chronically compensated (and unrecognized) obstruction of uterine venous return. This figure illustrates a situation that may occur with some frequency, especially in obese patients. There may frequently be some degree of obstruction of the inferior vena cava by the gravid uterus, but not so much as to cause maternal symptoms. The mother feels well (i.e., her blood pressure is well maintained) because of a combination of partial inferior vena cava flow, some collateral flow through the lumbar, vertebral venous, and azygos system, and cardiovascular compensation consisting of increased activity of the baroreceptor and sympathetic nervous systems in the short term and the renin–angiotensin–aldosterone and vasopressin systems in the longer term. But this "compensated" state that the mother tolerates well may not be so benign for the fetus, because of persistent and uncompensated increases in uterine venous pressure and decreases in intervillous space perfusion, both of which may cause placental insufficiency. During labor, such a mediocre but partially compensated hemodynamic situation might lead to myometrial hypoxia and acidosis, causing dysfunctional labor or postpartum uterine atony (see Chap. 6). *CV* cardiovascular, *BP* blood pressure, *CO* cardiac output, *IVC* inferior vena cava, *LVVA* lumbar, vertebral venous, and azygos collateral veins, *SVR* systemic vascular resistance, *UA* uterine arteries, *UBF* uterine blood flow, *UPP* uterine perfusion pressure, *UV* uterine veins, *UVP* uterine venous pressure, *VR* venous return

term, to maintain normal maternal blood pressure despite a reduction of cardiac output. Figure 1.8 is of key importance to the argument of this book: *that obstruction of uterine venous return may cause the following six major hemodynamic derangements for the mother, fetus, placenta, and myometrium* (Table 1.1)*: (1) reduced maternal cardiac output, (2) compensatory increased maternal systemic vascular resistance, resulting in (3) normal maternal blood pressure, but with the following three potentially harmful effects which are not corrected by the hemodynamic compensation: (4) decreased perfusion and oxygenation of the intervillous spaces and myometrium, (5) increased uterine venous and intervillous space pressure, and (6) decreased fetal perfusion of already-hypoxic chorionic villi. An irony of this supposedly "compensated" hemodynamic situation is that the pregnant woman feels well despite the fact that her fetus, placenta, and myometrium may be*

Table 1.1 How obstruction of uterine venous return may injure the mother, fetus, placenta, and myometrium

1. Reduced maternal cardiac output
2. Compensatory increased maternal systemic vascular resistance
3. Normal maternal blood pressure, mother feels well and does not change position
4. Decreased perfusion and oxygenation of intervillous spaces and myometrium
5. Increased uterine venous and intervillous space pressure
6. Decreased fetal perfusion of already-hypoxic chorionic villi

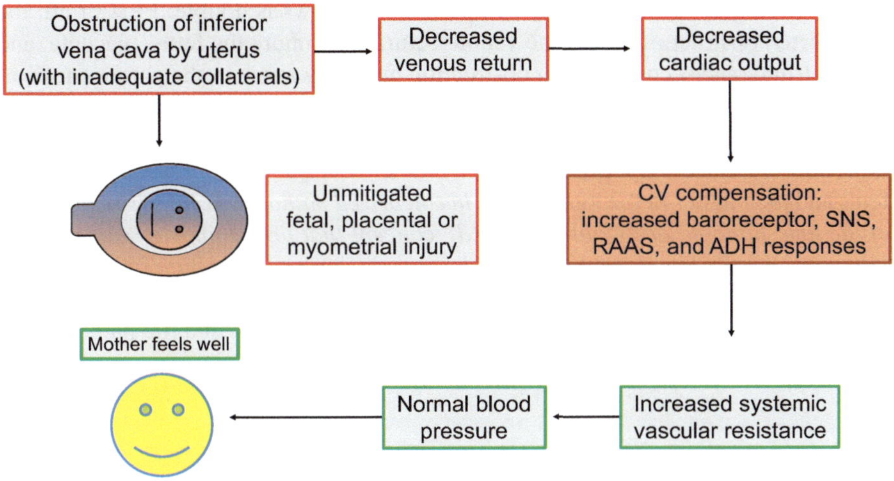

Fig. 1.9 Another view of incomplete hemodynamic compensation for obstruction of uterine venous return. This figure makes the same point as the preceding figure but emphasizes that the hemodynamic compensation for decreased cardiac output due to obstruction of uterine venous return may be incomplete, counterproductive, and harmful in the long term. When faced with a reduction in venous return and cardiac output, the maternal cardiovascular system increases the systemic vascular resistance to maintain the maternal blood pressure but does nothing to relieve the *cause* of the decreased cardiac output, which is obstruction of the inferior vena cava by the gravid uterus. The persisting, unrelieved, and unrecognized high uterine venous pressure and low uterine perfusion may then gradually injure the fetus, placenta, and myometrium over time, leading to fetal growth restriction, preeclampsia, preterm birth, dysfunctional labor, and postpartum uterine atony. Future research must determine whether this theory has any validity. *ADH* antidiuretic hormone (also known as vasopressin), *CV* cardiovascular, *RAAS* renin, angiotensin, and aldosterone system, *SNS* sympathetic nervous system

suffering ongoing injury. The fetus may suffer growth restriction or even stillbirth due to reduced placental intervillous perfusion and increased intervillous space pressure, and the mother may develop preeclampsia. But in the short term, the mother feels fine. *In other words, some pregnant women may spend some amount of time every day in body positions which impair uterine blood flow, harm their fetus, and threaten their own health, all without being aware that anything is wrong!* This "compensatory" but ultimately pathological result of obstruction of uterine venous return is further illustrated in Fig. 1.9.

"Cardiovascular Compensation" for Reduced Maternal Cardiac Output May Be a Doubly Harmful and Counterproductive "False Friend"

Figure 1.10 shows that the "cardiovascular compensation" for reduced maternal cardiac output shown in Figs. 1.8 and 1.9 may really be a "doubly false friend," or doubly counterproductive process, *because it does not correct the underlying cause of the reduced cardiac output—which is obstruction of the inferior vena cava.* The injury which this "cardiovascular compensation" allows is double: First of all, the uncorrected obstruction of uterine venous return may injure the fetus, placenta, and myometrium, and secondly, such obstruction may play a role in the pathogenesis of preeclampsia, thereby injuring the mother. For this reason, the theory presented in Fig. 1.10 is another key message of this book: that "cardiovascular compensation" for reduced cardiac output may help the mother in the short term but may hurt the fetus and the mother in the long term. *This theorized pathophysiology is reminiscent of the time-honored and "old-fashioned" concept that preeclampsia represents an "attempt" by the fetoplacental unit to increase its own oxygenation by means of a higher maternal blood pressure!* Perhaps obstruction of uterine venous return has a lot to do with both depriving the fetoplacental unit of oxygen and the pathogenesis of preeclampsia!

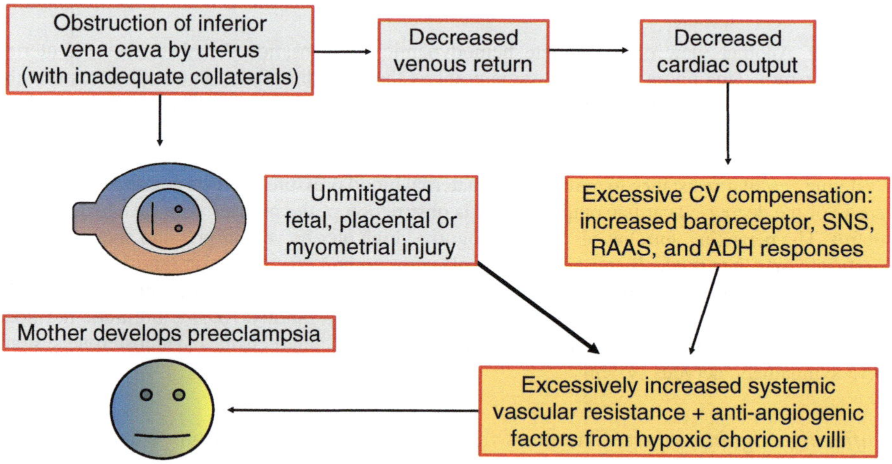

Fig. 1.10 Imperfect cardiovascular compensation for reduced maternal cardiac output may ultimately cause both fetal injury and preeclampsia. This figure makes explicit the implied "threat" of the previous Fig. 1.9. In the short term, increased systemic vascular resistance maintains maternal blood pressure, but long term does nothing to correct the placental ischemia and hypoxia which cause both fetal growth restriction and preeclampsia. *ADH* antidiuretic hormone (also known as vasopressin), *CV* cardiovascular, *RAAS* renin, angiotensin, and aldosterone system, *SNS* sympathetic nervous system

Four Distinct "Perfusion Pathways" Must Remain Open to Adequately Oxygenate the Fetus, Placenta, and Myometrium

Up to this point I have presented the theory that unrecognized obstruction of uterine venous return at the inferior vena cava may impair the maternal and uterine circulations in ways that injure the mother, fetus, placenta, or myometrium. But unobstructed uterine and lower body venous return is only one of the four essential perfusion pathways which enable a successful pregnancy. Figure 1.11 shows all four of these perfusion pathways in their favorable or "healthy" states: (1) normally remodeled spiral arteries, (2) a normal heart and underlying cardiovascular system, (3) unobstructed uterine venous return at the inferior vena cava accompanied by normal uterine venous pressure, and (4) normal myometrial tissue pressure which does not obstruct the uteroplacental circulation within the myometrium.

Figure 1.12 provides a simplified view of these four essential blood flow pathways which together—*and in series*—provide adequate perfusion and oxygenation of the fetus, placenta, and myometrium. When any of these component "pathways" becomes obstructed or restricted it becomes a "bottle-neck" or "choke point" to successful oxygenation, and this book explores possible pathogenic *combinations* among these four circulatory "choke points" which may contribute to preeclampsia, fetal growth restriction, preterm birth, dysfunctional labor, and postpartum uterine

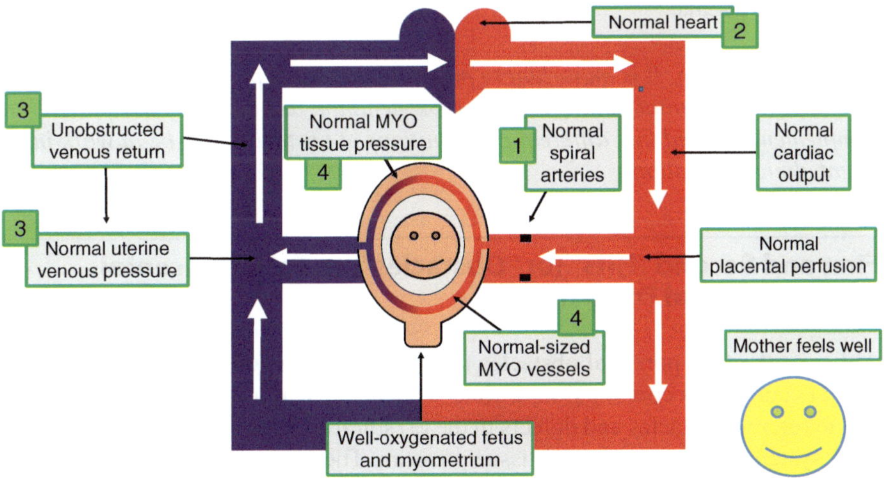

Fig. 1.11 Four interrelated and essential "perfusion pathways" that may malfunction during pregnancy—individually or in combinations. These four components of the maternal and uterine circulations may malfunction by themselves or in various combinations during pregnancy, causing hypoxic injury to the fetus, placenta, or myometrium. The four "perfusion pathways"—presented here in their normal and healthy states—are (1) normally remodeled spiral arteries, (2) a normal heart and underlying cardiovascular system, (3) unobstructed uterine venous return at the inferior vena cava, and (4) normal myometrial tissue pressure. *MYO* myometrial

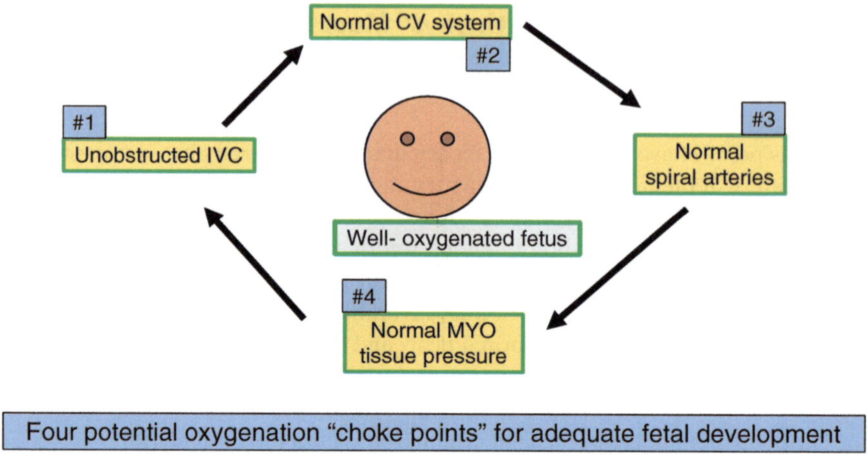

Fig. 1.12 Four potential oxygenation "choke points" for adequate fetal development. This figure makes the point that these four "perfusion pathways" which are essential for fetal oxygenation and development *are in series*. This means that if any one of the four pathways is blocked, fetal oxygenation and development are blocked. It also means that the harmful effects of a partial obstruction in one pathway might be gravely exacerbated by a partial obstruction in another pathway. In other words, the potential "choke points" can work in combination to deprive the fetus, placenta, and myometrium of oxygen, and *it may often be the case that the only choke point which can be "fixed" during pregnancy is positional obstruction of the inferior vena cava.* If this is true, the avoidance of obstruction of the inferior vena cava during gestation might significantly mitigate other obstacles to oxygenation which cannot be corrected. *CV* cardiovascular, *IVC* inferior vena cava, *MYO* myometrial

atony and infection. *It is important to point out that these possible obstacles to successful fetal, placental, and myometrial oxygenation are mutually compatible and complementary, and that different combinations of obstacles may be at work in different clinical situations.*

First and Second "Hits" (or "Obstacles") to Fetal, Placental, and Myometrial Oxygenation

Although the four potential obstacles to oxygenation shown in Figs. 1.11 and 1.12 could occur in any combination or time sequence, I will use the terminology "first hit" to refer to obstacles and defects in the (a) spiral arteries, (b) maternal cardiovascular system, or (c) myometrial tissue pressure. The term "second hit" will be used to refer to obstruction of uterine venous return, since it is potentially preventable. My idea is that generally little can be done to remove "first hits" (or "pre-existing conditions," if you will), but care-givers and mothers themselves may be able to prevent a "second hit" due to obstruction of uterine venous return.

The Healthy Fetus, Chorionic Villus, and Intervillous Space

Figure 1.13 is my representation of the healthy placenta: the spiral arteries have been appropriately remodeled and allow an abundant but gentle flow of maternal blood to bathe the chorionic villi and give up oxygen to the fetus across a well-oxygenated placental barrier. The hydrostatic pressure within the intervillous space is low, since there is no obstruction to venous outflow from the intervillous space into the uterine veins and then into a widely patent inferior vena cava. With Fig. 1.13 as our point of departure, we will now use preeclampsia and fetal growth restriction as examples of how obstruction of uterine venous return (as a "second hit") might combine with any of the other three "first hits" to make a bad situation worse.

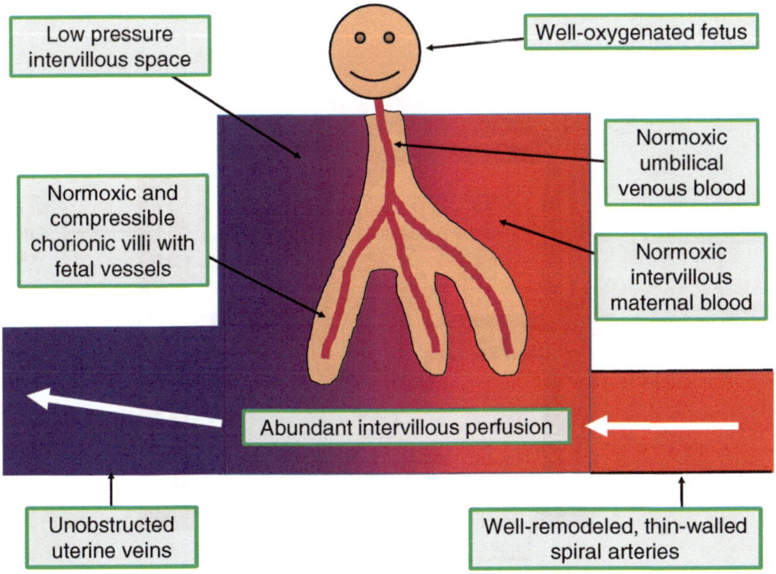

Fig. 1.13 The healthy fetus, chorionic villus, and intervillous space. In the ideal placenta, the spiral arteries have been appropriately remodeled and allow an abundant but gentle flow of maternal blood to bathe the chorionic villi and give up oxygen to the fetus across a well-oxygenated placental barrier. The hydrostatic pressure within the intervillous space is low, since there is no obstruction to venous outflow from the intervillous space into the uterine veins and then into a widely patent inferior vena cava

Defective Spiral Artery Remodeling Limits Placental Perfusion

As shown in Fig. 1.14, the classical model of preeclampsia and fetal growth restriction is that unremodeled (high-resistance) spiral arteries reduce intervillous perfusion, which causes hypoxia of both the chorionic villi and the fetus. Chorionic villus hypoxia causes the release of anti-angiogenic factors which cause preeclampsia and fetal hypoxia causes fetal growth restriction. In this model of the causation of preeclampsia and fetal growth restriction, defective spiral artery remodeling is "intrinsic" to the placenta, and the model does not include any "contributions" to preeclampsia and fetal growth restriction from the other three oxygenation choke points of the system.

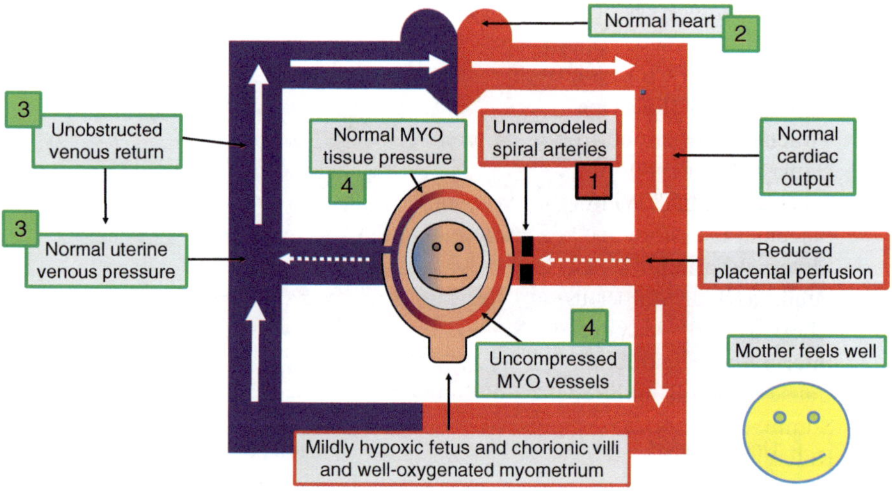

Fig. 1.14 Mildly defective spiral artery remodeling as a pre-existing vulnerability—a "first hit". This figure postulates that some patients have a relatively mild degree of defective spiral artery remodeling, which is causing mild and subclinical problems currently. In other words, we are postulating that this patient has some degree of reduced intervillous perfusion—a "first hit" or a "vulnerability"—which may or may not eventually lead to preeclampsia, but which may be exacerbated by obstruction of uterine venous return, the "second hit." In this example, we are assuming that there is no current obstruction of uterine venous return which further impedes intervillous perfusion. *MYO* myometrial

Obstruction of Uterine Venous Return Combines with Defective Spiral Artery Remodeling to Make a Bad Situation Worse

Figure 1.15 shows this same classical model of preeclampsia and fetal growth restriction from the closer perspective of the intervillous space. The hypothesized situation shown in Fig. 1.15 is that of an early, mild, or subclinical version of the disease state. Figure 1.15 shows that a small degree of impaired spiral artery remodeling is causing some small degree of fetal and chorionic villus hypoxia, perhaps with the release of a small quantity of anti-angiogenic factors from the hypoxic chorionic villi. But assume that at this stage the mother is asymptomatic and the fetus is only mildly stressed.

Figures 1.16 and 1.17 show the independent injurious effects of obstruction of uterine venous return when the spiral arteries are normal. In both Figs. 1.16 and 1.17, the fetus and thc chorionic villi are being subjected to modest hypoxic stress, but without any clinical manifestations so far.

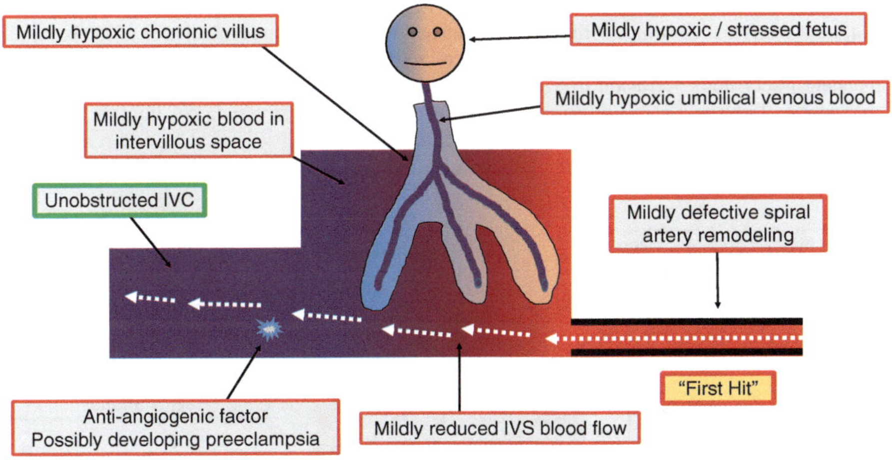

Fig. 1.15 Defective spiral artery remodeling—a "first hit" to chorionic villi and the fetus—as seen within the intervillous space. This figure shows the same situation as in the preceding figure, but from within the intervillous space. A mild degree of defective spiral artery remodeling has mildly reduced intervillous perfusion, creating a mild degree of intervillous hypoxia affecting both the chorionic villi and the fetus. The mildly hypoxic chorionic villi have begun to produce a small amount of anti-angiogenic factor and the patient is at risk of developing preeclampsia. This situation constitutes a "first hit"—a vulnerability whose injurious effects can be exacerbated by obstruction of uterine venous return if it occurs as the "second hit." *IVC* inferior vena cava, *IVS* intervillous space

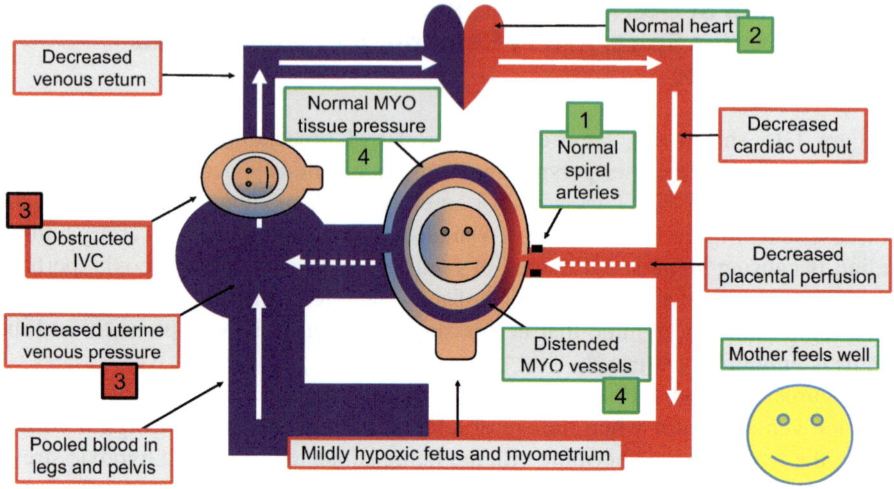

Fig. 1.16 Hemodynamic effects of obstruction of uterine venous return—*with normally remodeled spiral arteries.* This figure shows the "second hit" (obstruction of uterine venous return) in isolation—without the presence of the "first hit" (defective spiral artery remodeling). In this situation, both the fetus, chorionic villi, and myometrium are exposed to some degree of hypoxia, due to both reduced intervillous perfusion and increased intervillous pressure. But in this scenario, abundant intervillous perfusion from normal spiral arteries compensates for frequent episodes of obstruction of uterine venous return, and the fetus is only mildly stressed. *IVC* inferior vena cava, *MYO* myometrial

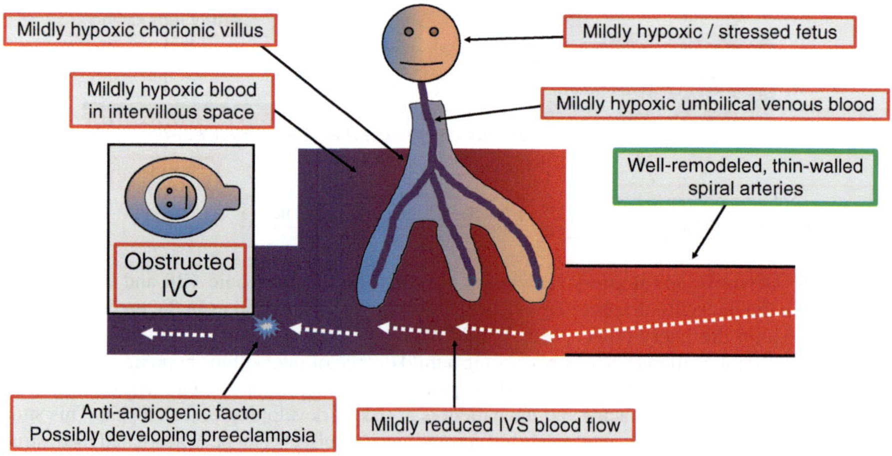

Fig. 1.17 Obstruction of uterine venous return can reduce intervillous perfusion too—just like unremodeled spiral arteries! If unremodeled spiral arteries can reduce intervillous perfusion and cause intervillous hypoxia, it would seem that obstruction to intervillous perfusion from the venous side could produce the same results (along with the added problem of increased intervillous space pressure). But in this figure, we are hypothesizing that, in this case, venous obstruction is only causing a minor problem, which is compensated by abundant but gentle intervillous perfusion from well-remodeled spiral arteries. *IVC* inferior vena cava, *IVS* intervillous space

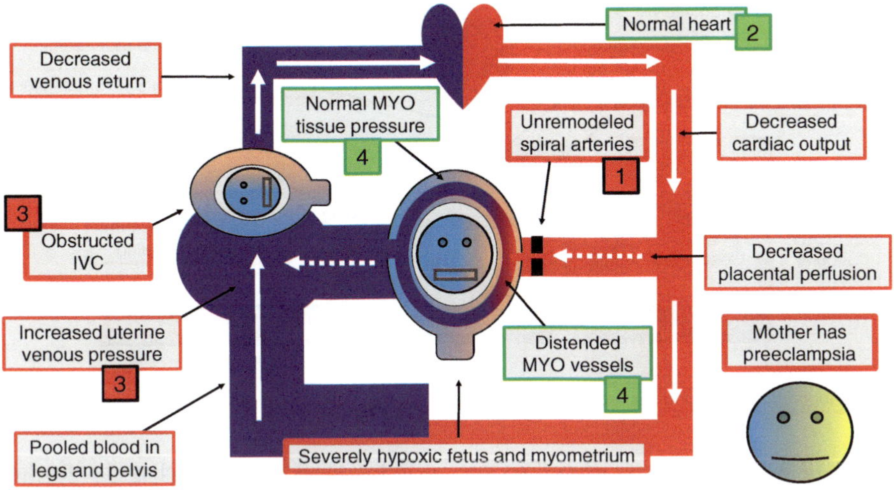

Fig. 1.18 Disaster from combined placental insults: obstruction of uterine venous return converts mild disease from mildly defective spiral artery remodeling into a grave problem for fetus and mother. This figure demonstrates one of the main points of this book: that obstruction of uterine venous return may act as a "second hit" to exacerbate the relatively mild effects of pre-existing vulnerabilities of uteroplacental perfusion. In this figure, the "first hit" is mildly defective spiral artery remodeling, but the "first hit" could also be maternal obesity, short maternal stature, diabetes, chronic hypertension, a globally defective maternal cardiovascular system, or a large uterus. In the situation shown, oxygenation of the fetus, chorionic villi, and myometrium is severely restricted from both the arterial and venous sides of the uterine circulation. The mother develops preeclampsia and the fetus may be severely growth restricted or die. Cardiac output-guided maternal positioning might have mitigated or prevented this outcome—but, of course, this theory requires further investigation. *IVC* inferior vena cava, *MYO* myometrial

Figures 1.18 and 1.19, however, show the dramatically increased injurious effect of obstruction of uterine venous return when it combines with defectively remodeled spiral arteries. When the two stressors are combined, the patient's clinical picture deteriorates quickly and dramatically. Intervillous perfusion slows greatly and intervillous hypoxia worsens, at the same time as intervillous space pressure increases and fetoplacental perfusion of the increasingly hypoxic chorionic villi decreases. Fetal growth restriction accelerates and the mother rapidly develops preeclampsia due to an outpouring of anti-angiogenic factors from the very hypoxic chorionic villi, as shown in Fig. 1.19. In this hypothetical example, we might theorize that if obstruction of uterine venous return had been recognized and prevented, then the appearance of preeclampsia and fetal growth restriction might have been delayed until later in gestation—or prevented altogether!

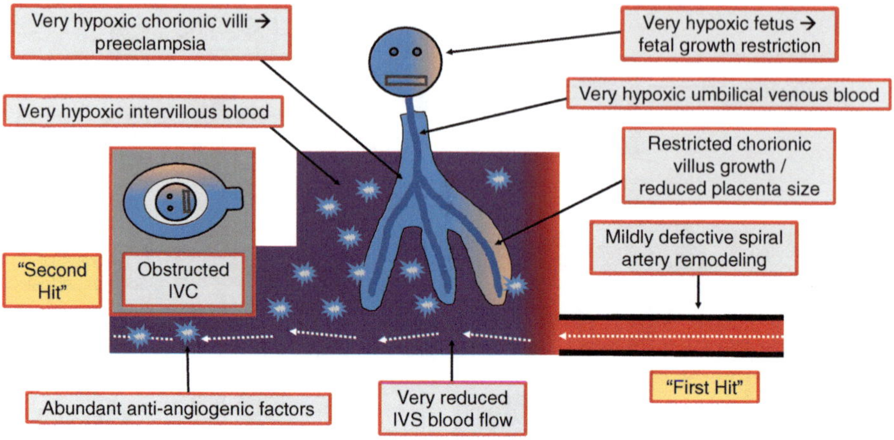

Fig. 1.19 Disaster within the intervillous space: defective spiral artery remodeling (the "first hit") *plus* obstruction of uterine venous return (the "second hit"). Obstruction of uterine venous return superimposed upon already precarious intervillous perfusion due to defective spiral artery remodeling has now created a grave threat to both fetus and mother. Intensely hypoxic chorionic villi now pour forth large quantities of anti-angiogenic factors, producing preeclampsia with severe features, and the fetus is exposed to severe hypoxia. Cardiac output-guided maternal positioning might have mitigated or prevented this outcome, but this is just a theory which requires further investigation. *IVC* inferior vena cava, *IVS* intervillous space

Defective Global Maternal Hemodynamics as a Cause of Preeclampsia and Fetal Growth Restriction

Defective or inappropriate global maternal hemodynamics—as described by systemic vascular resistance, cardiac output, and blood pressure—have also been proposed as playing a role in preeclampsia and fetal growth restriction. One global hemodynamic profile associated with fetal growth restriction is increased systemic vascular resistance and decreased cardiac output [27–33].

Another global hemodynamic profile—this one associated with preeclampsia—is a high maternal cardiac output in the presence of a normal systemic vascular resistance. Some authors believe that hypertension may be a relatively late sign of maternal hemodynamic deterioration in preeclampsia, and that earlier therapeutic hemodynamic intervention in normotensive women, based on their underlying high cardiac output and normal systemic vascular resistance, might lead to better outcomes [34–41].

This focus on global maternal hemodynamics seems appropriate and promising but appears to neglect the possible role of obstruction of uterine venous return in causing preeclampsia and fetal growth restriction. If obstruction of uterine venous return does play a role in these disease processes, it would seem short-sighted to manage these conditions by manipulating only the maternal cardiac output and systemic vascular resistance, without also correcting any underlying uterine venous obstruction—which may play a fundamental role in the development of the diseases in the first place, as suggested in Figs. 1.9 and 1.10. *A fundamental point of this book is to suggest that increased attention to obstruction of uterine venous return in future research might enable breakthroughs in our understanding of pregnancy-related diseases and in our ability to treat or prevent those diseases.* In the next section, we consider one possible future discovery, which (of course) is now just a theory.

Obstruction of Uterine Venous Return Combines with a Defective Maternal Cardiovascular System to Make a Bad Situation Worse

We now consider how superimposed obstruction of uterine venous return might exacerbate the effects of a globally impaired maternal cardiovascular system, due—for example—to a subtle cardiomyopathy. Figure 1.20 is my interpretation of what Gyselaers and Lees have described as a "maternal low-volume circulation [31]," a global maternal hemodynamic disorder characterized by low cardiac output and high systemic vascular resistance. Because of the low cardiac output in this theorized disorder (labeled here only as "heart disorder"), the perfusion of the placenta and the oxygenation of the fetus may already be somewhat precarious. But—in this hypothetical situation—the fetus is only under mild hypoxic stress.

Figure 1.21 shows the potentially catastrophic result of combining obstruction of uterine venous return with a "maternal low-volume circulation." As with the previous example of defective spiral artery remodeling, obstruction of uterine venous return makes a bad situation much worse—in this instance, by further decreasing maternal preload and cardiac output and by increasing uterine venous and intervillous space pressures. The combination of these two stressors may kill the fetus, whereas the fetus might have tolerated either stressor by itself.

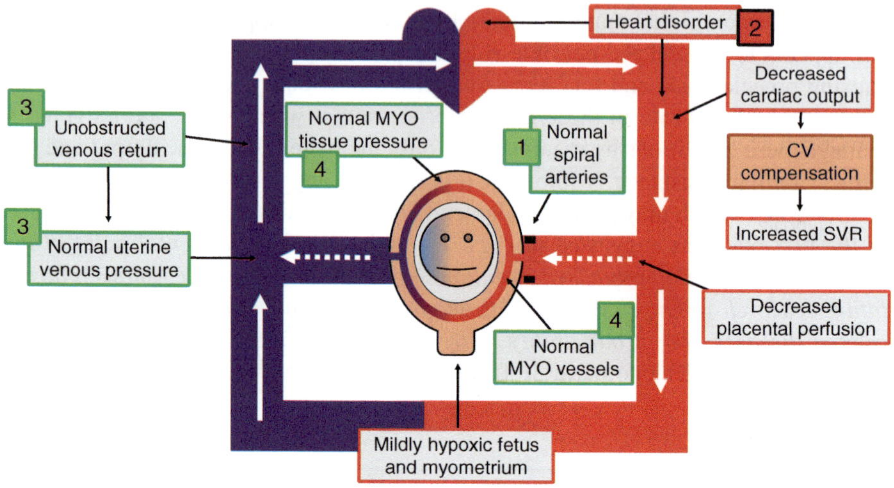

Fig. 1.20 A globally impaired maternal circulation as a "first hit" to the pregnancy, with high systemic vascular resistance and low cardiac output. This figure is an attempt to represent what Gyselaers and Lees have called a "maternal low-volume circulation" [31]. In this situation, maternal systemic vascular resistance is—for some reason—too high. Either the maternal heart does not generate sufficient cardiac output and the cardiovascular system compensates by increasing systemic vascular resistance, or increased systemic vascular resistance is the initiating cause and a reduced cardiac output is the compensatory response. A third possibility is that unrecognized obstruction of venous return at the inferior vena cava is reducing maternal cardiac output, which is then imperfectly compensated, as shown in Fig. 1.8. In any case, reduced cardiac output may cause placental and fetal hypoxia leading to fetal growth restriction or preeclampsia. In this model, a globally defective maternal circulation constitutes an initial threat to the pregnancy—a "first hit"—which puts the pregnancy at higher risk. But this threat may be amenable to hemodynamic therapy such as increased oral hydration, a calcium channel blocker such as nifedipine, or a nitric oxide donor such as nitroglycerin. However, if obstruction of venous return by the gravid uterus is one of the causes of this syndrome, then the first treatment should be avoidance of that obstruction. Pharmacologic and hydration therapy may have only limited benefits if the "maternal low-volume circulation" is due—at least in part—to obstruction of venous return, as shown in the next figure. *CV* cardiovascular, *MYO* myometrial, *SVR* systemic vascular resistance

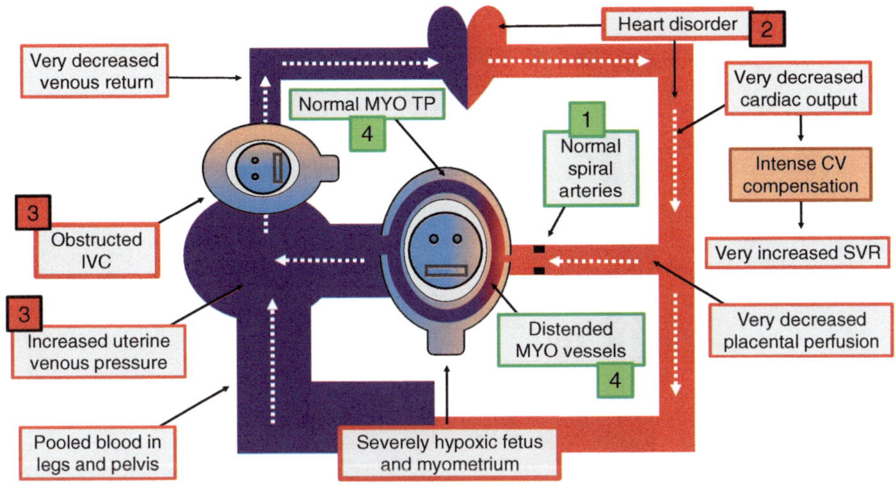

Fig. 1.21 Obstruction of uterine venous return makes a pre-existing "maternal low-volume circulation" much more harmful to the fetus, placenta, myometrium, and mother. If the maternal cardiac output is low and the systemic vascular resistance is high due to a global problem with the maternal cardiovascular system, superimposed obstruction of uterine venous return will reduce the cardiac output even further. Uterine venous pressure will also increase, thereby causing further deterioration of fetal, placental, and myometrial oxygenation, leading to fetal growth restriction, preeclampsia, or myometrial hypoxia. This is another example of how obstruction of uterine venous return can serve as a "second hit" which exacerbates the effects of a "first hit"—in this case, a globally impaired maternal cardiovascular system. Of course, it is possible that in some cases the only "problem" with the "maternal cardiovascular system" is that it is not receiving the venous return it needs to provide an adequate cardiac output! *CV* cardiovascular, *IVC* inferior vena cava, *MYO* myometrial, *TP* tissue pressure, *SVR* systemic vascular resistance

Obstruction of Uterine Venous Return Combines with Increased Myometrial Tissue Pressure to Make a Bad Situation Worse

Up to this point, I have emphasized that obstruction of uteroplacental perfusion can be caused by extra-uterine obstruction of the inferior vena cava by the gravid uterus or an obese abdominal wall. But there is another possible mechanism for the obstruction of uteroplacental perfusion: that of increased myometrial tissue pressure, as shown in Fig. 1.22. This increased tissue pressure may be created either by external compression due to obesity or short maternal stature (as shown in Fig. 1.22) or by the effects of Laplace's law within larger uteruses which are often characterized as being "overdistended." (The effects of Laplace's law are not shown in Fig. 1.22 but are discussed further in Chap. 7).

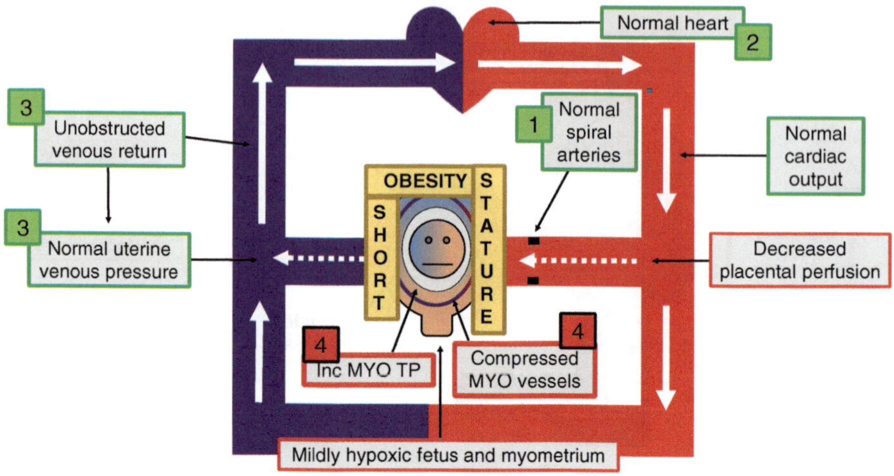

Fig. 1.22 Increased myometrial tissue pressure as another cause of decreased placental and myometrial perfusion—another "pre-existing vulnerability". The blood vessels serving both the placenta and the myometrium pass through the myometrium itself on the way to their respective intervillous spaces and capillary beds. Hence there is another possible mechanism for the obstruction of uteroplacental perfusion: that of increased myometrial tissue pressure, as shown in this figure. This increased tissue pressure can be created either by external compression due to obesity or short maternal stature or by the effects of Laplace's law within larger ("overdistended") uteruses. This is the basis for asserting that obesity, short maternal stature, or increased uterine size may constitute "first hits" or risk factors for placental and myometrial perfusion, whose effects can be exacerbated by obstruction of uterine venous return. (The effects of Laplace's law are not explicitly shown in this figure, but are discussed further in Chap. 7). *Inc* increased, *MYO* myometrial, *TP* tissue pressure

Figure 1.23 suggests that when obstruction of uterine venous return combines with increased myometrial tissue pressure, an already precarious uteroplacental perfusion can be made much worse. To use the terminology already introduced, obstruction of uterine venous return would constitute a "second hit" which would exacerbate the pre-existing effects of increased myometrial tissue pressure, which is the "first hit."

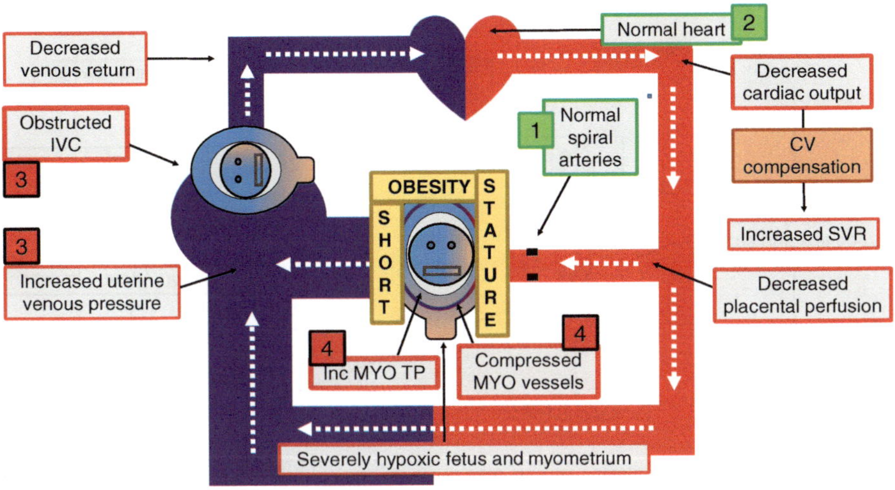

Fig. 1.23 As a "second hit," obstruction of uterine venous return may exacerbate the injury due to increased myometrial tissue pressure. In what should now be a familiar pattern, the "first hit" or "vulnerability" due to increased myometrial tissue pressure is exacerbated by the "second hit" of obstruction of uterine venous return. *CV* cardiovascular, *Inc* increased, *IVC* inferior vena cava, *MYO* myometrial, *SVR* systemic vascular resistance, *TP* tissue pressure

Positional Obstruction of the Inferior Vena Cava May Harm Only a Minority of Pregnancies

Figure 1.24 illustrates the idea that positional obstruction of the inferior vena cava may be harmful only in a subset of patients with one or more of the following "pre-existing conditions": (1) impaired spiral artery remodeling, (2) a global maternal hemodynamic disorder, (3) increased myometrial tissue pressure, (4) inadequate lumbar, vertebral venous, and azygos collaterals, (5) maternal obesity, (6) maternal short stature, (7) an "overdistended" (large) uterus, (8) chronic hypertension, or (9) diabetes.

As shown in Fig. 1.24, perhaps 80% of patients (an arbitrary figure) will be unaffected by positional obstruction of the inferior vena cava during pregnancy and labor, but perhaps 20% (an arbitrary figure) will be vulnerable to further injury because of pre-existing vulnerabilities, which I am calling "first hits." The additional stress or impact of obstruction of uterine venous return might constitute a "second hit" which converts the patient's vulnerability into actual injury. Some of the vulnerabilities—obesity, diabetes, and chronic hypertension, for example—are becoming more common, and this increasing vulnerability of the pregnant population might make obstruction of uterine venous return all that much more important to prevent.

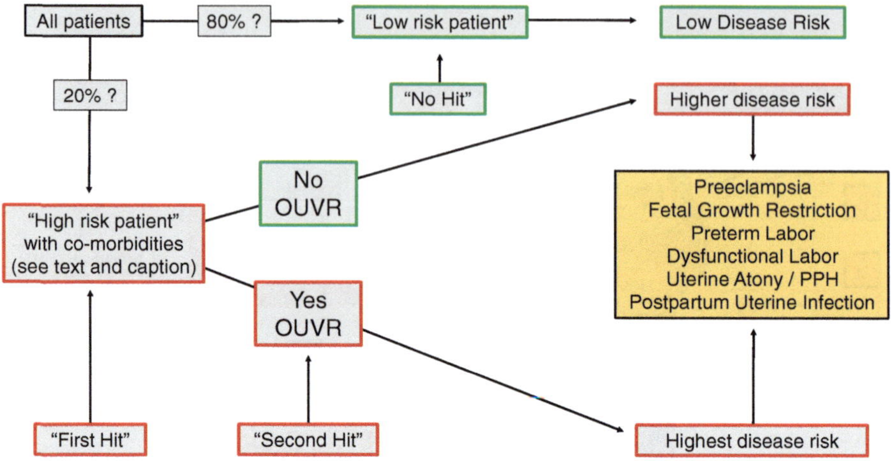

Fig. 1.24 Obstruction of uterine venous return—as a "second hit"—may cause problems mostly in patients who have significant pre-existing vulnerabilities ("first hits"). As suggested in this figure, healthy patients with no pre-existing vulnerabilities may be relatively immune to the deleterious effects of obstruction of uterine venous return. Obstruction of uterine venous return may function as a "second hit" which causes overt disease mostly in patients who are particularly vulnerable because of pre-existing conditions—or "first hits." Examples of such "first hit" pre-existing vulnerabilities might be (1) impaired spiral artery remodeling, (2) inadequate lumbar, vertebral venous, and azygos collaterals, (3) maternal obesity, (4) maternal short stature, (5) an "overdistended" (large) uterus due to multiple gestation or polyhydramnios, (6) chronic hypertension, (7) diabetes, or (8) a global maternal hemodynamic disorder. *OUVR* obstruction of uterine venous return, *PPH* postpartum hemorrhage

Clinical Examples of Asymptomatic Obstruction of Uterine Venous Return

Figures 1.25 [9] and 1.26 [10] show clinical examples of women who showed dramatic positional changes in cardiac output without feeling any symptoms. The patient shown in Fig. 1.25 was hospitalized at 26 + 3/7 weeks estimated gestational age for preterm labor, and the patient in Fig. 1.26 was hospitalized at 30 weeks estimated gestational age for fetal growth restriction. Both patients demonstrated dramatic positional changes in cardiac output without feeling any symptoms in any of the positions. Is it possible in their cases that unrecognized obstruction of uterine venous return originally caused the problems for which they were ultimately admitted to the hospital?

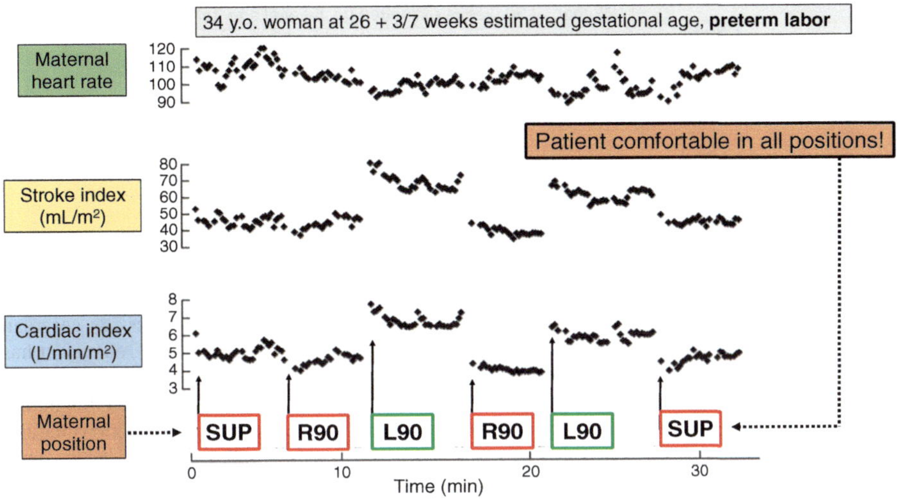

Fig. 1.25 Maternal cardiac output varies dramatically with changes in maternal position in a patient hospitalized for preterm labor. The 34-year-old patient from whom these hemodynamic measurements were obtained was hospitalized for preterm labor at 26 + 3/7 weeks' estimated gestational age. Measurements were taken with electrical cardiometry in the absence of contractions and the patient was awake, ambulatory, *and felt comfortable in all positions*. Fetal heart rate (not shown) was normal in all positions. Could chronic obstruction of uterine venous return have contributed to preterm labor in this patient by a variety of possible mechanisms? (see Chap. 7). Maternal position is indicated as follows: L90/R90, left/right side down with 90° tilt (full lateral decubitus position); S, supine. Figure 1.25 comes from reference [9]. The Figure and caption have been modified. Copyright (C) 2011 ISUOG. Published by John Wiley & Sons, Ltd

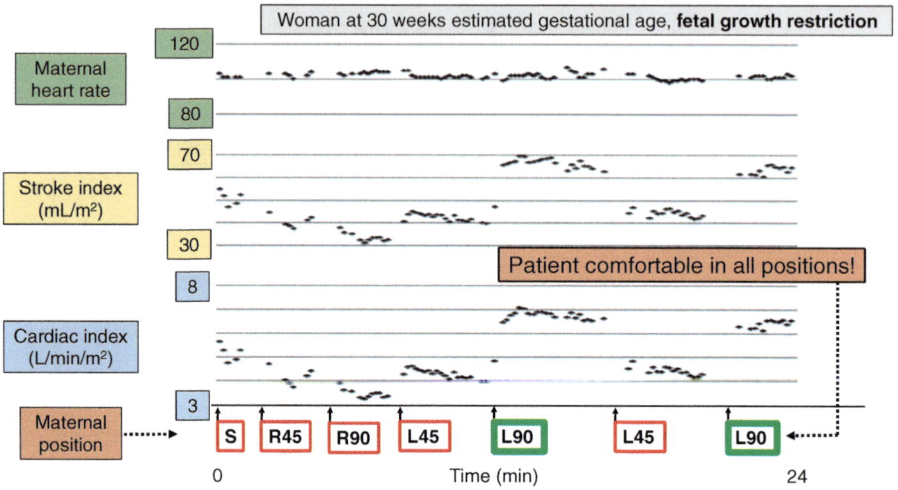

Fig. 1.26 Maternal cardiac output varies dramatically with changes in maternal position in a patient hospitalized for fetal growth restriction. This patient said that she felt comfortable in all positions, but her hemodynamic record shows that in order to maximize her cardiac output—and presumably minimize obstruction of the inferior vena cava—this patient has to be in the full left lateral position. Even with a 45° left tilt, her cardiac output was significantly decreased from its maximum seen in the full left lateral decubitus position. Common wisdom regarding positioning in pregnancy would be that a 45° tilt to the left should prevent obstruction of the inferior vena cava and decompress the uterine venous system—*but that appears not to have been the case in this patient. Could chronic obstruction of uterine venous return have contributed to fetal growth restriction in this patient?* (see Chaps. 3, 4, and 5). Maternal hemodynamics and abbreviations: *HR* heart rate, beats per minute, *SI* stroke index (mL/m^2), *CI* cardiac index (L/min/m^2), *S* supine position, *R* right side down, *L* left side down, *45* 45° tilt; *90* 90° tilt (full lateral decubitus position). Figure 1.26 comes from reference [10]. The Figure and caption have been modified. SAGE is the Publisher and this content is used under the STM guidelines

Positional Reduction of Maternal Cardiac Output May *Signal* the Presence of Other Associated Hemodynamic Conditions Which Are Just as Dangerous—Or Even More Dangerous—Than the Reduction of Cardiac Output Per Se

Figure 1.27 makes a very important point: Many people consider that the injury caused by "aortocaval compression" is due to the associated decrease in maternal cardiac output and blood pressure. Although compression of the inferior vena cava in the absence of adequate collateral venous return pathways will certainly decrease the maternal cardiac output and may decrease maternal blood pressure as well, *those results may not be its most harmful effect on the pregnancy! The primary*

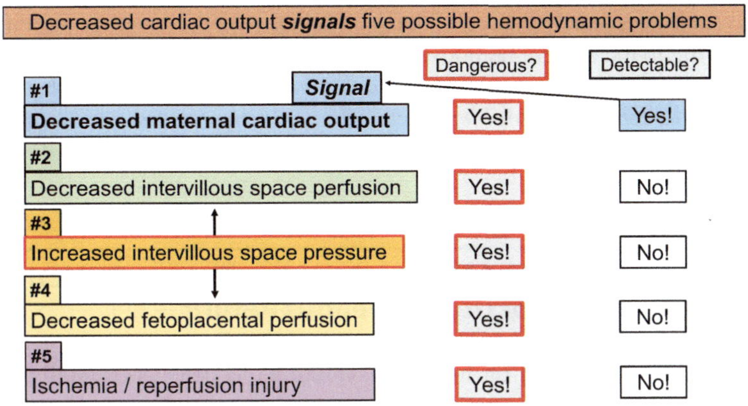

Fig. 1.27 Positional reduction of maternal cardiac output may *signal* the presence of other associated hemodynamic conditions which are just as dangerous—or even more dangerous—than the reduction of cardiac output per se. This figure makes a very important point: Many people consider that the injury caused by "aortocaval compression" is due to the associated decrease in maternal cardiac output and blood pressure. Although compression of the inferior vena cava in the absence of adequate collateral venous return pathways will certainly decrease the maternal cardiac output and may decrease maternal blood pressure as well, *those results may not be its most harmful effect on the pregnancy! The primary importance of a positional decrease in maternal cardiac output may be that it is an easily detectable signal or "marker" for the potentially disastrous but complicated hemodynamic situation set forth in this figure. Without an easily detectable signal or marker—such as a positional decrease in cardiac output—other aspects of this dangerous hemodynamic "complex"—such as increased intervillous space pressure—might be "silent" and undetectable*

importance of the decrease in maternal cardiac output associated with obstruction of the inferior vena cava may be that it constitutes an easily detectable signal or "marker" for a potentially disastrous hemodynamic situation which involves a multiplicity of otherwise undetectable harmful effects—as suggested in Fig. 1.27*!*

What Do Obstetricians Say?

When I have discussed this issue with obstetricians, most of them say they routinely advise their patients to avoid the supine position while resting, and that they encourage their patients to "listen to their bodies" and to change their body position if a given position does not seem comfortable either for themselves or for their baby. Some obstetricians have told me that some pregnant women seem to know what position is best for them and their baby, but even if that is true for some women, it may not be true for others whom we may be able to help via improved body positioning during pregnancy.

Without objective information about the presence, absence, or degree of obstruction of uterine venous return in each patient, obstetricians are probably doing all they can to prevent obstruction of uterine venous return from causing problems, but their advice is necessarily generic—that is, it is based on the "average patient"—and is not specific to the current hemodynamics of each patient. *It might be beneficial to know—in each pregnant patient and at each prenatal visit—whether obstruction of uterine venous return is a problem for uterine perfusion at that time or not, based on easily acquired, objective, and individualized positional cardiac output measurements.*

Positional Reductions of Maternal Cardiac Output Objectively Identify Obstruction of Uterine Venous Return

It is not reliable to depend on maternal symptoms to detect potentially injurious obstruction of uterine venous return. Will the mother always know when her uterus is obstructing its own venous return and causing hypoxic stress to the fetus, placenta, and myometrium? Probably not, and if we want to study the possible harmful effects of obstruction of uterine venous return during gestation—with the intention of preventing it—we need an objective, safe, and easy-to-use method for detecting it.

Our limited research suggests that positional reductions in maternal cardiac output may be useful as an objective marker indicating positional obstruction of uterine venous return. If the value of this approach is supported by further research, it might lead to maternal screening during gestation for significant "positionality" of maternal venous return and cardiac output. Each at-risk patient could then be advised to avoid those positions which significantly impair her uterine venous return, increase her uterine venous pressure, and decrease her cardiac output. This information could even be provided to the patient herself on an ongoing basis through the use of wearable technology that would detect positional reductions in cardiac output and give the patient appropriate and immediate feedback. The next chapter describes how our research group at the University of California San Diego began to develop these ideas starting in 2010.

Chapter Summary

1. Positional obstruction of the inferior vena cava by the gravid uterus can cause obstruction of uterine venous return and a well-known short-term problem for the mother near term: the "supine hypotensive syndrome of pregnancy." But if there are adequate lumbar, vertebral venous, and azygos collaterals, obstruction of the inferior vena cava by the gravid uterus does not necessarily obstruct uterine venous return, which can return to the heart via the collateral system.
2. When unrecognized and prolonged obstruction of uterine venous return occurs during gestation, it might play a role in causing or exacerbating preeclampsia, fetal growth restriction, preterm birth, dysfunctional labor, and postpartum uterine atony. These harmful effects may occur via three mechanisms: (a) reduced maternal perfusion of the intervillous space causing intervillous hypoxia, (b) increased intervillous space pressure compressing the chorionic

villi and the fetal vessels within them, and thereby reducing fetal perfusion of the chorionic villi, and (c) reduced myometrial perfusion, causing myometrial hypoxia, acidosis, and possible inflammation. Together, these results of obstruction of uterine venous return will reduce oxygen delivery to the fetus, placenta, and myometrium.

3. Four "perfusion pathways" are essential for a healthy pregnancy and the birth of a healthy baby: (a) well-remodeled spiral arteries, (b) a robust maternal cardiovascular system, (c) unobstructed uterine venous return, and (d) sufficiently low myometrial tissue pressure. Conditions which impair the health of pathways (a), (b), or (d) tend to be difficult to treat and can be considered fixed vulnerabilities of the reproductive system, or pre-existing "first hits." Pathway (c)—that of unobstructed uterine venous return—may be comparatively easy to protect via cardiac output-guided maternal positioning, and obstruction of this pathway may be considered as a preventable "second hit" which makes the effects of the unavoidable, fixcd "first hits" much worse.
4. Technology now exists to determine easily, quickly, non-invasively, and continuously, what maternal positions cause obstruction of uterine venous return sufficient to reduce the cardiac output. *A positional reduction in maternal cardiac output identifies body positions which cause obstruction of uterine venous return at the inferior vena cava.*
5. If found to be helpful in avoiding unfavorable pregnancy outcomes, this method of outpatient hemodynamic care during pregnancy might be called "cardiac output-guided maternal positioning."

References

1. McRoberts WA Jr. Postural shock in pregnancy. Am J Obstet Gynecol. 1951;62(3):627–32.
2. Howard BK, Goodson JH, Mengert WF. Supine hypotensive syndrome in late pregnancy. Obstet Gynecol. 1953;1(4):371–7. PMID: 13055188.
3. Wilkening RL, Knauer J, Larson RK. Postural shock in pregnancy. Calif Med. 1955;82(3):159–62. PMID: 14351983; PMCID: PMC1532751.
4. Scott DB. Inferior vena caval occlusion in late pregnancy and its importance in anaesthesia. Br J Anaesth. 1968;40(2):120–8. https://doi.org/10.1093/bja/40.2.120.
5. Kinsella SM, Whitwam JG, Spencer JA. Reducing aortocaval compression: how much tilt is enough? BMJ. 1992;305(6853):539–40. https://doi.org/10.1136/bmj.305.6853.539. PMID: 1393031; PMCID: PMC1883291.
6. Robson SC, Boys RJ, Rodeck C, Morgan B. Maternal and fetal haemodynamic effects of spinal and extradural anaesthesia for elective caesarean section. Br J Anaesth. 1992;68(1):54–9. https://doi.org/10.1093/bja/68.1.54. PMID: 1739568.
7. Katz VL, Hansen AR. Complications in the emergency transport of pregnant women. South Med J. 1990;83(1):7–10. https://doi.org/10.1097/00007611-199001000-00004.
8. De-Giorgio F, Grassi VM, Vetrugno G, d'Aloja E, Pascali VL, Arena V. Supine hypotensive syndrome as the probable cause of both maternal and fetal death. J Forensic Sci. 2012;57(6):1646–9. https://doi.org/10.1111/j.1556-4029.2012.02165.x.
9. Archer TL, Suresh P, Ballas J. Don't forget aortocaval compression when imaging abdominal veins in pregnant patients. Ultrasound Obstet Gynecol. 2011;38(4):479–80; author reply 480-1. https://doi.org/10.1002/uog.10065. Erratum in: Ultrasound Obstet Gynecol. 2021;57(3):516. PMID: 21837755.

10. Archer TL, Suresh P, Shapiro AE. Cardiac output measurement, by means of electrical velocimetry, may be able to determine optimum maternal position during gestation, labour and caesarean delivery, by preventing vena caval compression and maximising cardiac output and placental perfusion pressure. Anaesth Intensive Care. 2011;39(2):308–11. PMID: 21485686.
11. Archer TL, Shapiro AE, Suresh PJ. Maximisation of maternal cardiac output during labour might help to prevent not only foetal hypoxaemia but also myometrial ischaemia, dysfunctional labour, uterine atony and postpartum endometritis. Anaesth Intensive Care. 2011;39(4):774–5. PMID: 21823407.
12. Archer TL. Cardiac output-guided resuscitation of the *uterus*: an obese patient has dysfunctional labor which resolves with position change. Coincidence or possible therapy? In: Archer TL, editor. Obstetric anesthesia: a case-based and visual approach. 1st ed. Switzerland: Springer; 2020. Ch 32, p. 293–301. https://doi.org/10.1007/978-3-030-26478-9_32.
13. Archer TL. Cardiac output-guided maternal position therapy for preterm labor-it's time for a trial. Acta Obstet Gynecol Scand. 2022;101(8):931–2. https://doi.org/10.1111/aogs.14365. Epub 2022 May 6. PMID: 35514219; PMCID: PMC9564800.
14. Archer TL. Obstructed uterine venous return: a preventable cause of dysfunctional labor? Reproduction. 2021;161(4):V15–7. https://doi.org/10.1530/REP-21-0002. PMID: 33617462.
15. Archer TL. Position therapy in pregnancy: can trending maternal cardiac output put it on a more objective foundation? Acta Obstet Gynecol Scand. 2021;100(8):1539–40. https://doi.org/10.1111/aogs.14167. Epub 2021 Jun 13. PMID: 34121190.
16. Archer TL, Conrad BE. Electrical velocimetry follows the hemodynamics of drug therapy and aortocaval compression in preeclampsia. Int J Obstet Anesth. 2011;20(1):91–2. https://doi.org/10.1016/j.ijoa.2010.08.001. Epub 2010 Dec 3. PMID: 21126865.
17. Archer TL. Neuraxial anesthesia and the supine position cause non-reassuring fetal status. In: Archer TL, editor. Obstetric anesthesia: a case-based and visual approach. 1st ed. Switzerland: Springer; 2020. Ch 2, Figure 2.4, p. 25. https://doi.org/10.1007/978-3-030-26478-9_2.
18. Humphries A, Stone P, Mirjalili SA. The collateral venous system in late pregnancy: a systematic review of the literature. Clin Anat. 2017;30(8):1087–95. https://doi.org/10.1002/ca.22959.
19. Humphries A, Mirjalili SA, Tarr GP, Thompson JMD, Stone P. Hemodynamic changes in women with symptoms of supine hypotensive syndrome. Acta Obstet Gynecol Scand. 2020;99(5):631–6. https://doi.org/10.1111/aogs.13789. Epub 2019 Dec 29. PMID: 31856296. Figure is from data provided in the article. Caption is mine.
20. Jani D, Clark A, Couper S, Thompson JMD, David AL, Melbourne A, Mirjalili A, Lydon AM, Stone PR. The effect of maternal position on placental blood flow and fetoplacental oxygenation in late gestation fetal growth restriction: a magnetic resonance imaging study. J Physiol. 2023;601(23):5391–411. https://doi.org/10.1113/JP284269. Epub ahead of print. PMID: 37467072.
21. Couper S, Clark A, Thompson JMD, Flouri D, Aughwane R, David AL, Melbourne A, Mirjalili A, Stone PR. The effects of maternal position, in late gestation pregnancy, on placental blood flow and oxygenation: an MRI study. J Physiol. 2021;599(6):1901–15. https://doi.org/10.1113/JP280569. Epub 2021 Jan 18. PMID: 33369732; PMCID: PMC7613407.
22. Rossi A, Cornette J, Johnson MR, Karamermer Y, Springeling T, Opic P, Moelker A, Krestin GP, Steegers E, Roos-Hesselink J, van Geuns RJ. Quantitative cardiovascular magnetic resonance in pregnant women: cross-sectional analysis of physiological parameters throughout pregnancy and the impact of the supine position. J Cardiovasc Magn Reson. 2011;13(1):31. https://doi.org/10.1186/1532-429X-13-31. PMID: 21708015; PMCID: PMC3148552.
23. Humphries A, Mirjalili SA, Tarr GP, Thompson JMD, Stone P. The effect of supine positioning on maternal hemodynamics during late pregnancy. J Matern Fetal Neonatal Med. 2019;32(23):3923–30. https://doi.org/10.1080/14767058.2018.1478958. Epub 2018 Jun 3. PMID: 29772936.
24. Fujita N, Higuchi H, Sakuma S, Takagi S, Latif MAHM, Ozaki M. Effect of right-lateral versus left-lateral tilt position on compression of the inferior vena cava in pregnant women determined by magnetic resonance imaging. Anesth Analg. 2019;128(6):1217–22. https://doi.org/10.1213/ANE.0000000000004166. PMID: 31094791.

25. Hughes EJ, Price AN, McCabe L, Hiscocks S, Waite L, Green E, Hutter J, Pegoretti K, Cordero-Grande L, Edwards AD, Hajnal JV, Rutherford MA. The effect of maternal position on venous return for pregnant women during MRI. NMR Biomed. 2021;34(4):e4475. https://doi.org/10.1002/nbm.4475. Epub 2021 Jan 21. PMID: 33480110.
26. Kerr MG. The mechanical effects of the gravid uterus in late pregnancy. J Obstet Gynaecol Br Commonw. 1965;72:513–29. https://doi.org/10.1111/j.1471-0528.1965.tb00061.x. PMID: 14341106.
27. Easterling TR, Benedetti TJ. Preeclampsia: a hyperdynamic disease model. Am J Obstet Gynecol. 1989;160(6):1447–53. https://doi.org/10.1016/0002-9378(89)90869-7. PMID: 2567574.
28. Mulder EG, de Haas S, Mohseni Z, Schartmann N, Abo Hasson F, Alsadah F, van Kuijk S, van Drongelen J, Spaanderman M, Ghossein-Doha C. Cardiac output and peripheral vascular resistance during normotensive and hypertensive pregnancy - a systematic review and meta-analysis. BJOG. 2022;129(5):696–707. https://doi.org/10.1111/1471-0528.16678. Epub 2021 Apr 6. PMID: 33630403; PMCID: PMC9291763.
29. Masini G, Foo LF, Tay J, Wilkinson IB, Valensise H, Gyselaers W, Lees CC. Preeclampsia has two phenotypes which require different treatment strategies. Am J Obstet Gynecol. 2022;226(2S):S1006–18. https://doi.org/10.1016/j.ajog.2020.10.052. Epub 2021 Jun 10. PMID: 34774281.
30. Tay J, Masini G, McEniery CM, Giussani DA, Shaw CJ, Wilkinson IB, Bennett PR, Lees CC. Uterine and fetal placental Doppler indices are associated with maternal cardiovascular function. Am J Obstet Gynecol. 2019;220(1):96.e1–8. https://doi.org/10.1016/j.ajog.2018.09.017. Epub 2018 Sep 19. PMID: 30243605.
31. Gyselaers W, Lees C. Maternal low volume circulation relates to normotensive and preeclamptic fetal growth restriction. Front Med (Lausanne). 2022;9:902634. https://doi.org/10.3389/fmed.2022.902634. PMID: 35755049; PMCID: PMC9218216.
32. Valensise H, Farsetti D, Pometti F, Vasapollo B, Novelli GP, Lees C. The cardiac-fetal-placental unit: fetal umbilical vein flow rate is linked to the maternal cardiac profile in fetal growth restriction. Am J Obstet Gynecol. 2023;228(2):222.e1–222.e12. https://doi.org/10.1016/j.ajog.2022.08.004. Epub 2022 Aug 6. PMID: 35944606.
33. Foo FL, Mahendru AA, Masini G, Fraser A, Cacciatore S, MacIntyre DA, McEniery CM, Wilkinson IB, Bennett PR, Lees CC. Association between prepregnancy cardiovascular function and subsequent preeclampsia or fetal growth restriction. Hypertension. 2018;72(2):442–50. https://doi.org/10.1161/HYPERTENSIONAHA.118.11092. Epub 2018 Jul 2. PMID: 29967040.
34. Easterling TR. Individualized management of maternal hemodynamics to prevent preeclampsia: improvement in maternal outcomes without adverse fetal effects. Hypertension. 2021;77(6):2054–6. https://doi.org/10.1161/HYPERTENSIONAHA.121.17202. Epub 2021 May 12. PMID: 33979186.
35. Easterling TR. Post-control of hypertension in pregnancy study (CHIPS): what is the optimal strategy to manage hypertension during pregnancy? Hypertension. 2016;68(1):36–8. https://doi.org/10.1161/HYPERTENSIONAHA.116.07190. Epub 2016 May 16. PMID: 27185752.
36. Mulder EG, Ghossein-Doha C, Cauffman E, Lopes van Balen VA, Schiffer VMMM, Alers RJ, Oben J, Smits L, van Kuijk SMJ, Spaanderman MEA. Preventing recurrent preeclampsia by tailored treatment of nonphysiologic hemodynamic adjustments to pregnancy. Hypertension. 2021;77(6):2045–53. https://doi.org/10.1161/HYPERTENSIONAHA.120.16502. Epub 2021 Apr 5. PMID: 33813842.
37. Valensise H, Vasapollo B, Novelli GP, Giorgi G, Verallo P, Galante A, Arduini D. Maternal and fetal hemodynamic effects induced by nitric oxide donors and plasma volume expansion in pregnancies with gestational hypertension complicated by intrauterine growth restriction with absent end-diastolic flow in the umbilical artery. Ultrasound Obstet Gynecol. 2008;31(1):55–64. https://doi.org/10.1002/uog.5234. PMID: 18098350.

38. Tiralongo GM, Pisani I, Vasapollo B, Khalil A, Thilaganathan B, Valensise H. Effect of a nitric oxide donor on maternal hemodynamics in fetal growth restriction. Ultrasound Obstet Gynecol. 2018;51(4):514–8. https://doi.org/10.1002/uog.17454. PMID: 28295749.
39. Vasapollo B, Novelli GP, Farsetti D, Pometti F, Frantellizzi R, Maellaro F, Silvestrini M, Pais M, Valensise H. NO donors on top of anti-hypertensive therapy reduces complications in chronic hypertensive pregnancies with hypodynamic circulation. Eur J Obstet Gynecol Reprod Biol. 2023;291:219–24. https://doi.org/10.1016/j.ejogrb.2023.10.033. Epub ahead of print. PMID: 37924629.
40. Easterling TR, Brateng D, Schmucker B, Brown Z, Millard SP. Prevention of preeclampsia: a randomized trial of atenolol in hyperdynamic patients before onset of hypertension. Obstet Gynecol. 1999;93(5 pt 1):725–33. https://doi.org/10.1016/s0029-7844(98)00522-5.
41. Easterling TR, Carr DB, Brateng D, Diederichs C, Schmucker B. Treatment of hypertension in pregnancy: effect of atenolol on maternal disease, preterm delivery, and fetal growth. Obstet Gynecol. 2001;98:427–33. https://doi.org/10.1016/s0029-7844(01)01477-6.

2 Cardiac Output-Guided Maternal Positioning

Personal Note

One afternoon late in 2010, the anesthesia resident and I were called to place an epidural in an obese patient whose labor was being induced because of preeclampsia. We had already consented the patient for our hemodynamic research and were already trending her cardiac output using electrical cardiometry.

When we arrived at her bedside she was in severe pain and her mean arterial pressure (MAP) was 143 mmHg. We gave her intravenous fentanyl for the pain and had her sit up for epidural placement. Her next blood pressure reading showed a mean arterial pressure of 113. Epidural placement went smoothly and the resident gave the epidural dose of local anesthetic and fentanyl in three divided injections, starting at 1545. At 1550, after the epidural dosing was complete, we lay the patient onto her right side to tape the epidural catheter in place (at "R90" in Fig. 2.1) [1, 2]. At 1555, her mean arterial pressure was 86 mmHg and immediately thereafter we obtained a reading of 72 mmHg. As we expected, the sympathectomy from the epidural was lowering her blood pressure and—with the patient tipped 30° to her right—we gave her one intravenous dose of the vasopressor phenylephrine at 1557, another dose at 1602, and a dose of ephedrine at 1607. But despite these three doses of two different vasopressors, her mean arterial pressure stayed low.

The mother had received excellent pain relief by now and was beginning to relax and converse amiably with us despite the dramatic decrease in her blood pressure. It was also reassuring that the fetal heart rate and beat-to-beat variability were normal. Despite the fact that both she and her baby appeared to be OK, we would have liked to see a higher mean arterial pressure—especially since the patient was preeclamptic and probably accustomed to much higher blood pressures. We were also bothered by the fact that vasopressors were needed to maintain an adequate blood pressure.

T. L. Archer, *Threats to Fetal, Placental and Myometrial Oxygenation*,
https://doi.org/10.1007/978-3-031-60364-8_2

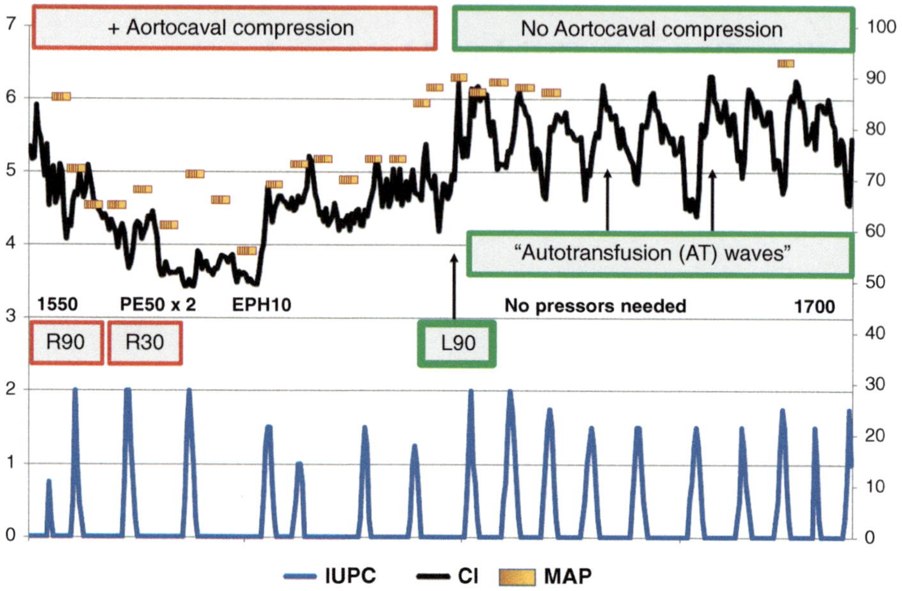

Fig. 2.1 Our first visualization of "autotransfusion waves": the increases in maternal cardiac output caused by uterine contractions. For me and my colleagues, caring for this patient was a "Eureka moment." Everyone taking care of pregnant women knows about the importance of avoiding the supine position to prevent aortocaval compression, but with this patient my colleagues and I were able to *see* the hemodynamics of aortocaval compression in real time. Furthermore, this record demonstrates what is often forgotten: obstruction of the inferior vena cava by the uterus occurs in various positions—not just in the supine position. For this reason, it may be best to use cardiac output-guided maternal positioning to make sure that a pregnant woman is avoiding positions in which her baby and myometrium are not receiving the maximum amount of oxygen—even though, for the moment, the baby and myometrium might appear to be doing well. *CI* cardiac index (L/min/m^2, left axis), *EPH10* ephedrine 10 mg intravenously, *IUPC* pressure from intrauterine pressure catheter (arbitrary units, right axis), *L90* patient tipped into full left lateral decubitus position, *MAP* mean arterial pressure (mmHg, right axis), *PE50* phenylephrine 50 μg intravenously (vasopressor), *R30* patient tipped 30° to the right, *R90* patient tipped into full right lateral decubitus position [1, 2]

We thought that obstruction of the inferior vena cava—along with the sympathectomy from the epidural—might explain the hypotension and we therefore had the patient turn herself into the full left lateral decubitus position at 1628 (marked "L90" in Fig. 2.1) [3–5]. With the adoption of the full left lateral decubitus position, the patient's mean arterial pressure stabilized around 90 mmHg without the need for further vasopressor administration and—to our delight and amazement—her baseline cardiac output increased substantially, as shown in Fig. 2.1 at "L90." Also—as we watched with growing excitement—each uterine contraction was followed immediately by an increase in cardiac output, as shown in the right half of Fig. 2.1.

Turning the patient into the left lateral decubitus position appeared to have caused two key events: (1) an increase in baseline cardiac output and (2) the appearance of additional increases in cardiac output immediately following each uterine contraction which we called "autotransfusion waves." *We realized that we were seeing autotransfusion in real time!* Autotransfusion had always seemed to be a somewhat theoretical or even mythical process—interesting to imagine but never really seen. Now we were seeing it as it occurred—and we were seeing it with commercially available technology that was U.S. Food and Drug Administration-approved, non-invasive, hands-free, and continuous!

Furthermore, when we put the cardiac output data together with the uterine contraction data from external tocometry, we saw that when the patient had been lying on her right side there had been no increases in cardiac output following uterine contractions! The contractions had occurred—since we could see them in the time-stamped external tocometry strip—but there were no corresponding increases in cardiac output, as seen in Fig. 2.1. We were very excited: perhaps we had discovered a means of detecting aortocaval compression in real time! Perhaps the increase in baseline cardiac output in the left lateral decubitus position, together with the additional increases in cardiac output following uterine contractions, showed that we had relieved obstruction of the inferior vena cava by changing her position! From then on the patient's course was unremarkable. We kept her tipped over to her left side and she required no further vasopressors. Her pain relief continued to be excellent and she delivered a healthy infant some time later. *But perhaps most remarkable of all was the fact that during the entire episode of maternal hypotension and reduced cardiac output, the fetal heart rate and variability had continued to be normal—not giving us any indication that anything was wrong with uterine perfusion!* We thought that perhaps we had discovered a new way of detecting and intervening *early* in a situation of deteriorating maternal hemodynamics, which might cause fetal heart rate changes or dysfunctional labor only much later, if it were allowed to continue.

Cardiac Output-Guided Maternal Positioning to Optimize Uteroplacental Perfusion

Figure 2.2 [1] shows another example of positional changes in baseline maternal cardiac output as well as the positional appearance and disappearance of what we began to call "autotransfusion waves"—the normal increases in maternal cardiac output caused by uterine contractions when the inferior vena cava is unobstructed. We were seeing aortocaval compression appear and disappear with position change!

We immediately started to study more laboring patients and routinely saw hemodynamic tracings like the one shown in Fig. 2.3 [1], in which maternal cardiac output increases after each uterine contraction when the inferior vena cava is

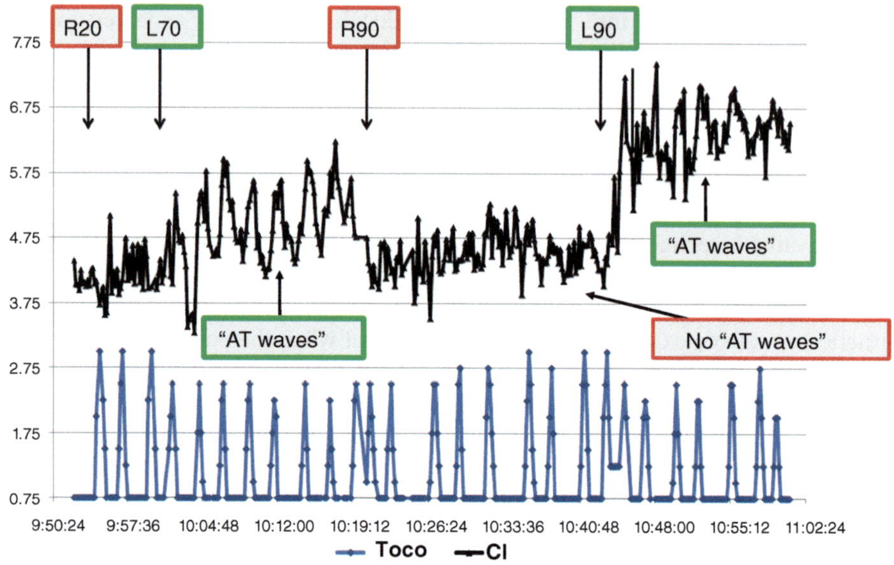

Fig. 2.2 Autotransfusion waves in another laboring patient. We found that positional decreases in baseline cardiac output and the disappearance of "autotransfusion waves" were common in laboring patients with epidurals in place. Epidurals may make obstruction of uterine venous return more common because the sympathectomy they produce (along with pain relief) reduces venous tone in the lower half of the body, reducing the venous pressure available to overcome an obstruction to the flow of venous blood. Note in this patient that the maternal cardiac output is reduced and autotransfusion waves are blunted or abolished even in the full right lateral decubitus position. This example helps make the point that obstruction of uterine venous return is highly variable—between patients and probably within the same patient over time, due to changes in (1) maternal position, (2) station of the fetus within the birth canal, (3) patient fluid and medication administration, and (4) degree of sympathetic blockade produced by neuraxial anesthesia. These considerations make the point that obstruction of uterine venous return is a dynamic process—which argues for monitoring maternal cardiac output continuously during labor. *CI* cardiac index (L/min/m^2), *Toco* tocometry tracing (external contraction monitor), *R90/L90* full right and left lateral decubitus positions, respectively, *R20* patient tipped 20 degrees to the right, *L70* patient tipped 70 degrees to the left [1]

unobstructed. We also realized that autotransfusion during labor provides a "homemade," intrinsic, and repetitive volume challenge to the heart, which may have diagnostic value, as shown in Fig. 2.4 [1]. Some years later we obtained the hemodynamic record shown in Fig. 2.5 [6], which shows intrauterine pressure and cardiac output measured simultaneously by transthoracic echocardiography and electrical cardiometry. Figure 2.5 shows that the two simultaneous measurements of cardiac output by different techniques trend together, confirming that what we were seeing with electrical cardiometry was not some sort of artifact.

In summary, we saw the positional behavior of maternal cardiac output that one might have expected from a knowledge of aortocaval compression: in some

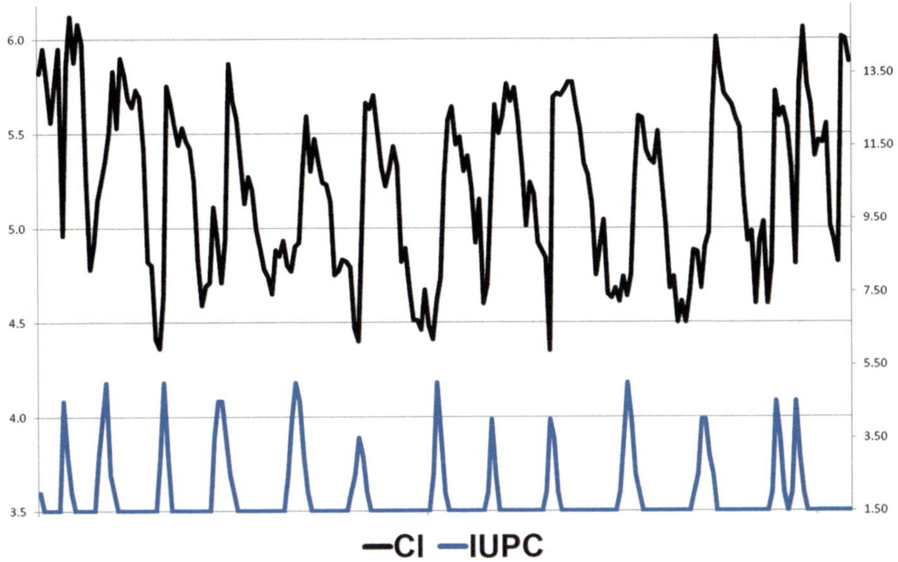

Fig. 2.3 "Autotransfusion waves" of increased cardiac output reach their maximum approximately 20–40 s after intrauterine pressure reaches its maximum. This figure shows the cardiac output as it changes during autotransfusion. This patient was in painless labor at 3 cm of cervical dilation. Peaks of cardiac index follow peaks of intrauterine pressure by about 40 s. 50 min of data are shown. Autotransfusion provides a "homemade" volume challenge to the maternal left ventricle, and the pain-free laboring patient's cardiovascular response to autotransfusion might yield valuable information about her cardiac function—specifically, the heart's position on its Starling Curve, as suggested by the next Fig. 2.4, in which the maternal heart is shown to be "fluid responsive" because the stroke volume increases when the autotransfusion occurs. *CI* cardiac index (L/min/m^2, left axis), *IUPC* pressure, intrauterine pressure catheter (arbitrary units, right axis) [1]

positions, patients had robust blood pressure and cardiac output and we saw autotransfusion waves after each uterine contraction, whereas in other positions the blood pressure and cardiac output both decreased and the autotransfusion waves either looked dampened or disappeared altogether, as shown in Figs. 2.1 and 2.2. This hemodynamic behavior is summarized schematically in Figs. 2.6 and 2.7: when the inferior vena cava is unobstructed, the cardiac output is high and autotransfusion waves occur after each uterine contraction (Fig. 2.6), but when the patient changes position, the cardiac output decreases and the autotransfusion waves disappear (Fig. 2.7).

But even more important than our ability to finally see the hemodynamic effects of aortocaval compression in real time was the fact that *these positional changes in maternal hemodynamics usually occurred without any immediate changes in the fetal heart rate or variability*, as shown in Fig. 2.8 [7]. Additionally, as also seen in Fig. 2.8, *uterine contractions did not appear to be affected (at least immediately) by the apparent obstruction of uterine venous return.*

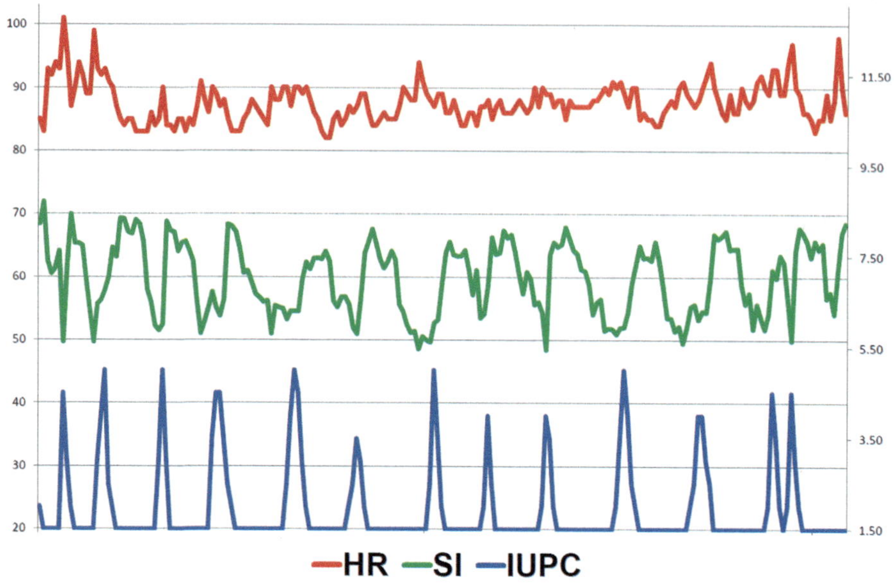

Fig. 2.4 This patient is "fluid responsive" because her stroke volume increases markedly in response to the "fluid challenge" of autotransfusion. This figure shows the same patient and time period as the preceding figure, but with the cardiac index broken up into its two components—heart rate and stroke index. In pain-free labor—as in this example—the maternal heart rate tends to stay relatively constant during contractions and therefore it is the stroke volume which increases—if it can!—in order to "handle" or "process" the volume challenge produced by autotransfusion. But the stroke volume will increase only if the patient's heart is on the steep "fluid-responsive" portion of its Starling Curve. If the heart is already functioning at its maximum end-diastolic volume before it receives the increased venous return caused by autotransfusion, the heart will be unable to increase its stroke volume any further and either the heart rate will increase—or the heart will fail! *HR* heart rate (beats per minute, left axis), *SI* stroke index (mL/m^2, left axis), *IUPC* pressure, intrauterine pressure catheter (arbitrary units, right axis) [1]

At least in the short term, it appeared that both the fetus and the myometrium continued to function as though nothing was wrong—even though uterine venous return was obstructed, cardiac output had decreased and uterine venous pressure had probably increased. It appeared that the fetus and myometrium were often sufficiently resilient to continue functioning normally for a while despite the gradual development of a growing threat to their oxygenation! We theorized further that eventually the fetus and myometrium would show the effects of growing hypoxia, but that these later changes might have been prevented if we had intervened earlier to change patient position on the basis of reductions in maternal cardiac output. In Fig. 2.9, the fetus shows the effects of hypoxia before the myometrium does and a cesarean delivery is performed for fetal distress, while in Fig. 2.10, it is the myometrium that fails first, and a cesarean delivery is performed for dysfunctional labor. **But in both cases, a cesarean delivery is performed which might have been avoided by recognizing and promptly correcting the fundamental cause of the fetal and myometrial hypoxia—obstruction of uterine venous return.**

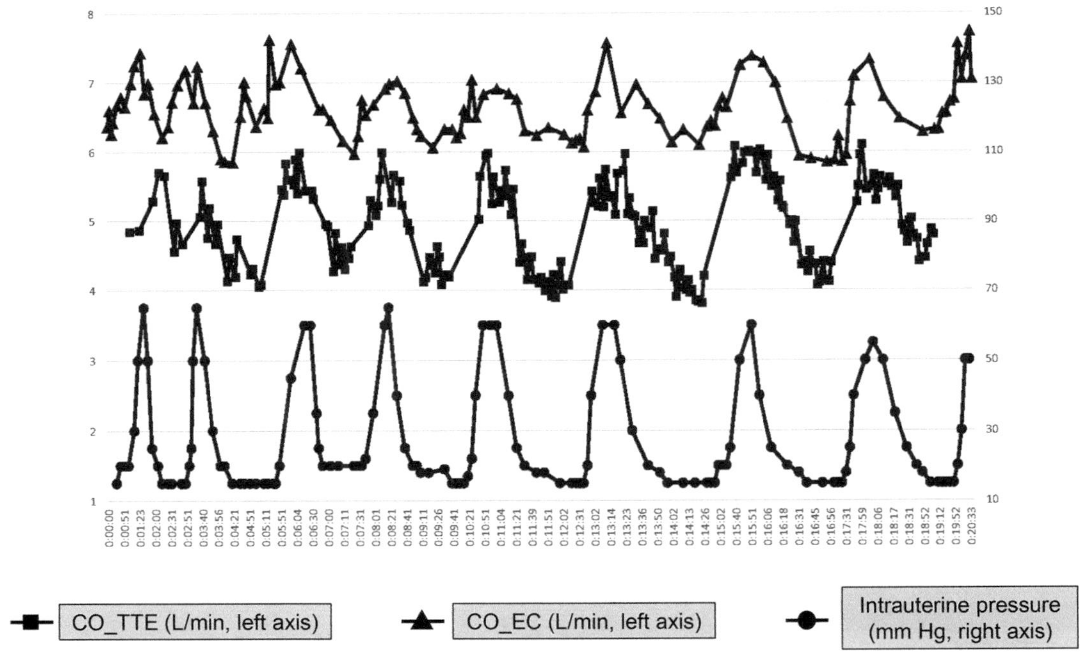

Fig. 2.5 "Autotransfusion waves" of increased cardiac output demonstrated simultaneously by electrical cardiometry and transthoracic echocardiography. This healthy patient in normal labor had an epidural in place and was tipped approximately 45° to her left to facilitate both venous return and imaging with transthoracic echocardiography. The values from electrical cardiometry are averages of the preceding 10 heartbeats, whereas each transthoracic echocardiography value is derived from one heartbeat. Chapter 8 gives an explanation of how electrical cardiometry works and shows how this impedance cardiography technique derives cardiac output in a way that is conceptually similar to that used in echocardiography. *CO_TTE* cardiac output measured by transthoracic echocardiography, *CO_EC* cardiac output measured by electrical cardiometry. Figure reference [6]. Published by Elsevier and used with permission. The caption has been modified

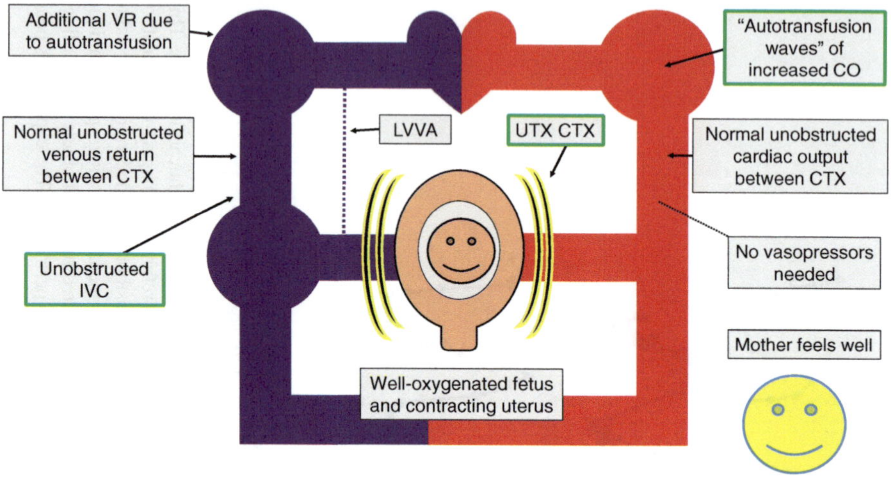

Fig. 2.6 Schematic diagram of "autotransfusion waves". This is the normal process of autotransfusion produced by uterine contractions in the presence of unobstructed pathways for the rapid return of venous blood to the heart. *CO* cardiac output, *CTX* contractions, *IVC* inferior vena cava, *LVVA* lumbar, vertebral venous, and azygos collateral pathways for venous return from the lower half of the body, including the uterus, *UTX* uterine, *VR* venous return

Of course, it is true that in current practice when the fetal heart rate slows, changes of maternal position are often applied empirically, but what I am suggesting is that we may be able to intervene much earlier in a deteriorating hemodynamic situation if we reposition the patient as soon as her cardiac output decreases, rather than waiting until the fetus becomes bradycardic or the myometrium starts to contract less frequently and with less force, in the process which we usually call "dysfunctional labor," but which might better be called (at least in some patients) "hypoxic myometrial failure."

We also realized that we could now detect obstruction of the inferior vena cava before it might be reflected in the recorded maternal blood pressure, which might be taken only every 15 min during a routine labor. In routine labor, blood pressures are not measured continuously, and decreases in blood pressure related to maternal position could easily be missed—or their recognition delayed. But by trending maternal cardiac output continuously, we seemed to be able to detect obstruction of the inferior vena cava as soon as it occurred, and to detect it independently of its effect on blood pressure. Vasopressors or the patient's sympathetic nervous system might be capable of maintaining an adequate blood pressure even in the face of a reduced maternal cardiac output, as shown in Fig. 2.11, and this maintenance of the maternal blood pressure might create a false sense of security. In contrast to the misleading maternal blood pressure, however, the decrease in maternal cardiac output would constitute a reliable early warning sign that a potentially dangerous hemodynamic situation was developing.

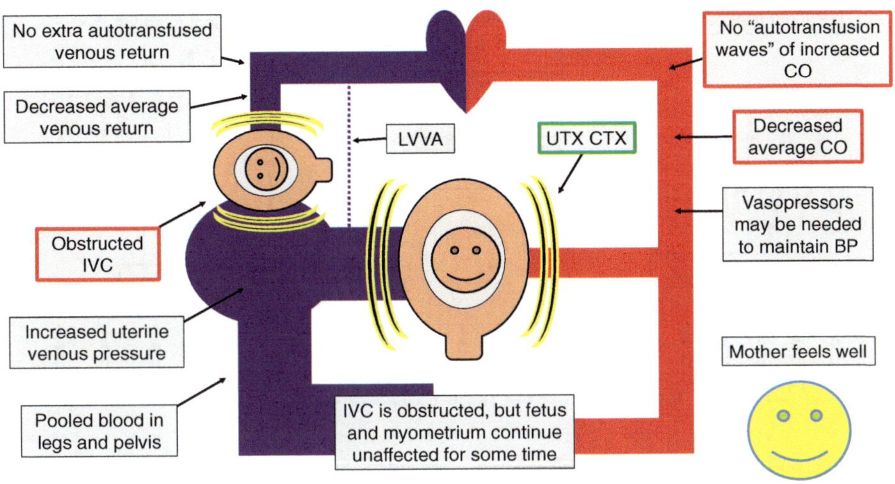

Fig. 2.7 The fetal heart and myometrium may continue to function normally for a while despite reduction of placental and myometrial perfusion. The obstetricians, nurses, and anesthesiologists taking care of the laboring patient may be so focused on the fetal heart rate as an indicator of adequate overall uterine perfusion that they may not realize that fetal heart rate changes and myometrial dysfunction may occur many minutes after obstruction of uterine venous return has occurred. Therefore, positional reductions of maternal cardiac output may serve as an *early warning* during labor of developing problems with fetal or myometrial oxygenation. If this is true, trending maternal cardiac output during labor—as well as the fetal heart rate—might allow the care team to reposition the patient as soon as reductions in maternal cardiac output occur, rather than having to wait until the fetal heart rate deteriorates in rate or variability or dysfunctional labor develops. *BP* blood pressure, *CO* cardiac output, *CTX* contractions, *IVC* inferior vena cava, *LVVA* lumbar, vertebral venous, and azygos collateral pathways for venous return from the lower half of the body, including the uterus, *UTX* uterine

So we began to think that the fetal heart rate may not be the most sensitive indicator of the safety of the fetal environment, or the well-being of the uterus as a whole during pregnancy. On the contrary, decreases in fetal heart rate or myometrial contractility may be relatively late signs in the sequence of events leading up to fetal or myometrial injury and a cesarean delivery either for fetal distress or dysfunctional labor.

The fetal heart rate is obviously very important and there are many important causes of fetal heart rate changes other than aortocaval compression, such as obstruction of the umbilical cord or placental abruption. But perhaps it is time to add another monitoring modality to labor—maternal cardiac output—as a warning indicator for obstruction of uterine venous return. Vasopressors may give us a false sense of security by restoring the blood pressure despite poor uterine perfusion, as shown in Fig. 2.11. This physiology is similar—on a short-term basis—to what we have theorized the maternal sympathetic nervous system may do during gestation on a chronic basis, as shown in Fig. 1.8.

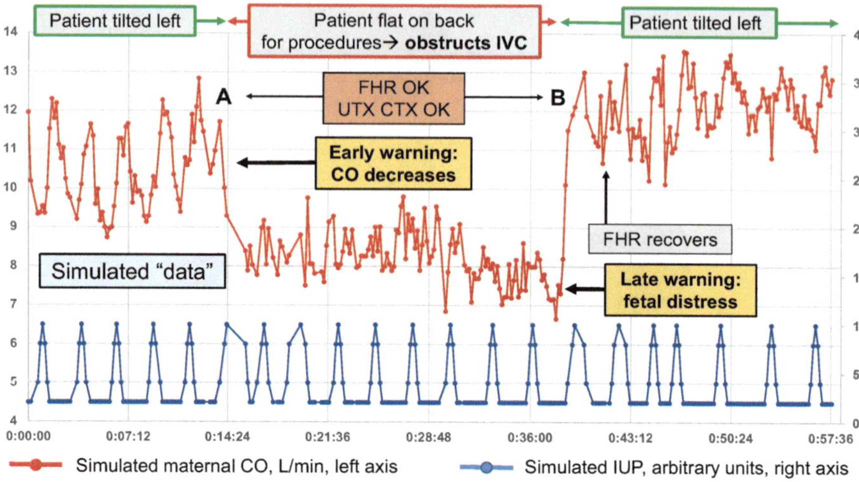

Fig. 2.8 Fetal bradycardia can be delayed after obstruction of uterine venous return occurs. (This is simulated "data" based on the author's unpublished clinical research experience). This figure uses simulated data to describe the essence of a patient care episode which I witnessed during our clinical research. We were following the cardiac output of a woman in labor who required the placement of urinary and intrauterine pressure catheters because her labor was not progressing satisfactorily. The patient was comfortable because she had an epidural in place, and she had been positioned on her left side to prevent obstruction of the inferior vena cava by the uterus, but in order to facilitate the placement of the two catheters, the patient was placed into the supine position. The placement of both catheters was delayed due to a temporary absence of personnel, but the fetal heart rate continued to show good rate and variability. For this reason, it was considered acceptable to allow the patient to remain supine since "the baby was tolerating the position." The urinary catheter was finally placed, but the resident obstetrician had trouble placing the intrauterine pressure catheter, and in the middle of her attempts the fetus became bradycardic. The patient was immediately turned onto her left side, oxygen was applied, and the fetal heart rate promptly returned to normal. Review of the hemodynamic data revealed that the patient's cardiac output had decreased significantly in the supine position and had remained in a downward trend for over 20 min before the fetus became bradycardic, as shown in this visual description using simulated data. *CO* cardiac output, *CTX* contractions, *FHR* fetal heart rate, *IUP* intrauterine pressure, *IVC* inferior vena cava, *UTX* uterine. Figure reference: [7]. Figure and modified caption used with permission

As we continued to think about the usefulness of trending maternal cardiac output in labor, we began to think that unrecognized obstruction of uterine venous return might also occur much earlier in gestation. If cardiac output-guided maternal positioning could help us in labor management, perhaps it could help in obstetric management throughout gestation! This possibility is the subject of succeeding chapters.

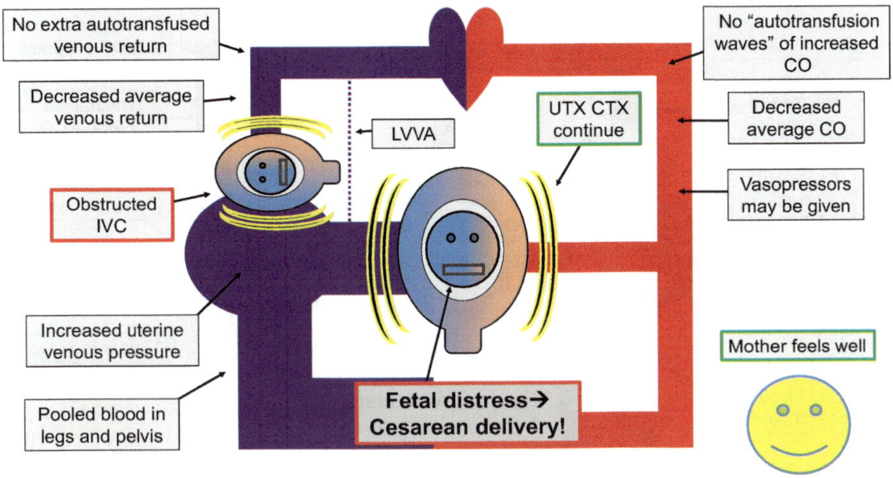

Fig. 2.9 Unrecognized obstruction of uterine venous return may cause unnecessary cesarean deliveries for fetal distress. In practice, when there is fetal bradycardia, one of the first interventions performed is maternal position change, but this change is made on an empirical basis and results might be better if position change were (1) performed earlier, i.e., as soon as maternal cardiac output decreases and (2) performed with cardiac output maximization, to ensure that obstruction of uterine venous return was being maximally relieved by the maneuver. This figure postulates that unrecognized obstruction of uterine venous return can sometimes precipitate "fetal distress" when the myometrium is still able to contract adequately despite partial blockage of its venous return and some degree of myometrial hypoxia. In other words, under the effects of the generalized hypoxia produced by obstruction of uterine venous return, it may be that sometimes the fetus "fails" before the myometrium does. *CO* cardiac output, *CTX* contractions, *IVC* inferior vena cava, *LVVA* lumbar, vertebral venous, and azygos collateral venous system, *UTX* uterine

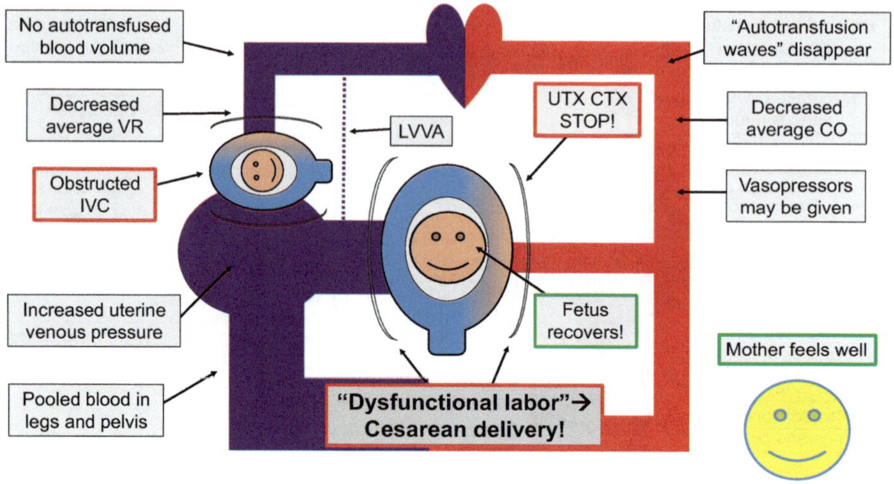

Fig. 2.10 Unrecognized obstruction of uterine venous return may cause unnecessary cesarean deliveries for dysfunctional labor. As an anesthesiologist practicing in Labor and Delivery, it has often seemed that labor is a race between the uterus and the fetus to see which will have problems first. This figure shows the opposite situation to that shown in the preceding figure. In this figure, it is the myometrium which "fails" first—and the fetus fully recovers! Uterine contractions require the myometrium to consume more oxygen, but the contractions themselves deprive the myometrium of the oxygen it needs! Obviously, too, the fetus requires oxygen, and uterine contractions cut off blood flow to the placenta, threatening fetal oxygenation as well. Both of these processes are unavoidable, but what may be avoidable is the role that obstruction of uterine venous return may play in making both fetal and myometrial oxygenation much less efficient. The figure shows a not uncommon situation: the fetus has not been "tolerating labor," as manifested by late decelerations (not shown), but the myometrium—whose contractions have been "augmented" with oxytocin—is failing as well, and uterine contractions have weakened or stopped, as shown in the figure. The fetal heart rate has recovered, because myometrial contractions have stopped and continuous fetal oxygenation has been restored, but since sufficient progress down the birth canal has not occurred, the decision is made for cesarean delivery due to "failure to progress." The oxytocin is turned off and the hypoxic myometrium stops contracting altogether. A cesarean delivery is performed and a healthy, well-oxygenated infant is delivered. But was it possible that unrecognized obstruction of uterine venous return had set the stage for the problem in the first place? Perhaps cardiac output-guided maternal positioning would have allowed better oxygenation of both fetus and myometrium throughout labor and allowed a vaginal delivery, rather than a cesarean. *CO* cardiac output, *CTX* contractions, *IVC* inferior vena cava, *LVVA* lumbar, vertebral venous, and azygos collateral venous system, *UTX* uterine, *VR* venous return

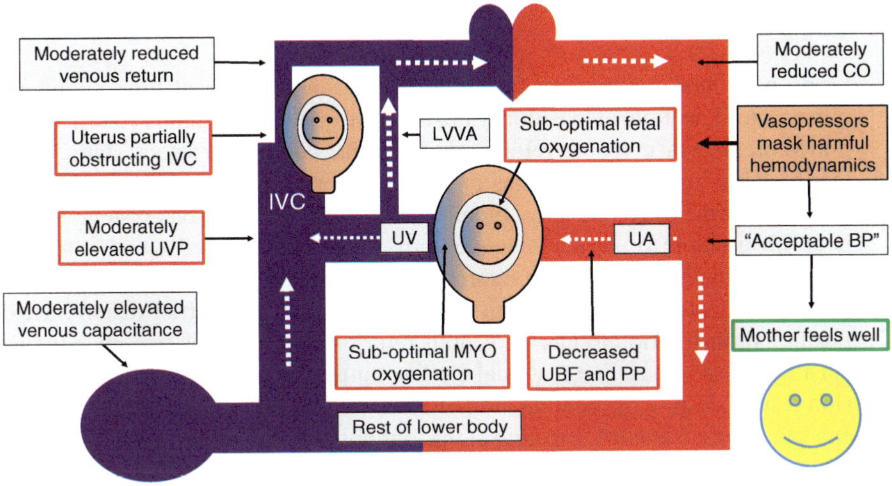

Fig. 2.11 Hemodynamic mediocrity in labor, with multiple weak links in oxygen delivery. This is the highly imperfect situation we should avoid in labor: the inferior vena cava is partially obstructed, but not completely, and some venous return from the uterus is able to arrive at the heart via the lumbar, vertebral venous, and azygos system—but not enough to fully compensate for the partial obstruction of the inferior vena cava. The fetus may be showing early signs of hypoxia, but the maternal blood pressure is being maintained in an "acceptable" (though suboptimal) range with vasopressors. Would it not be better to use cardiac output-guided maternal positioning to ensure that the inferior vena cava is completely unobstructed so that venous return to the heart, maternal blood pressure, and uteroplacental perfusion were all maximized? *Without cardiac output-guided maternal positioning, we may be "flying blind" with respect to maternal and uterine hemodynamics, and we may be accepting a "good enough" labor course (with or without a cesarean delivery), even though it may not be the optimal labor course.* *BP* blood pressure, *CO* cardiac output, *IVC* inferior vena cava, *LVVA* lumbar, vertebral venous, and azygos collateral venous system, *MYO* myometrial, *PP* perfusion pressure, *UA* uterine artery, *UBF* uterine blood flow, *UTX* uterine, *UV* uterine vein, *UVP* uterine venous pressure

Summary

1. Using a method for trending maternal cardiac output in real time allows the immediate detection of positional obstruction of uterine venous return by the gravid uterus, since venous return equals cardiac output in a steady state.
2. During labor, uterine contractions produce autotransfusion of maternal blood. In other words, the uterus squeezes blood out of itself into the venous system. If there is no obstruction to uterine venous return, this autotransfused blood enters the central circulation and rapidly returns to the heart all at once, causing periodic increases in maternal cardiac output which we have called "autotransfusion waves."
3. Positional obstruction to uterine venous return in labor causes two phenomena: (1) a decrease in baseline maternal cardiac output and (2) a loss of autotransfusion waves, despite the continuation of uterine contractions. These two phenomena can be used as *early warning signs* to reposition the patient before the fetus or myometrium begins to be negatively affected by the decreased uteroplacental perfusion and the increase in uterine venous pressure which accompany obstruction to uterine venous return.
4. This use of reductions in maternal cardiac output as a signal to reposition the patient may be termed "cardiac output-guided maternal positioning" and its practice might result in fewer episodes of fetal distress and fewer cesarean deliveries for dysfunctional labor.
5. Cardiac output-guided maternal positioning might also prevent serious problems earlier in gestation, as we will discuss in the following chapters.

References

1. Ballas J, Mantell K, Archer TL. Electrical cardiometry demonstrates the hemodynamics of aortocaval compression and autotransfusion during labor. Poster and oral presentation at Society for Obstetric Anesthesia and Perinatology (SOAP) meeting, May 2–5, 2012, Monterey, California.
2. Archer TL, Suresh P, Shapiro AE. Cardiac output measurement, by means of electrical velocimetry, may be able to determine optimum maternal position during gestation, labour and caesarean delivery, by preventing vena caval compression and maximising cardiac output and placental perfusion pressure. Anaesth Intensive Care. 2011;39(2):308–11. PMID: 21485686.
3. Kerr MG, Scott DB, Samuel E. Studies of the inferior vena cava in late pregnancy. Br Med J. 1964;1(5382):522–33. PMID: 20790097; PMCID: PMC1813561.
4. Scott DB. Inferior vena caval occlusion in late pregnancy and its importance in anaesthesia. Br J Anaesth. 1968;40(2):120–8. https://doi.org/10.1093/bja/40.2.120. PMID: 5645758.
5. Higuchi H, Takagi S, Zhang K, Fruit I, Ozaki M. Effect of lateral tilt angle on the volume of the abdominal aorta and inferior vena cava in pregnant and nonpregnant women determined by magnetic resonance imaging. Anesthesiology. 2015;122(2):286–93. https://doi.org/10.1097/ALN.0000000000000553. PMID: 25603203.
6. Archer TL. Transthoracic echocardiography and electrical cardiometry elucidate the hemodynamics of autotransfusion during labor under epidural analgesia. Int J Obstet Anesth. 2017;31:113–5. https://doi.org/10.1016/j.ijoa.2017.03.010. Epub 2017 Mar 24. PMID: 28676402.
7. Archer TL. Neuraxial anesthesia and the supine position cause non-reassuring fetal status. In: Archer TL, editor. Obstetric anesthesia: a case-based and visual approach. 1st ed. Cham: Springer; 2020. https://doi.org/10.1007/978-3-030-26478-9_2.

Preeclampsia and Fetal Growth Restriction: Intervillous Space *Flow*

3

Personal Note

Every morning, the anesthesia team sat in on Obstetrical Board Rounds led by the maternal-fetal medicine professor assigned to Labor and Delivery that day. For me, it was a wonderful experience, since I not only got to learn about the specific patients for the day but also learned a lot of obstetrics and maternal-fetal medicine, along with the residents and medical students. Figure 3.1 shows the normal placental circulation in an anatomically accurate way. Figure 3.2 focuses on a healthy intervillous space in what is (at least for me) an easy-to-understand way of thinking about intervillous space blood flow, pressure, and oxygenation of the chorionic villi and fetus.

At Board Rounds during 2010—as our anesthesia research team was learning that reductions in maternal cardiac output could be used as a marker for obstruction of uterine venous return—I began to learn about the umbilical artery Doppler velocimetry changes seen in fetal growth restriction. I was also beginning to understand how preeclampsia and fetal growth restriction might be separate disorders. Until then I had thought that both disorders were tightly associated (if not two aspects of the same process), as shown in Fig. 3.3. I believed that defective spiral artery remodeling reduced perfusion of the intervillous space, thereby producing hypoxia of the maternal blood in that space. This hypoxia then caused the fetus to be growth restricted and the chorionic villi to release anti-angiogenic factors into the mother's circulation—which then caused the preeclampsia syndrome. This seemed to be the "classical" theory of preeclampsia—that one lesion (defective spiral artery remodeling) produced both fetal growth restriction and preeclampsia [1–4].

In light of our ongoing research which seemed to allow us to detect obstruction of uterine venous return—and as I tried to imagine the placenta's "point of view" regarding its own perfusion—I began to ask myself, "Couldn't uterine *venous* obstruction reduce perfusion of the intervillous space and cause preeclampsia and fetal growth restriction in the same way?" [5–7]. The reduction of intervillous space

T. L. Archer, *Threats to Fetal, Placental and Myometrial Oxygenation*,
https://doi.org/10.1007/978-3-031-60364-8_3

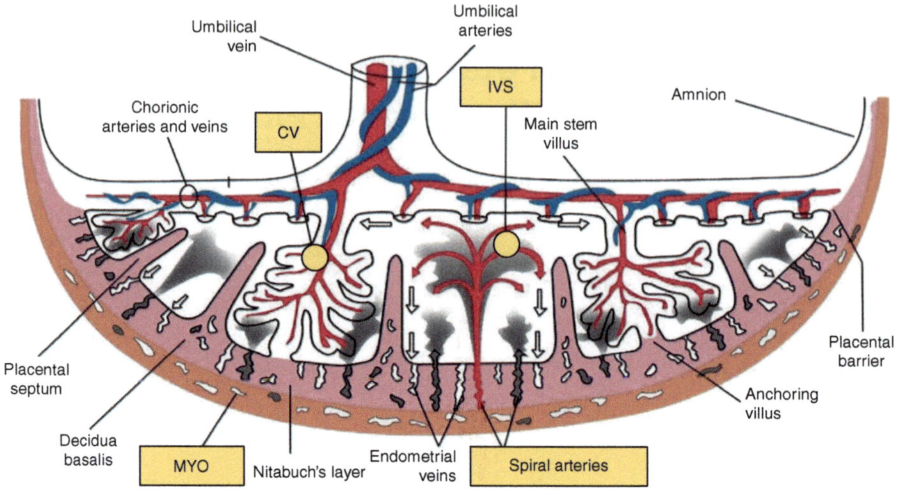

Fig. 3.1 Anatomic view of the normal placenta. The intervillous space is the "main stage" of the placenta, where the crucial work of matching maternal and fetal perfusion occurs. Without adequate perfusion from both sides—and without the successful matching up of those two blood flows—the fetus either suffers growth restriction or dies. Slow-moving but voluminous streams of maternal blood enter the intervillous spaces through spiral arteries which have gone through a process of "remodeling," which means that they have been converted from high-resistance thick-walled vessels into flaccid and widely dilated vessels which allow more voluminous but less violent blood flow through the intervillous space. The fetal circulation is confined within the chorionic villus trees, with each separate tree being called a "cotyledon" (labeled "CV" for "chorionic villus" in the figure). A placenta has approximately 15–28 cotyledons [35]. The maternal blood exits the intervillous space through decidual endometrial veins which empty into the uterine veins and then into the inferior vena cava to return to the heart. *Obstruction of uterine venous return at any point from the myometrium itself to the inferior vena cava will increase pressure within the intervillous space and tend to reduce maternal intervillous perfusion. The increased intervillous space pressure may also compress chorionic villi and reduce fetoplacental perfusion, but consideration of the pressure effects of obstruction of uterine venous return on fetal oxygenation is deferred until the next chapter.* This chapter concentrates on intervillous *flow*. *CV* chorionic villus (also called "cotyledon" to refer to the entire villus "tree"), *IVS* intervillous space, *MYO* myometrium [36]. Caption has been changed and figure has been modified by addition of labels. © 2020 The Authors. Acta Obstetricia et Gynecologica Scandinavica published by John Wiley & Sons Ltd on behalf of Nordic Federation of Societies of Obstetrics and Gynecology (NFOG). This is an open access article distributed under the terms of the Creative Commons CC BY license

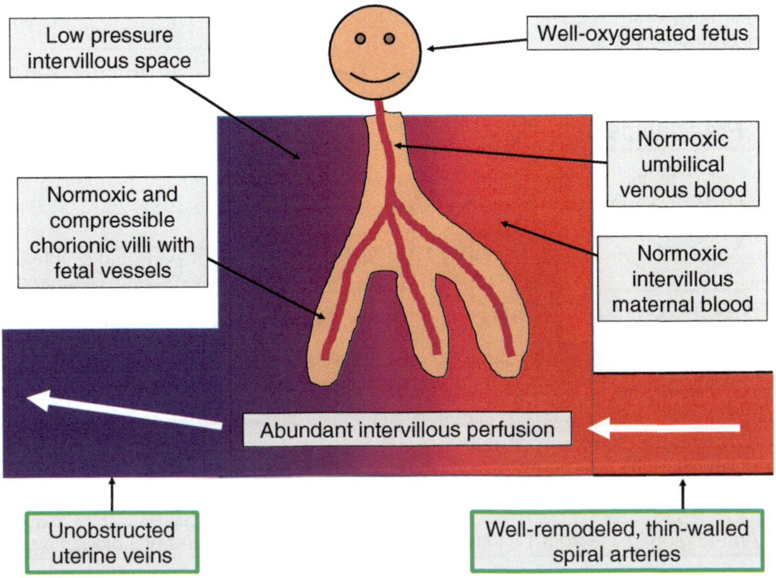

Fig. 3.2 Schematic view of the intervillous space. This schematic view helps me think about perfusion and pressure within the intervillous space. Blood flows from right to left, entering through well-remodeled and widely patent spiral arteries and exiting through a uterine venous system that is not blocked in any way—either at the inferior vena cava or by increased tissue pressure within the myometrium itself. Blood flow through the intervillous space is brisk but not violent, and the fetus is well oxygenated. The pressure within the intervillous space is low and therefore the chorionic villi are not compressed by the maternal blood around them

flow would be similar between the two lesions: defective spiral artery remodeling would restrict intervillous space flow from the arterial side of the intervillous space, whereas obstruction of uterine venous return would restrict flow from the venous side. Figures 3.3 and 3.4 together represent this similarity. I also thought that perhaps the obstruction of uterine venous return could act as a "second hit" acting in synergy with defective spiral artery remodeling (the "first hit"), to accelerate the onset of preeclampsia or exacerbate its effects, as shown in Fig. 3.5. If this were true, prevention of obstruction of uterine venous return during gestation could decrease the rate of development and final impact of fetal growth restriction or preeclampsia which had been set in motion by other less treatable conditions such as a mild degree of impaired spiral artery remodeling, obesity, chronic hypertension or diabetic vasculopathy. In other words, prevention of obstruction of uterine venous return might mitigate the development of preeclampsia or fetal growth restriction even if such obstruction were not the sole or even primary cause of those disorders.

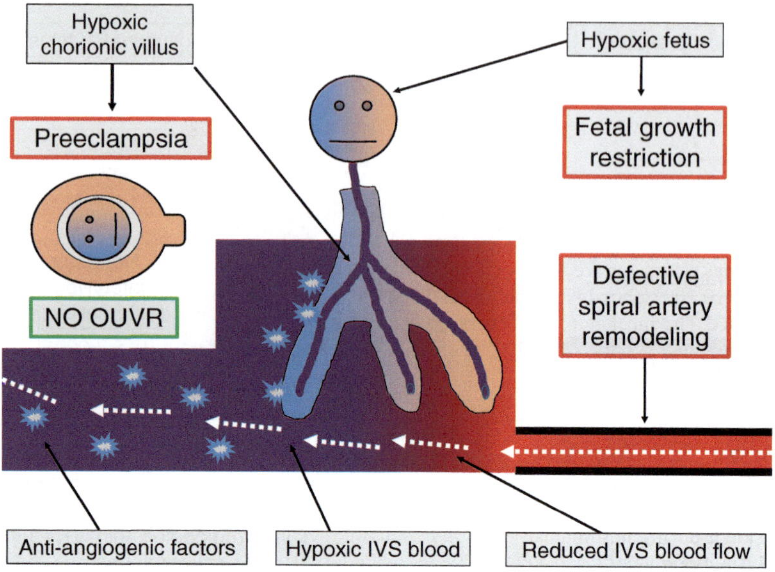

Fig. 3.3 The "classical" theory of preeclampsia and fetal growth restriction, as I understood it in 2010. Defective spiral artery remodeling at 16–18 weeks of gestation fails to convert the normally thick-walled and high-resistance spiral arteries into the thin-walled and low-resistance arteries that are needed to provide abundant but gentle maternal blood flow through the intervillous spaces. Reduced intervillous perfusion through these high-resistance arteries reduces the pO_2 in the intervillous space, making the chorionic villi hypoxic and making them release anti-angiogenic factors into the maternal circulation. These factors then damage maternal endothelium and cause the preeclampsia syndrome. Fetal growth restriction—a closely related result—occurs because the fetus does not get enough oxygen from the hypoxic intervillous space in order to realize its full growth potential. In this "classic" view of preeclampsia and fetal growth restriction, obstruction of uterine return is not considered to be a factor in causing either condition nor is increased intervillous space pressure a part of the model. *OUVR* obstruction of uterine venous return, *IVS* intervillous space

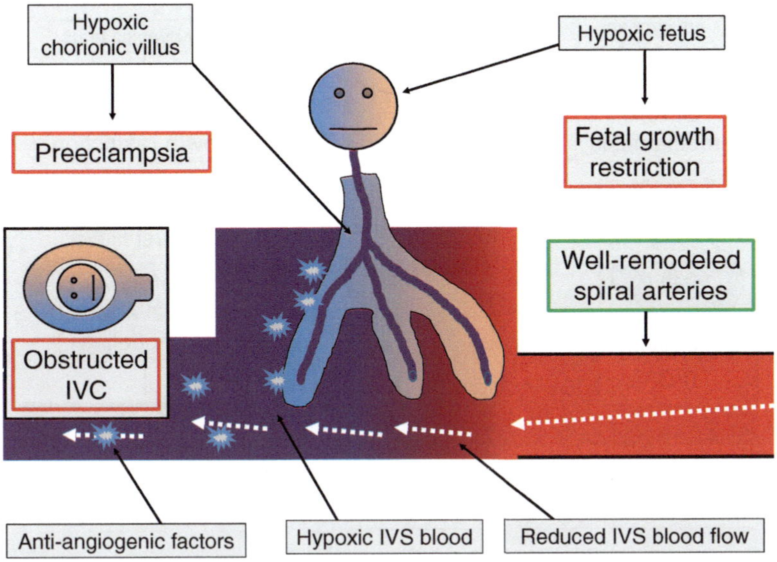

Fig. 3.4 Could obstruction of uterine venous return reduce intervillous perfusion and cause preeclampsia or fetal growth restriction? Prolonged obstruction of uterine venous return might accelerate the development of preeclampsia or fetal growth restriction set in motion by other causes or even cause those conditions by itself. As we proceeded with our research at the University of California San Diego, this became more than a theoretical question since my colleagues and I felt we were developing a method of knowing when obstruction of uterine venous return was taking place. If obstruction of uterine venous return in the second half of gestation could cause or accelerate injury, then preventing it might prevent or mitigate that injury. *IVC* inferior vena cava, *IVS* intervillous space

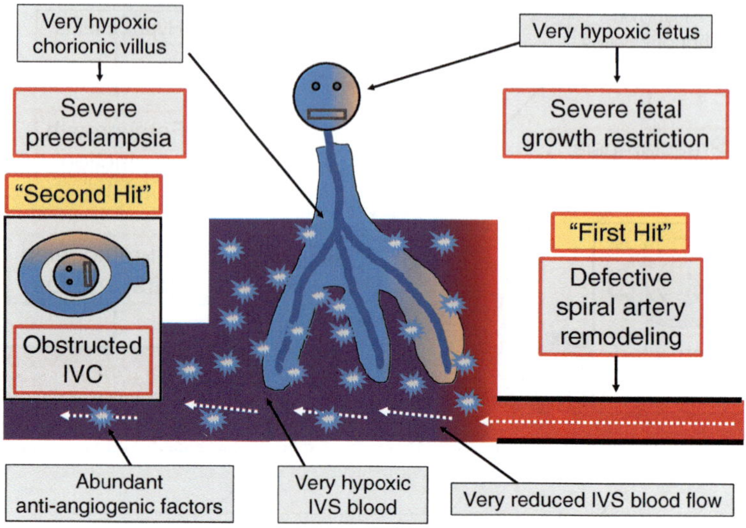

Fig. 3.5 Obstruction of uterine venous return may aggravate other fetal, placental, or myometrial vulnerabilities. Obstruction of uterine venous return might cause placental perfusion problems on its own or in synergy with other risk factors, such as diabetes, chronic hypertension, multiple gestation, obesity, short maternal stature, or defective spiral artery remodeling, as shown here. Any structure or process that either decreased the oxygen supply or increased the oxygen demand of the fetus, placenta or myometrium would be a "first hit" whose impact could be increased by a "second hit" from obstruction of uterine venous return. *IVC* inferior vena cava, *IVS* intervillous space

Uterine Perfusion Is "Pressure Passive"

Perfusion of the uterus is "pressure passive," as shown in Fig. 3.6 [8]. This term means that the uterus has neither the autoregulation of the brain nor the metabolic regulation of muscle. The purpose of autoregulation for the brain is to keep cerebral perfusion constant despite changing blood pressure, and the purpose of the metabolic regulation of perfusion to muscle is to provide blood flow to muscle cells only when they need it. But the uterus has no mechanism for regulating its own perfusion to meet its own needs or those of the fetus. Uterine perfusion is at the mercy of three simple factors: (1) uterine artery pressure, (2) uterine venous pressure, and (3) myometrial tissue pressure, when it exceeds uterine venous pressure.

The simple determination of uterine perfusion shown in Fig. 3.6 highlights the importance of uterine venous pressure in determining uterine perfusion and suggests that obstruction of uterine venous return with increased uterine venous pressure might harm both placental and myometrial function. Reduction of intervillous

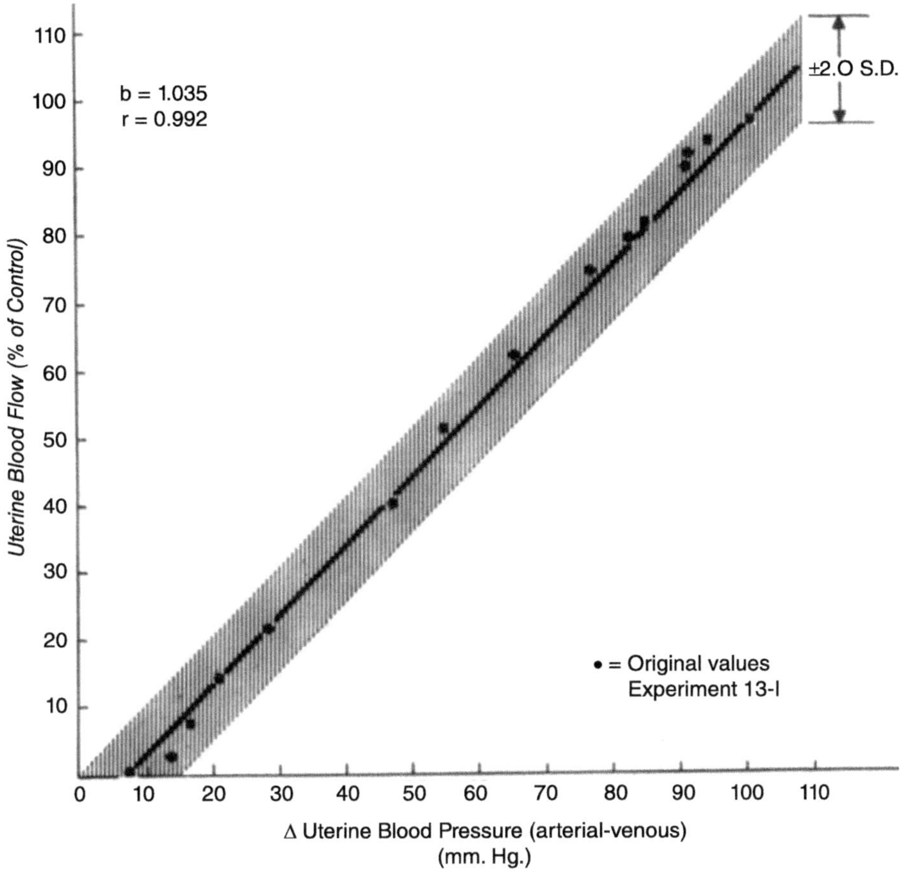

Fig. 3.6 Perfusion of the uterus is "pressure passive". The uterus has neither the autoregulation of cerebral perfusion nor the metabolic regulation of muscle perfusion. Uterine perfusion is at the mercy of three factors: (1) uterine artery pressure, (2) uterine venous pressure, and (3) myometrial tissue pressure, when it exceeds uterine venous pressure. The simple "pressure passive" determination of uterine perfusion shown in Fig. 3.6 highlights the importance of uterine venous pressure in determining uterine perfusion and suggests that obstruction of uterine venous return could easily reduce placental and myometrial perfusion and function. *Δ* difference [8]: Publisher is Elsevier. Used with permission

space perfusion could be due to obstruction of uterine venous return alone or in combination with other causes such as maternal arterial disease from diabetes or chronic hypertension—or maternal arterial hypotension, such as that due to hemorrhage or neuraxial anesthesia.

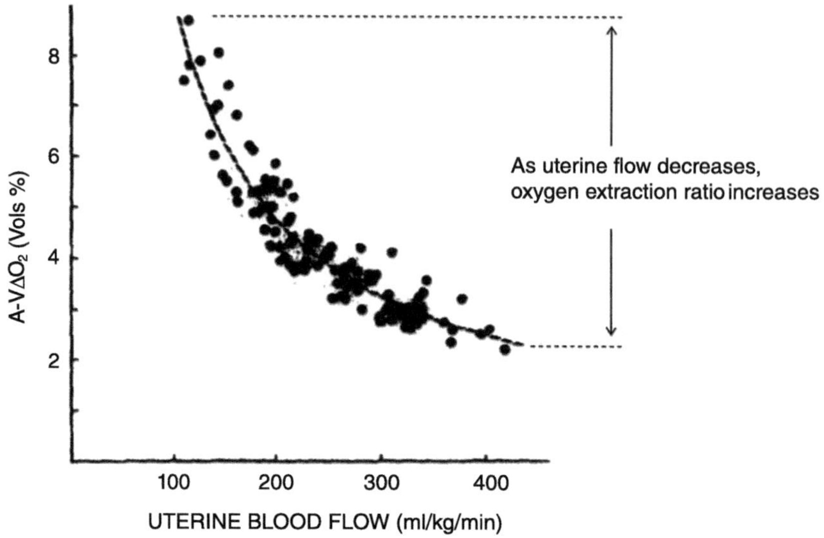

Fig. 3.7 The oxygenation of maternal blood in the intervillous space decreases as uterine perfusion decreases. This experiment was performed in sheep, but it is believed that its results apply to humans as well. Uterine blood flow was artificially controlled in living pregnant sheep and uterine venous blood samples were obtained as uterine perfusion was changed. When uterine (and presumably placental) perfusion was experimentally decreased, the arterial-uterine venous oxygen content difference increases. This experiment makes use of the "series" model of placental perfusion (see the next figure) which assumes that all uterine perfusion passes through the IVS, and therefore that a reduction in uterine venous pO_2 reflects a comparable reduction in intervillous space pO_2. Some uterine perfusion passes through the myometrium and other perfusion may pass through arteriovenous shunts [12], but since most uterine perfusion does pass through the placenta, the following conclusion can be drawn from the experiment: reduction of uterine perfusion—by whatever means—will reduce intervillous pO_2, which in turn might cause preeclampsia and/or fetal growth restriction. *A-V* O_2 Δ arteriovenous oxygen content difference in vols % [13]. Publisher is Elsevier. Used with permission

As shown in Fig. 3.7, experimentally reduced uterine perfusion in sheep does, as would be expected, result in decreased uterine venous oxygen tension, which is taken to reflect a reduced oxygen tension within the intervillous space. Therefore, it appears plausible that reduced uterine perfusion will cause intervillous space hypoxia, and that this reduced perfusion could be imposed either from the arterial or the venous side.

Decreased Intervillous Perfusion Leads to Decreased Intervillous Oxygen Tension

Figure 3.8 shows healthy and abundant maternal perfusion of the intervillous space. Well-remodeled maternal spiral arteries gently release large quantities of maternal blood into the intervillous space where it percolates around the chorionic villi without damaging them with the force of its stream [9].

This gentle flow—perhaps aided by a "utero-placental pump"—creates a well-mixed lake of intervillous blood with a pO_2 adequate for fetal oxygenation [10]. The chorionic tissue and fetal vessels within that space could be compressed and deformed by external pressure if it were elevated [11], but in the absence of uterine venous obstruction the intervillous space pressure is low and compression of the chorionic villi does not occur.

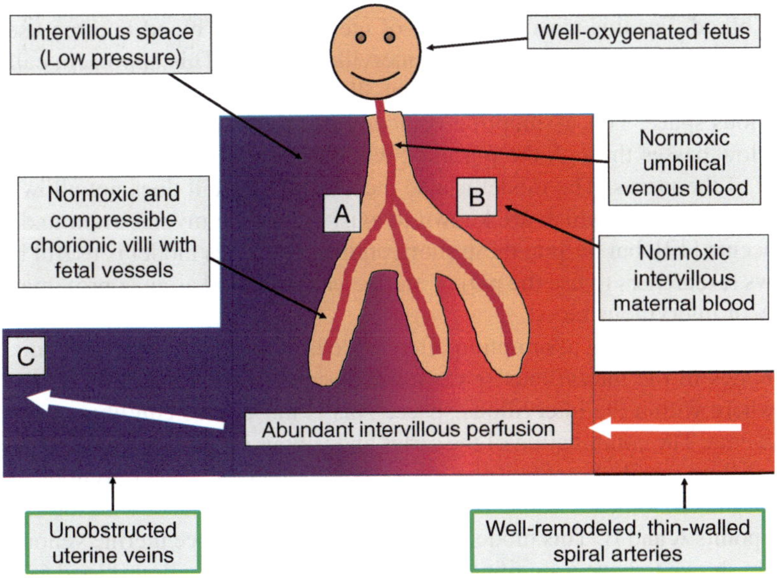

Fig. 3.8 The series model for uterine perfusion: uterine venous pO_2 = intervillous space pO_2. We would like to know the pO_2 of the maternal blood within the intervillous spaces and intervillous blood can be drawn from the placenta at the time of cesarean delivery, but historically in animal research, serial blood samples have been drawn from the uterine veins. We would like to know the oxygen tension at point A because that is the "driving pressure" for diffusion of oxygen from the intervillous space into fetal blood. For practical reasons, we must use the oxygen tension in uterine venous blood as a proxy for the oxygen tension within the intervillous space. This practical compromise is the combination of the series and venous equilibrator models (see the next figure), which assumes that all uterine perfusion passes through intervillous spaces, and that the mixing of blood within the IVS is instantaneous. Blood oxygen level dependent (BOLD) MRI imaging is an emerging non-invasive technique for measuring hemoglobin oxygen saturation in vivo, which allows the completely non-invasive assessment of placental and fetal oxygenation [10]

Point A in Fig. 3.8 represents maternal blood in contact with the chorionic villi, and the oxygen tension (pO_2) at this point is of interest for three reasons: first, it is the pO_2 which drives diffusion of oxygen across the placental barrier into fetal blood; second, it is the pO_2 which—if low—probably triggers the release of anti-angiogenic factors from the syncytiotrophoblast layer of the chorionic villus into the maternal circulation to cause preeclampsia; and third, it is the pO_2 which—when low— triggers the vasoconstriction of the fetoplacental circulation which is known as "hypoxic fetoplacental vasoconstriction." But blood from point A is merely a theoretical construct. The best we can do is to sample intervillous blood from one or multiple intervillous spaces, as shown in Fig. 3.8 as point B.

The blood sample from point B has participated in two processes: (1) it has given up oxygen to the fetal circulation by diffusion across the placental barrier and (2) it has mixed with fresh spiral artery blood. Although it is possible to acquire blood samples from the intervillous space, it is much easier in instrumented sheep to acquire serial samples of uterine venous blood (point C in Fig. 3.8) instead of intervillous blood. For this reason, the pO_2 of uterine venous blood is often used as a surrogate for the pO_2 of blood in the intervillous space. This approach, called the series model of the placenta, assumes that all uterine blood flow passes through the intervillous space. This assumption is incorrect since, at term, only 80% of uterine blood flow passes through the placenta, while 20% perfuses the myometrium and the rest of the uterus. The model is also incorrect because it does not allow for the arteriovenous shunts which are known to exist within the myometrium underneath the placenta [12], but despite these shortcomings the series model is useful because it allows researchers to use the pO_2 of uterine venous blood as an approximation for the pO_2 of intervillous blood.

Another simplifying assumption often made is that spiral artery blood mixes and equilibrates in the intervillous space instantaneously, so that the pO_2 is the same everywhere within the intervillous space. This is the venous equilibrator model of the placenta. The combination of the series and venous equilibrator models is shown in Fig. 3.9, in which the pO_2 of the more easily obtainable uterine venous blood at point C is taken to be the same as that of blood in actual contact with the chorionic villi at points A and B. This model is not exactly correct, since uterine venous blood has been shown to have a significantly higher pO_2 than intervillous blood (as shown in Fig. 3.10), but despite the shortcomings of the series and venous equilibrator models, they have served well to establish an essential and generally accepted point: decreased perfusion of the intervillous space decreases the pO_2 of the blood in that space. By the Fick principle, as intervillous space flow decreases, more and more oxygen will be extracted from the available maternal blood to satisfy the relatively

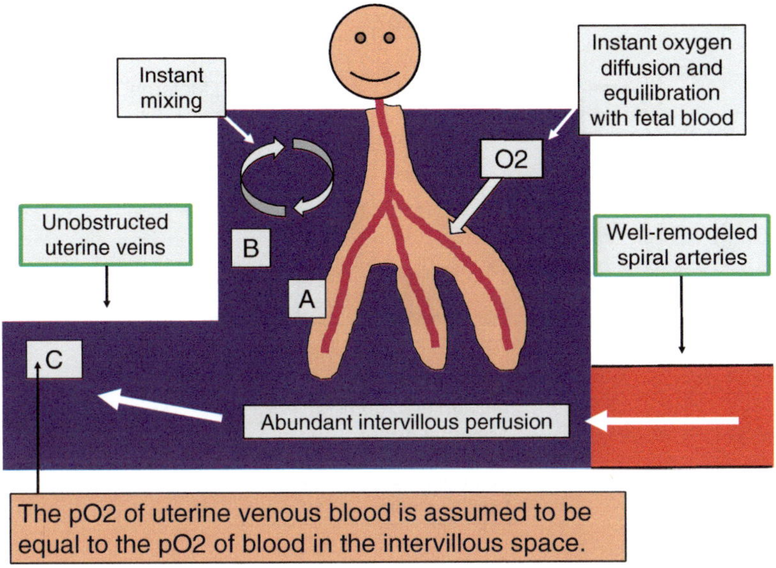

Fig. 3.9 The "venous equilibrator" model: instant equilibration of intervillous space blood with fetal blood and instant mixing of intervillous space blood. The assumption of this model is that the maternal blood within the intervillous space instantly (1) equilibrates its oxygen tension with that of fetal blood and (2) mixes completely. If this "venous equilibrator" assumption—and the "series" assumption described in the previous figure—were true, then the pO_2 of intervillous blood would be the same throughout the intervillous space, and the pO_2 of uterine venous blood would be the same as that of mixed intervillous space blood. O_2 oxygen, pO_2 partial pressure of oxygen (mm Hg)

fixed oxygen requirements of the fetus and the placenta itself. This point was verified experimentally in 1978 in chronically instrumented sheep in which uterine arteriovenous (AV) oxygen content differences were measured at different controlled rates of overall uterine perfusion. These experiments resulted in the data shown in Fig. 3.7, where the arteriovenous oxygen content difference across the uterus increases as the rate of uterine perfusion decreases [13]. *Obstruction of uterine venous return could cause the rate of uterine perfusion to decrease and the resulting decreased intervillous space oxygen tension would not only decrease the amount of oxygen available to the fetus within the intervillous space but might also trigger hypoxic fetoplacental vasoconstriction in a generalized and counterproductive way, as discussed later in this chapter.*

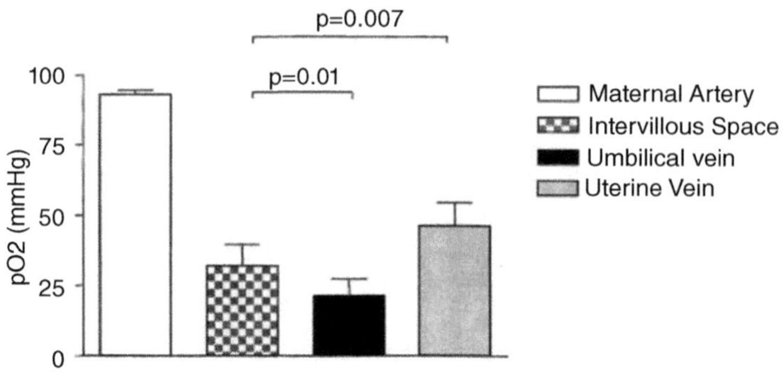

Median pO2 (mmHg)	
Maternal Artery	93
Uterine Vein	46.1
Intervillous space	29.2
Umbilical vein	19

Fig. 3.10 The oxygen tension of uterine venous blood is higher than that of intervillous space blood—disproving the series model. This human data obtained during cesarean delivery shows that uterine venous blood had a higher oxygen tension than intervillous space blood, suggesting that maternal blood was somehow being shunted around the intervillous spaces—either through myometrial capillary beds or through myometrial arteriovenous shunts within which no gas exchange occurs. pO_2 partial pressure of oxygen [12]. Figure has been modified. Used with permission. Publisher is Elsevier

Can We Prevent Fetal Growth Restriction and Preeclampsia?

If uterine venous obstruction does play a role in fetal growth restriction and preeclampsia, it may be preventable. By avoiding obstruction of uterine venous return, obstetricians, midwives and pregnant women themselves might be able to prevent or delay the development of preeclampsia, rather than just managing the disorder when it occurs. In 1983, Spinapolice et al. published a study in which 4 h/day of maternal rest in the left lateral decubitus position reduced the incidence of preeclampsia in a group of patients at high risk for the disease [14]. The rationale for that treatment was to avoid obstruction of uterine venous return during the rest period.

More recently, there have been attempts to prevent or palliate fetal growth restriction and preeclampsia using the nitric oxide donor nitroglycerin and supplemental intravascular volume expansion to improve global maternal hemodynamics by reducing systemic vascular resistance and increasing cardiac output [15–18]. These studies appear promising, but they have not considered the possible importance of obstruction of uterine venous return in the pathogenesis of preeclampsia and fetal growth restriction and the possible conflicting roles that nitroglycerin may play in hemodynamic processes related to that obstruction.

Specifically, nitroglycerin dilates vascular smooth muscle at multiple sites, including maternal capacitance veins [19], non-uterine maternal resistance arterioles [19], and chorionic fetoplacental vessels [20–22]. The vasodilation of capacitance veins occurs at very low doses, and this effect may not only require fluid loading to counteract it (as is performed in some of the studies) but may also potentiate the reduction of venous return and cardiac output caused by obstruction of the inferior vena cava. At higher doses, nitroglycerin does dilate systemic resistance arterioles, and this reduction in systemic vascular resistance may be helpful in increasing cardiac output—*but only if venous return is adequate.*

Does Nitroglycerin Dilate Unremodeled Spiral Arteries?

It is also possible—although speculative—that nitroglycerin dilates any remaining smooth muscle in unremodeled spiral arteries and thereby increases intervillous perfusion.

Does Nitroglycerin Dilate the Lumbar, Vertebral Venous, and Azygos Collateral System?

One can also speculate that nitroglycerin might prevent or palliate preeclampsia or fetal growth restriction by dilating the lumbar, vertebral venous, and azygos collateral system or contributing to its growth. Increased maternal venous return and cardiac output and decreased uterine venous pressure could then allow both a reflex decrease in systemic vascular resistance and an increase in uteroplacental perfusion.

Nitroglycerin, Preeclampsia, and Fetal Growth Restriction

The purpose of raising these questions about possible nitroglycerin therapy is not to detract from its possible utility in preventing or palliating preeclampsia or fetal growth restriction but rather to point out that the hemodynamic environment in which these disorders occur is highly complex and that it is important to clarify the possible role of obstruction of uterine venous return in such a complicated picture. In my opinion, *future trials of nitric oxide donors, fluid loading, and other therapies need to be conducted in a way which objectively documents and accounts for the presence or absence of obstruction of uterine venous return in the study participants.* Studies should no longer be performed in which it is simply assumed that the maternal supine position causes obstruction of uterine venous return at the inferior vena cava and that lateral positions prevent such obstruction.

Hypoxic Fetoplacental Vasoconstriction—A Gatekeeper for Fetoplacental Perfusion and a Possible Therapeutic Target

Hypoxic fetoplacental vasoconstriction is a mechanism whereby the primary stem villus artery perfusing each chorionic villous "tree" constricts in response to intervillous space hypoxia [23–26]. Hypoxic fetoplacental vasoconstriction has an analog in the lung—hypoxic pulmonary vasoconstriction—which matches pulmonary blood flow with alveolar ventilation, and it is known that the nitric oxide donor nitroglycerin interferes with both hypoxic fetoplacental vasoconstriction and hypoxic pulmonary vasoconstriction [27–33].

Hypoxic Fetoplacental Vasoconstriction—Beneficial When Acting Locally

Hypoxic fetoplacental vasoconstriction is usually thought of as a beneficial response which functions locally to match fetoplacental perfusion with uteroplacental perfusion. When one intervillous space and its corresponding chorionic villus become hypoxic due to a lack of maternal perfusion, localized hypoxia triggers vasoconstriction of the primary stem villus artery of that one hypoxic chorionic villus. The result is that fetal cardiac output is re-directed away from that single hypoxic intervillous space and towards other spaces which contain more oxygen.

Hypoxic Fetoplacental Vasoconstriction: Harmful When Acting Globally

But hypoxic fetoplacental vasoconstriction may be profoundly harmful if it restricts the perfusion of all chorionic villi at once, as might occur when globally decreased intervillous perfusion creates generalized intervillous hypoxia. This generalized restriction of all fetoplacental perfusion would deprive the fetus of even the small amount of oxygen which remains within all the hypoxic intervillous spaces.

Hypoxic Fetoplacental Vasoconstriction Appears to Occur Slowly

In ex vivo experiments on double-perfused isolated human cotyledons, fetal arterial vasoconstriction begins after about 12–15 min of experimentally imposed intervillous space anoxia and increases progressively after that time [23]. Normoxia was restored after approximately 30 total minutes of hypoxia, at which time the fetal vascular resistance was still increasing, and after restoration of normoxia approximately 20 min was required for the anoxia-induced vasoconstriction to gradually dissipate and fetal arterial resistance to return toward baseline. This series of experiments also demonstrated that chorionic (fetal) arterial resistance increased with increasing degrees of hypoxia, showing that hypoxic fetoplacental vasoconstriction is a relatively slow and graduated process which becomes more intense as the intervillous space oxygen level is reduced [23]. These results suggest that hypoxic fetoplacental vasoconstriction responds slowly and gradually to changes in uteroplacental (maternal) perfusion over time, and one might theorize that longer periods of obstruction of uterine venous return in a patient would establish a lower average intervillous space oxygen tension throughout the day, leading to a higher average level of fetal arterial vasoconstriction.

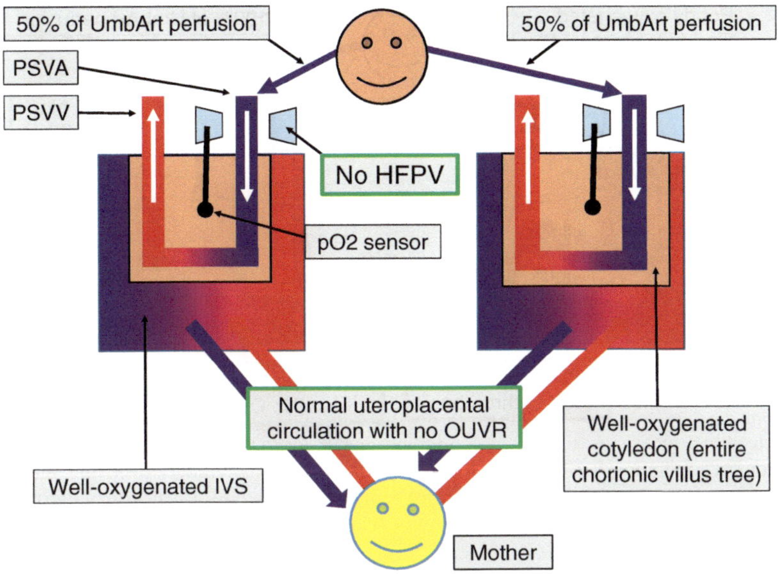

Fig. 3.11 Hypoxic fetoplacental vasoconstriction: beneficial when local, but harmful when global? This figure shows the basic "machinery" of hypoxic fetoplacental vasoconstriction in a non-activated state. The usual conception of hypoxic fetoplacental vasoconstriction is that it works locally—within each cotyledon to match fetal and maternal blood flows within the placenta. With this mechanism, cotyledons within hypoxic intervillous spaces restrict their own fetal perfusion via the mechanism of hypoxic fetoplacental vasoconstriction. This figure shows an imaginary placenta consisting of just two cotyledons and two intervillous spaces (real placentas have 15–28 cotyledons). In this example, there is no obstruction of uterine venous return and therefore there is no venous obstruction to intervillous perfusion and the oxygen tension in both intervillous spaces is normal. The primary stem villus arteries at the base of each cotyledon are sensitive to the oxygen tension within the intervillous space and will gradually constrict if the intervillous space is hypoxic, thereby reducing fetal perfusion to that intervillous space. But in this example, the intervillous spaces are well oxygenated and hypoxic fetoplacental vasoconstriction has not been activated. Since both intervillous spaces are well perfused, the fetus is sending 50% of its umbilical artery flow to each of the two cotyledons through the two primary stem villus arteries. *HFPV* hypoxic fetoplacental vasoconstriction, *IVS* intervillous spaces, *OUVR* obstruction of uterine venous return, pO_2 oxygen tension in mm Hg, *PSVA* primary stem villus artery, *PSVV* primary stem villus vein, UmbArt umbilical artery

As explained further below, hypoxic fetoplacental vasoconstriction is helpful in matching fetal to maternal perfusion when it occurs within single cotyledons exposed to hypoxic maternal blood [23–26], but this vasoconstriction may become profoundly counterproductive when it occurs in all cotyledons at once, due to generalized intervillous space hypoxia caused by obstruction of uterine venous return. The fact that nitroglycerin reduces umbilical artery pulsatility indices is consistent with the theory that hypoxic fetoplacental vasoconstriction plays a role in fetal growth restriction and preeclampsia [20–22].

Figure 3.11 shows the "machinery" of hypoxic fetoplacental vasoconstriction in an inactive state, in a simplified model of the placenta consisting of only two

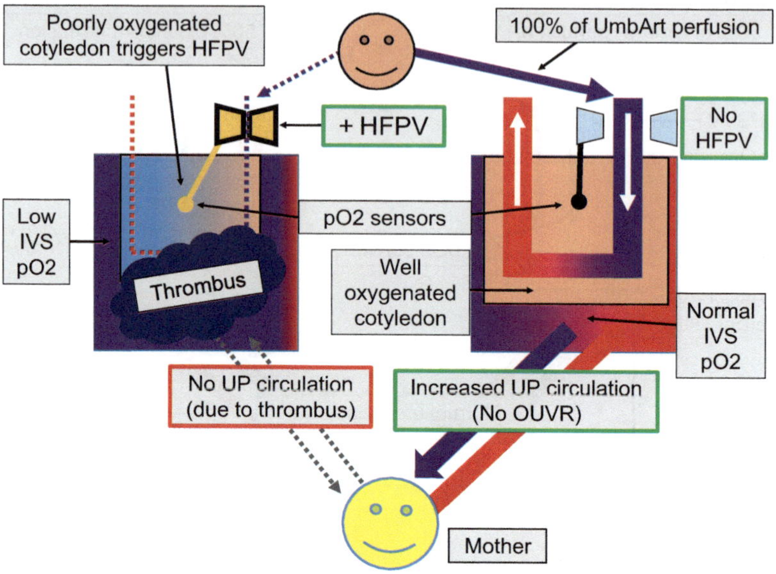

Fig. 3.12 Hypoxic fetoplacental vasoconstriction is beneficial to fetal oxygenation when it occurs locally. Hypoxic fetoplacental vasoconstriction is a mechanism whereby the primary stem villus artery of each placental cotyledon constricts in response to hypoxia within its own intervillous space. On a local basis, it is highly efficient for the fetus to send its precious cardiac output only to cotyledons located within oxygen-containing intervillous spaces. Due to thrombus formation (as shown in the figure) or other causes, a given intervillous space may be relatively hypoxic, and hypoxic fetoplacental vasoconstriction prevents the fetus from wasting cardiac output on the perfusion of cotyledons within hypoxic intervillous spaces. *HFPV* hypoxic fetoplacental vasoconstriction, *IVS* intervillous space, *OUVR* obstruction of uterine venous return, pO_2 oxygen tension mm Hg, *UmbArt* umbilical artery, *UP* uteroplacental

intervillous spaces. Both intervillous spaces are well oxygenated, and the primary stem villus arteries of both chorionic villi are widely patent. The primary stem villus arteries do possess, however, a mechanism for sensing the pO_2 within the intervillous space, and if the intervillous space pO_2 decreases to a sufficient degree, hypoxic fetoplacental vasoconstriction will be activated and the primary stem villus arteries will constrict, reducing or eliminating fetal perfusion of that specific chorionic villus. As shown in Fig. 3.12, hypoxic fetoplacental vasoconstriction is beneficial when it acts locally, within single chorionic villi, to shunt fetal cardiac output away from hypoxic intervillous spaces and toward intervillous spaces that are better oxygenated. But we can hypothesize that when obstruction of uterine venous return makes all intervillous spaces hypoxic, hypoxic fetoplacental vasoconstriction may act globally—that is, throughout the placenta—in a profoundly counterproductive

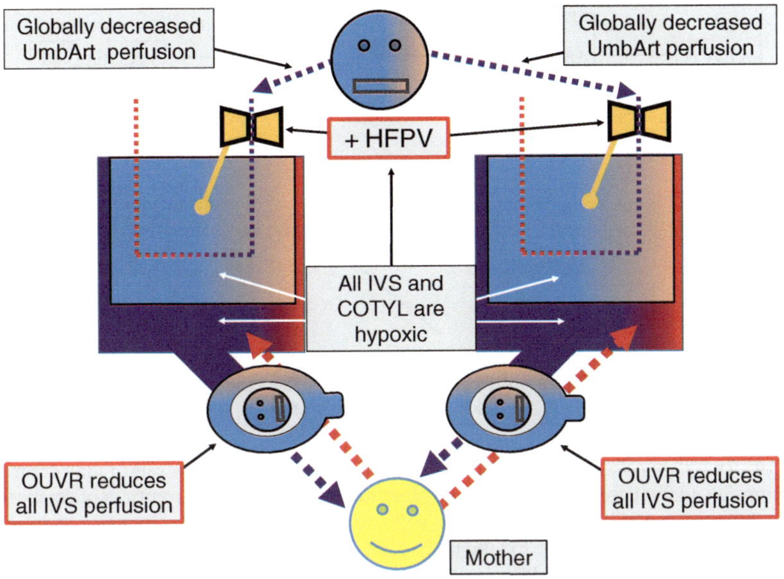

Fig. 3.13 Hypoxic fetoplacental vasoconstriction may be counterproductive when it occurs globally—that is, if all intervillous spaces are hypoxic. If all intervillous spaces are hypoxic due to obstruction of uterine venous return, then hypoxic fetoplacental vasoconstriction restricts perfusion of all cotyledons, making a bad situation worse! This figure shows how hypoxic fetoplacental vasoconstriction may become highly counterproductive *when intervillous space hypoxia occurs globally throughout the placenta due to obstruction of uterine venous return.* In that situation, hypoxic fetoplacental vasoconstriction may restrict the perfusion of *all* cotyledons, with the result that it is even harder for the fetus to get the oxygen it needs. This postulated mechanism is a theory which (to my knowledge) has not been investigated. *COTYL* cotyledon, *HFPV* hypoxic fetoplacental vasoconstriction, *IVS* intervillous space, *OUVR* obstruction of uterine venous return, *UmbArt* umbilical artery

manner, by reducing all fetoplacental perfusion, as shown in Fig. 3.13. But, as noted previously, hypoxic fetoplacental vasoconstriction appears to be slow to develop and slow to dissipate. Therefore, it may tend to reflect the average level of intervillous space oxygenation over time. Since hypoxic fetoplacental vasoconstriction is a gradual and graduated process—and not an "all or nothing" response—it may allow the fetus to survive when there is frequent obstruction of uterine venous return, but with the fetus surviving under suboptimal conditions which lead to fetal growth restriction. This slow and gradual response may also explain why some fetuses appear to "tolerate" the supine position for some time—perhaps approximately 23 min [34].

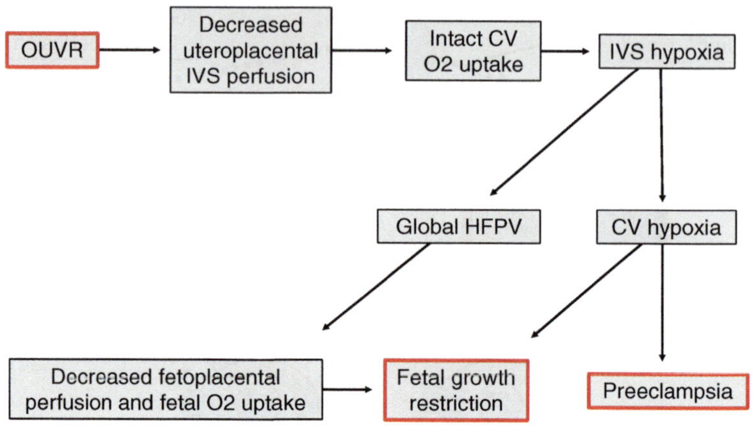

Fig. 3.14 Two *flow-related* ways in which obstruction of uterine venous return may contribute to preeclampsia and fetal growth restriction. Obstruction of uterine venous return may decrease intervillous ("uteroplacental") perfusion, which will cause intervillous space hypoxia as long as the chorionic villi are intact and able to take up oxygen. Intervillous space hypoxia may then damage the chorionic villi, causing preeclampsia, and initiate fetal growth restriction as well. But intervillous space hypoxia—which is generalized throughout the placenta—may also trigger generalized hypoxic fetoplacental vasoconstriction, thereby reducing *fetoplacental* perfusion and exacerbating the fetus' oxygen deficit, making fetal growth restriction even more likely. *CV* chorionic villus, *HFPV* hypoxic fetoplacental vasoconstriction, *IVS* intervillous space, O_2 oxygen, *OUVR* obstruction of uterine venous return

This chapter has considered two mechanisms by which obstruction of uterine venous return may cause chorionic villous and fetal hypoxia: (1) reduction of intervillous space oxygen tension due to a reduction in maternal intervillous space perfusion, and (2) the global activation of hypoxic fetoplacental vasoconstriction which—slowly and gradually over a time course approximating 30 min—may progressively reduce fetal perfusion of all of the already-hypoxic chorionic villi in a counterproductive and massive (but slow) "over-reaction." Figure 3.14 summarizes those two mechanisms as a flow chart. In the next chapter, we will examine a third way in which obstruction of uterine venous return may impair both fetal and chorionic villous oxygenation: increased intervillous space pressure.

Since obstruction of uterine venous return may impair chorionic villous and fetal oxygenation by three separate mechanisms, it might not be an exaggeration to say—using blunt but accurate language—that **some cases of preeclampsia or fetal growth restriction may result from the uterus strangling itself by obstruction of its own venous return!**

Summary

1. An important current model of fetal growth restriction and preeclampsia is that it is due to defective spiral artery remodeling which reduces intervillous perfusion and oxygenation. In this model, intervillous space hypoxia damages chorionic villi and the fetus, causing preeclampsia and fetal growth restriction, respectively.
2. Obstruction of uterine venous return could similarly reduce intervillous space perfusion from the venous side of the intervillous space and cause similar hypoxia of both the chorionic villi and the fetus, providing another mechanism to explain fetal growth restriction and preeclampsia. Obstruction of uterine venous return could act on its own or in combination with maternal arterial disease to reduce intervillous space perfusion.
3. Uterine perfusion is "pressure passive," that is, it is determined solely by the difference between uterine artery and uterine venous pressure (unless myometrial tissue pressure is higher than venous pressure, in which case uterine perfusion pressure is arterial pressure minus myometrial tissue pressure).
4. The dominant model for placental perfusion is a combination of the "series" model and the "venous equilibrator" model. The former assumes that all uterine perfusion passes through intervillous spaces, and the latter assumes that the mixing of blood within the intervillous space is instantaneous. Together, the two models allow investigators to accept the pO_2 of uterine venous blood as an approximation of the pO_2 of the blood within intervillous spaces.
5. Nitroglycerin therapy combined with volume loading may prevent or mitigate preeclampsia and fetal growth restriction, but further research needs to take the possible effects of concurrent obstruction of uterine venous return into account. Generalized intervillous hypoxia due to obstruction of uterine venous return may trigger generalized hypoxic fetoplacental vasoconstriction, and nitroglycerin may prevent this response, among its many other hemodynamic effects.
6. Hypoxic fetoplacental vasoconstriction (HFPV) is a mechanism by which the primary stem villus artery (which perfuses the entire cotyledon, or "chorionic villous tree") gradually constricts when the intervillous space is hypoxic, perhaps over a time course approximating 30 min. This mechanism is useful to the fetus when it acts locally, since it tends to match fetal perfusion with maternal perfusion. The author theorizes that obstruction of uterine venous return might create generalized intervillous space hypoxia sufficient to trigger a massive and counterproductive hypoxic fetoplacental vasoconstriction response which would reduce fetoplacental perfusion throughout the placenta and impair oxygenation of the fetus even further. But this over-reaction would take time to develop and might reflect the average intervillous space oxygenation over time.

7. Since it occurs on the venous side of the placental circulation, obstruction of uterine venous return not only decreases intervillous space perfusion and intervillous space pO_2, but increases intervillous space pressure as well. This increased pressure could be an important cause of chorionic villous and fetal damage which will be addressed in the next chapter.

References

1. Burton GJ, Jauniaux E. Pathophysiology of placental-derived fetal growth restriction. Am J Obstet Gynecol. 2018;218(2S):S745–61. https://doi.org/10.1016/j.ajog.2017.11.577. PMID: 29422210.
2. Erez O, Romero R, Jung E, Chaemsaithong P, Bosco M, Suksai M, Gallo DM, Gotsch F. Preeclampsia and eclampsia: the conceptual evolution of a syndrome. Am J Obstet Gynecol. 2022;226(2S):S786–803. https://doi.org/10.1016/j.ajog.2021.12.001. PMID: 35177220; PMCID: PMC8941666.
3. Redman CWG, Staff AC, Roberts JM. Syncytiotrophoblast stress in preeclampsia: the convergence point for multiple pathways. Am J Obstet Gynecol. 2022;226(2S):S907–27. https://doi.org/10.1016/j.ajog.2020.09.047. Epub 2021 Feb 2. PMID: 33546842.
4. Schoots MH, Gordijn SJ, Scherjon SA, van Goor H, Hillebrands JL. Oxidative stress in placental pathology. Placenta. 2018;69:153–61. https://doi.org/10.1016/j.placenta.2018.03.003. Epub 2018 Mar 16. PMID: 29622278.
5. Archer TL, Suresh P, Shapiro AE. Cardiac output measurement, by means of electrical velocimetry, may be able to determine optimum maternal position during gestation, labour and caesarean delivery, by preventing vena caval compression and maximising cardiac output and placental perfusion pressure. Anaesth Intensive Care. 2011;39(2):308–11. PMID: 21485686.
6. Archer TL, Shapiro AE, Suresh PJ. Maximisation of maternal cardiac output during labour might help to prevent not only foetal hypoxaemia but also myometrial ischaemia, dysfunctional labour, uterine atony and postpartum endometritis. Anaesth Intensive Care. 2011;39(4):774–5. PMID: 21823407.
7. Archer TL, Suresh P, Ballas J. Don't forget aortocaval compression when imaging abdominal veins in pregnant patients. Ultrasound Obstet Gynecol. 2011;38(4):479–80. https://doi.org/10.1002/uog.10065. Erratum in: Ultrasound Obstet Gynecol. 2021;57(3):516. PMID: 21837755.
8. Greiss FC Jr. Pressure-flow relationship in the gravid uterine vascular bed. Am J Obstet Gynecol. 1966;96(1):41–7. https://doi.org/10.1016/s0002-9378(16)34639-7. PMID: 5950264. Accessed at: https://derangedphysiology.com/main/cicm-primary-exam/required-reading/cardiovascular-system/Chapter%20480/uteroplacental-blood-flow, on September 14, 2023.
9. Burton GJ, Woods AW, Jauniaux E, Kingdom JC. Rheological and physiological consequences of conversion of the maternal spiral arteries for uteroplacental blood flow during human pregnancy. Placenta. 2009;30(6):473–82. https://doi.org/10.1016/j.placenta.2009.02.009. Epub 2009 Apr 17. PMID: 19375795; PMCID: PMC2697319.
10. Dellschaft NS, Hutchinson G, Shah S, Jones NW, Bradley C, Leach L, Platt C, Bowtell R, Gowland PA. The haemodynamics of the human placenta in utero. PLoS Biol. 2020;18(5):e3000676. https://doi.org/10.1371/journal.pbio.3000676. PMID: 32463837; PMCID: PMC7255609.
11. Karimu AL, Burton GJ. The effects of maternal vascular pressure on the dimensions of the placental capillaries. Br J Obstet Gynaecol. 1994;101(1):57–63. https://doi.org/10.1111/j.1471-0528.1994.tb13011.x. PMID: 8297870.
12. Schaaps JP, Tsatsaris V, Goffin F, Brichant JF, Delbecque K, Tebache M, Collignon L, Retz MC, Foidart JM. Shunting the intervillous space: new concepts in human uteroplacental

vascularization. Am J Obstet Gynecol. 2005;192(1):323–32. https://doi.org/10.1016/j.ajog.2004.06.066. PMID: 15672043.
13. Clapp JF 3rd. The relationship between blood flow and oxygen uptake in the uterine and umbilical circulations. Am J Obstet Gynecol. 1978;132(4):410–3. https://doi.org/10.1016/0002-9378(78)90776-7. PMID: 707583.
14. Spinapolice RX, Feld S, Harrigan JT. Effective prevention of gestational hypertension in nulliparous women at high risk as identified by the rollover test. Am J Obstet Gynecol. 1983;146(2):166–8. https://doi.org/10.1016/0002-9378(83)91047-5. PMID: 6846433.
15. Lees C, Valensise H, Black R, Harrington K, Byiers S, Romanini C, Campbell S. The efficacy and fetal-maternal cardiovascular effects of transdermal glyceryl trinitrate in the prophylaxis of pre-eclampsia and its complications: a randomized double-blind placebo-controlled trial. Ultrasound Obstet Gynecol. 1998;12(5):334–8. https://doi.org/10.1046/j.1469-0705.1998.12050334.x. PMID: 9819872.
16. Valensise H, Vasapollo B, Novelli GP, Giorgi G, Verallo P, Galante A, Arduini D. Maternal and fetal hemodynamic effects induced by nitric oxide donors and plasma volume expansion in pregnancies with gestational hypertension complicated by intrauterine growth restriction with absent end-diastolic flow in the umbilical artery. Ultrasound Obstet Gynecol. 2008;31(1):55–64. https://doi.org/10.1002/uog.5234. PMID: 18098350.
17. Tiralongo GM, Pisani I, Vasapollo B, Khalil A, Thilaganathan B, Valensise H. Effect of a nitric oxide donor on maternal hemodynamics in fetal growth restriction. Ultrasound Obstet Gynecol. 2018;51(4):514–8. https://doi.org/10.1002/uog.17454. PMID: 28295749.
18. Vasapollo B, Novelli GP, Farsetti D, Pometti F, Frantellizzi R, Maellaro F, Silvestrini M, Pais M, Valensise H. NO donors on top of anti-hypertensive therapy reduces complications in chronic hypertensive pregnancies with hypodynamic circulation. Eur J Obstet Gynecol Reprod Biol. 2023;291:219–24. https://doi.org/10.1016/j.ejogrb.2023.10.033. Epub ahead of print. PMID: 37924629.
19. Abrams J. Hemodynamic effects of nitroglycerin and long-acting nitrates. Am Heart J. 1985;110(1 Pt 2):216–24. PMID: 3925741.
20. Gupta S, Chauhan M, Sen J, Nanda S. Effect of transdermal nitroglycerine on Doppler velocity waveforms of the uterine, umbilical and fetal middle cerebral arteries in patients with chronic placental insufficiency: a prospective RCT. J Clin Diagn Res. 2017;11(7):QC13–7. https://doi.org/10.7860/JCDR/2017/21438.10282. Epub 2017 Jul 1. PMID: 28892981; PMCID: PMC5583822.
21. Trapani A Jr, Gonçalves LF, Trapani TF, Franco MJ, Galluzzo RN, Pires MM. Comparison between transdermal nitroglycerin and sildenafil citrate in intrauterine growth restriction: effects on uterine, umbilical and fetal middle cerebral artery pulsatility indices. Ultrasound Obstet Gynecol. 2016;48(1):61–5. https://doi.org/10.1002/uog.15673. PMID: 26279411.
22. Trapani A Jr, Gonçalves LF, Pires MM. Transdermal nitroglycerin in patients with severe pre-eclampsia with placental insufficiency: effect on uterine, umbilical and fetal middle cerebral artery resistance indices. Ultrasound Obstet Gynecol. 2011;38(4):389–94. https://doi.org/10.1002/uog.8983. PMID: 21374750.
23. Ramasubramanian R, Johnson RF, Downing JW, Minzter BH, Paschall RL. Hypoxemic fetoplacental vasoconstriction: a graduated response to reduced oxygen conditions in the human placenta. Anesth Analg. 2006;103(2):439–42. https://doi.org/10.1213/01.ane.0000222468.76942.d8. PMID: 16861430.
24. Hampl V, Jakoubek V. Regulation of fetoplacental vascular bed by hypoxia. Physiol Res. 2009;58(Suppl 2):S87–94. https://doi.org/10.33549/physiolres.931922. PMID: 20131940.
25. Howard RB, Hosokawa T, Maguire MH. Hypoxia-induced fetoplacental vasoconstriction in perfused human placental cotyledons. Am J Obstet Gynecol. 1987;157(5):1261–6. https://doi.org/10.1016/s0002-9378(87)80307-1. PMID: 3688085.
26. Howard RB. Control of human placental blood flow. Med Hypotheses. 1987;23(1):51–8. https://doi.org/10.1016/0306-9877(87)90180-0. PMID: 3614003.

27. Byrne BM, Howard RB, Morrow RJ, Whiteley KJ, Adamson SL. Role of the L-arginine nitric oxide pathway in hypoxic fetoplacental vasoconstriction. Placenta. 1997;18(8):627–34. https://doi.org/10.1016/s0143-4004(97)90003-5. PMID: 9364597.
28. Bednov A, Espinoza J, Betancourt A, Vedernikov Y, Belfort M, Yallampalli C. L-arginine prevents hypoxia-induced vasoconstriction in dual-perfused human placental cotyledons. Placenta. 2015;36(11):1254–9. https://doi.org/10.1016/j.placenta.2015.08.012. Epub 2015 Aug 31. PMID: 26342955.
29. King RG, Gude NM, Di Iulio JL, Brennecke SP. Regulation of human placental fetal vessel tone: role of nitric oxide. Reprod Fertil Dev. 1995;7(6):1407–11. https://doi.org/10.1071/rd9951407. PMID: 8743139.
30. D'Oliveira M, Sykes MK, Chakrabarti MK, Orchard C, Keslin J. Depression of hypoxic pulmonary vasoconstriction by sodium nitroprusside and nitroglycerine. Br J Anaesth. 1981;53(1):11–8. https://doi.org/10.1093/bja/53.1.11. PMID: 6779843.
31. Annest SJ, Gottlieb ME, Rhodes GR, Paloski WH, Barie P, Newell JC, Shah DM. Nitroprusside and nitroglycerine in patients with posttraumatic pulmonary failure. J Trauma. 1981;21(12):1029–31. https://doi.org/10.1097/00005373-198112000-00004. PMID: 6798221.
32. Weygandt GR, Kopman EA, Ludbrook PA. Mechanism of nitroglycerin-induced hypoxemia. Cathet Cardiovasc Diagn. 1980;6(4):387–95. https://doi.org/10.1002/ccd.1810060407. PMID: 6781754.
33. Benoit A, Ducas J, Girling L, Schick U, Prewitt RM. Acute cardiopulmonary effects of nitroglycerin in canine oleic acid pulmonary edema. Anesthesiology. 1985;62(6):754–8. https://doi.org/10.1097/00000542-198506000-00009. PMID: 3923869.
34. Archer TL. Neuraxial anesthesia and the supine position cause non-reassuring fetal status. In: Archer TL, editor. Obstetric anesthesia: a case-based and visual approach. 1st ed, Ch 2, Figure 2.4. Cham: Springer; 2020. p. 25. https://doi.org/10.1007/978-3-030-26478-9_2.
35. Vascular biology of the placenta. https://www.ncbi.nlm.nih.gov/books/NBK53254/.
36. Jansen CHJR, Kastelein AW, Kleinrouweler CE, Van Leeuwen E, De Jong KH, Pajkrt E, Van Noorden CJF. Development of placental abnormalities in location and anatomy. Acta Obstet Gynecol Scand. 2020;99(8):983–93. https://doi.org/10.1111/aogs.13834. Epub 2020 Mar 18. PMID: 32108320; PMCID: PMC7496588.

Preeclampsia and Fetal Growth Restriction: Intervillous Space *Pressure*

4

Preeclampsia and Fetal Growth Restriction: Intervillous Space *Pressure*

In the previous chapter, we saw that obstruction of uterine venous return might impair placental function by two *flow-related mechanisms*: (1) decreased maternal perfusion of the intervillous space, causing generalized intervillous hypoxia due to continued fetal oxygen uptake from the under-perfused intervillous spaces and (2) the triggering by that intervillous hypoxia of generalized hypoxic fetoplacental vasoconstriction, thereby decreasing fetoplacental perfusion.

In this chapter, we consider three additional *pressure-related mechanisms* by which obstruction of uterine venous return might impair placental function: (1) immediate reduction of fetoplacental perfusion by direct compression of chorionic villi and the fetal vessels within them, in what has been described as "sluice flow" [1, 2]; (2) interference with future "downstream" chorionic villus growth by reduction of beneficial flow shear stress within chorionic vessels; and (3) the opening of subplacental myometrial arteriovenous shunts which may deprive both the fetus and the myometrium of oxygen.

Intervillous Space Pressure: Normal and Elevated

Figure 4.1 shows an intervillous space to which well-remodeled spiral arteries admit a gentle flow of well-oxygenated maternal blood. There is no obstruction of uterine venous return, with the result that the pressure within the space is low and the compressible chorionic villi (not shown) are not compressed [1]. Due to this lack of compression, there is no *current* impediment to fetoplacental perfusion of the villi. Furthermore, fetoplacental *flow shear stress* within the chorionic vessels (not shown and explained below) is adequate for the promotion of *future* chorionic villus growth. Figure 4.2 shows that obstruction of uterine venous return both decreases the rate of intervillous perfusion and increases intervillous pressure.

T. L. Archer, *Threats to Fetal, Placental and Myometrial Oxygenation*,
https://doi.org/10.1007/978-3-031-60364-8_4

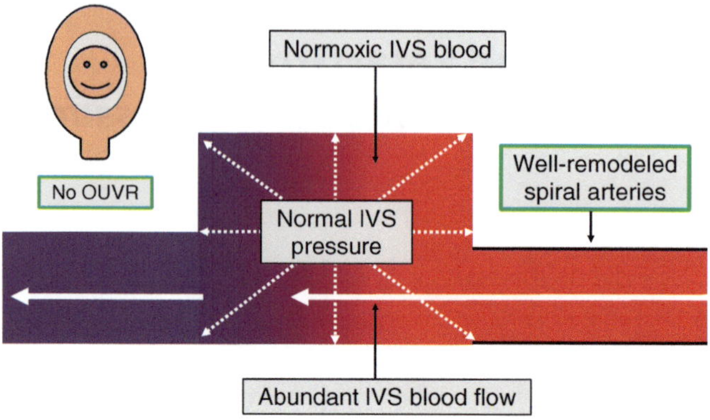

Fig. 4.1 The healthy intervillous space. This intervillous space has normal pressure and abundant perfusion because there is no obstruction to uterine venous return and the spiral arteries have been remodeled to provide a voluminous but gentle flow of maternal blood throughout the space. The chorionic villi are not shown, but this intervillous space is the perfect environment in which they can grow and successfully perform their job of supporting the growth of the developing fetus. *IVS* intervillous space, *OUVR* obstruction of uterine venous return

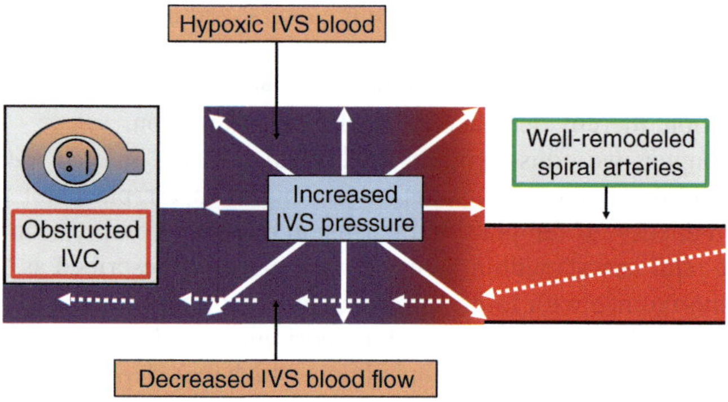

Fig. 4.2 The double threat of obstruction of uterine venous return: decreased intervillous space perfusion and increased intervillous space pressure. In the previous chapter, we deliberately ignored the effects of pressure within the intervillous space in order to focus on blood flow, but of course the two processes occur simultaneously, making the situation complex. In this chapter, we examine the possibility that increased intervillous space pressure could restrict *fetal* perfusion of the placenta by compressing chorionic villi and the fetal vessels within them, in addition to limiting *maternal* perfusion of the space. *IVC* inferior vena cava, *IVS* intervillous space

The Current and Future Benefits of a Low-Pressure Intervillous Space

Figure 4.3 presents another view of a healthy intervillous space, which now includes the presence of a highly simplified (rectangular) chorionic villus "tree." The low pressure within the intervillous space allows abundant *current* fetoplacental

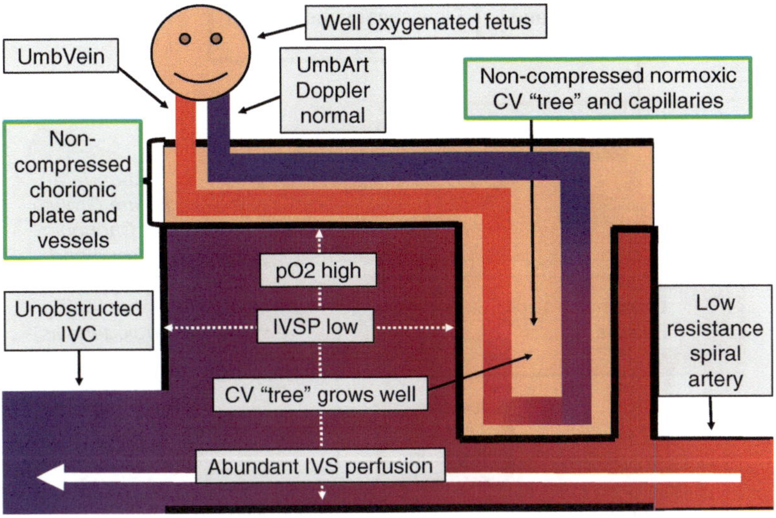

Fig. 4.3 The low-pressure, unobstructed intervillous space with an uncompressed chorionic villus and a well-oxygenated fetus. The chorionic villi can be compressed by increased hydrostatic pressure [5], but that is not happening in this figure. The fetal heart easily pumps deoxygenated blood through the low-resistance and highly compliant umbilical and chorionic arteries, resulting in the low pulsatility index umbilical artery Doppler waveforms characteristic of a healthy placenta. The vigorous fetal blood flow within the chorionic villi also supports future chorionic villous growth due to the beneficial effects of flow shear stress [3–6]. *CV* chorionic villus, *IVC* inferior vena cava, *IVS* intervillous space, *IVSP* intervillous space pressure, pO_2 partial pressure of oxygen (mm Hg), *UmbArt* umbilical artery, *UmbVein* umbilical vein

perfusion, since the chorionic villi and the vessels within them are not being compressed, and vigorous fetal blood flow within the chorionic villi also supports future chorionic villous growth due to the beneficial effects of flow shear stress [3–6].

Flow Shear Stress Promotes Branching and Non-branching Angiogenesis Downstream

As shown in Fig. 4.4, chorionic vascular endothelial cells have flow sensors on their luminal surfaces which are activated by the shear force of flowing blood, which is termed "flow shear stress." Sensor activation causes the release of vascular growth factors which then support future angiogenesis and chorionic villus growth. *It is a positive feedback system in which robust blood flow through an existing villus tree paves the way for further growth of that same tree!*

Hence, low intervillous space pressure promotes fetal survival and growth in two different time frames: (1) *immediately*, by allowing abundant *current* fetal perfusion of chorionic villi to meet *current* needs and (2) *in the future*, because adequate flow shear stress from *current* perfusion lays the foundation for vigorous *future* chorionic villus growth "downstream."

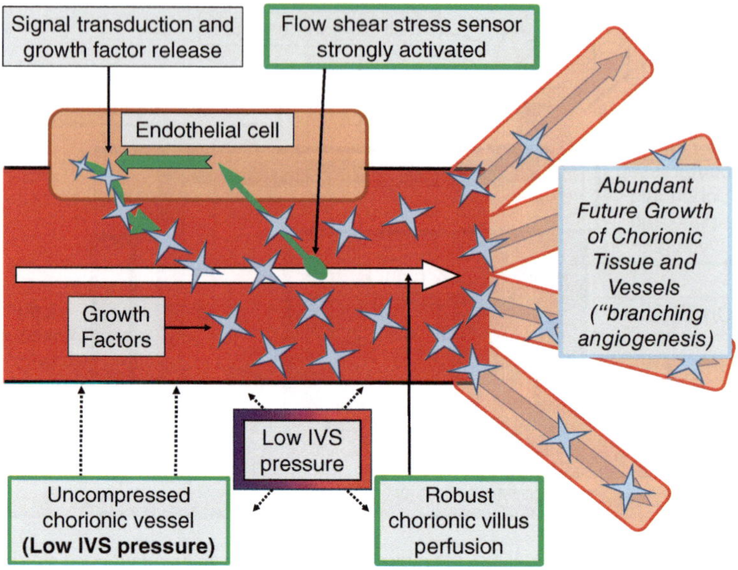

Fig. 4.4 Flow shear stress encourages downstream branching and non-branching angiogenesis, which is necessary for chorionic villus growth. Chorionic vascular endothelium has flow sensors which detect flow shear stress. The endothelial cells transduce that flow signal into the release of vascular growth factors into the flowing stream of blood, and these growth factors encourage more chorionic villus growth, or angiogenesis "downstream." In this fanciful portrayal, intervillous space pressure is low and chorionic villus perfusion is vigorous, resulting in the abundant release of vascular growth factors which will stimulate future chorionic villus growth. (The chorionic villus stroma located between the intervillous space and the fetal vessel is not shown). *IVS* intervillous space

The Opportunistic Placenta

The mechanism of flow shear stress makes the placenta *opportunistic*—where there is growth and blood flow, flow shear stress promotes more growth and more blood flow, and *this virtuous cycle allows the placenta to meet both the current and future needs of the growing fetus.* This process is illustrated figuratively in Figs. 4.4 and 4.5, in which uncompressed chorionic villi within well-perfused and low-pressure intervillous spaces "encourage themselves" to proliferate in order to support ongoing fetal growth.

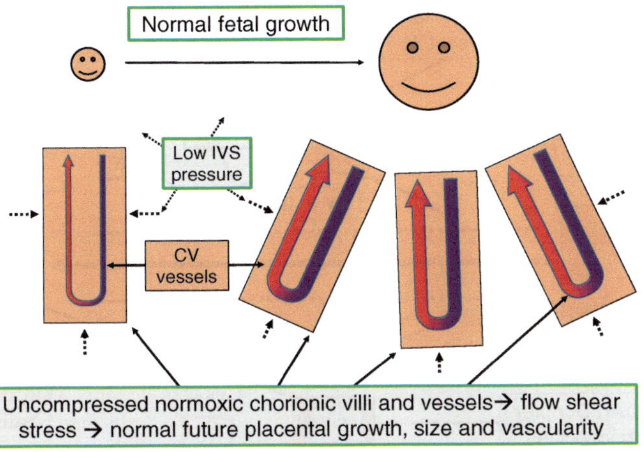

Fig. 4.5 Another fanciful portrayal of healthy chorionic villus growth. Here we see that one small but uncompressed chorionic villus grows and multiplies due to the effects of high flow shear stress. The key to vigorous chorionic villus growth is healthy flow shear stress within a low-pressure and well-oxygenated intervillous space. *CV* chorionic villus, *IVS* intervillous space

Umbilical Artery Doppler Waveforms in a Healthy Placenta with Low Intervillous Space Pressure

Low intervillous space pressure does not compress the fetal vessels of the chorionic plate or villi, and this lack of external compression allows the low-resistance and highly compliant arteries to behave as shown in Figs. 4.6 and 4.7. Their high compliance allows the vessels to expand markedly during fetal systole, during which time they store a substantial volume of blood which they then release during diastole. High vascular compliance results in umbilical artery Doppler velocity waveforms with a low *pulsatility index*, as shown at the bottom of the two figures. The key feature of this umbilical artery Doppler waveform is that *there is substantial blood flow during diastole*. The formula for pulsatility index is as follows: Pulsatility Index = (Systolic Flow Velocity − Diastolic Flow Velocity)/Mean Flow Velocity.

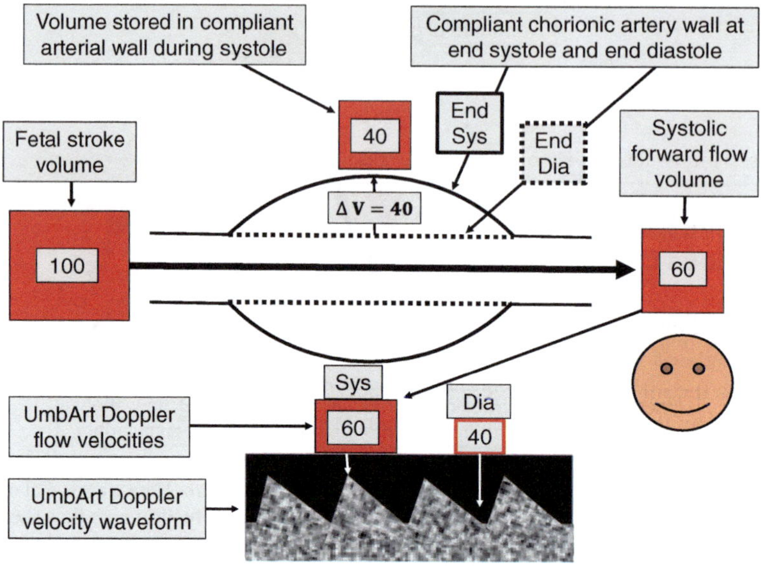

Fig. 4.6 Low-resistance and highly compliant umbilical and chorionic arteries expand markedly during systole, absorbing a large fraction of the fetal stroke volume, which is then released during diastole. Uncompressed umbilical and chorionic arteries have low resistance and are highly compliant. In this numerical example with arbitrary units, out of a total fetal stroke volume of 100, the arteries expand during systole to "absorb" 40 units and only 60 units flow forward during systole. During diastole (shown in Fig. 4.7), the compliant arterial walls release those 40 units, supplying an abundant diastolic flow of 40 units. This high diastolic flow results in a low pulsatility index, or difference between systolic and diastolic flows, as reflected in the normal umbilical artery Doppler velocity waveform shown at the bottom of the figure. This is often called a "low–resistance" waveform, but it really should be called a "low resistance and high compliance" or "low–impedance" waveform. *Dia* diastole, *Sys* systole, *UmbArt* umbilical artery, ΔV change in volume

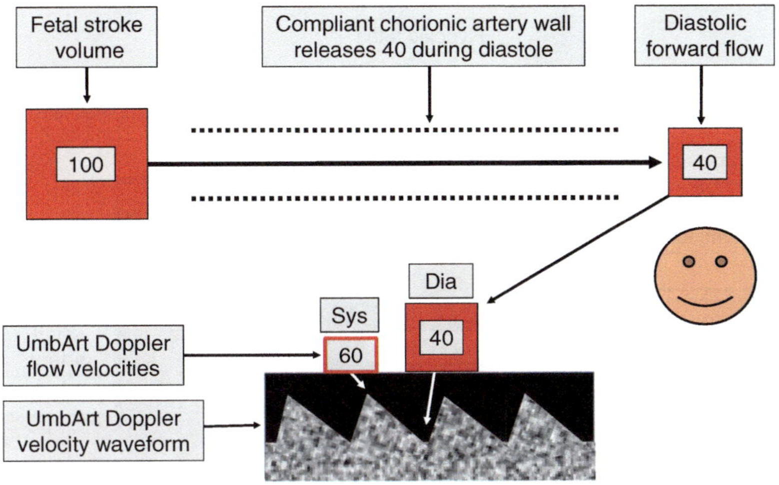

Fig. 4.7 During diastole, compliant umbilical and chorionic arteries release the blood which had been stored between their distended walls during systole. During diastole, the distended arterial walls contract, resulting in the forward flow of the 40 units of volume which had been stored between their walls during systole. This high diastolic flow results in the "low resistance and high compliance" waveform shown at the bottom of the figure. *Dia* diastole, *Sys* systole, *UmbArt* umbilical artery, ΔV change in volume

Umbilical Artery Doppler Waveforms in Placental Insufficiency

Figure 4.8 shows what may happen when obstruction of uterine venous return increases the pressure within the hypoxic intervillous space. Increased hydrostatic pressure compresses the blood vessels within the chorionic plate and villi and tends to literally *squeeze* fetal blood out of the chorionic vessels [1, 2]. This limitation of tissue perfusion by tissue pressure rather than by downstream venous pressure—in this case, by umbilical venous pressure—has been termed "sluice flow." Based on known data, this scenario is entirely plausible. The pressure within the obstructed inferior vena cava of a woman in the supine position approximates 25 mmHg [7], and pressure within the intervillous spaces of the placenta at that same time should be higher. In a large series of extremely premature newborns at 23–26 weeks gestational age, the mean arterial blood pressure approximated 30 mmHg [8]. From these two data points, it seems entirely plausible that obstruction of the inferior vena cava and uterine venous return could raise the intervillous space pressure high enough to seriously compromise fetoplacental perfusion of the chorionic villi within the intervillous spaces and thereby cause severe fetal hypoxia.

This external compression of chorionic vessels increases chorionic vascular resistance, decreases compliance, and may also reduce the beneficial flow shear stress needed for further villous growth, as suggested figuratively in Fig. 4.9.

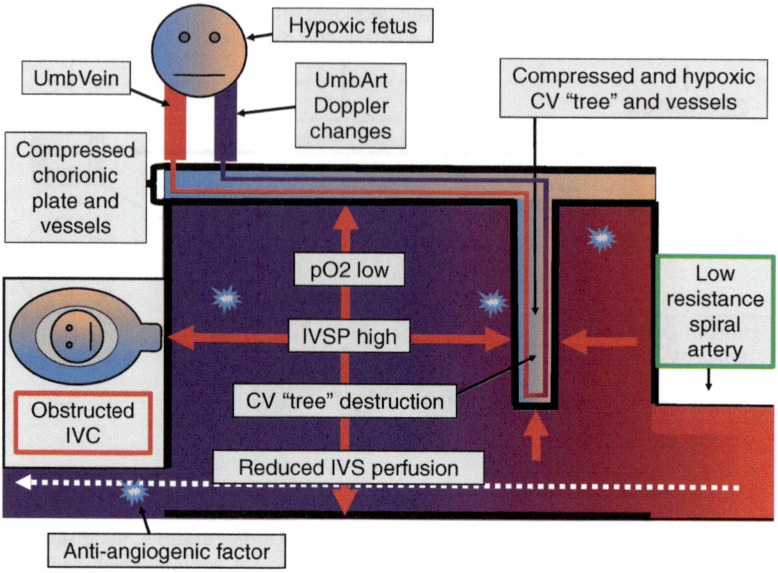

Fig. 4.8 Obstruction of uterine venous return increases intervillous pressure, compressing chorionic vessels and increasing their resistance and reducing their compliance. This figure shows the "double damage" that obstruction of uterine venous return may do to placental function and structure by decreasing intervillous flow and increasing intervillous pressure. Decreased uteroplacental flow creates intervillous hypoxia and the increased pressure literally "squeezes" fetal perfusion out of the chorionic vessels while increasing their resistance and decreasing their compliance. This limitation of tissue perfusion (in this case fetoplacental perfusion) by external tissue pressure rather than by downstream venous pressure (in this case umbilical venous pressure) has been termed "sluice flow." By itself, obstruction of uterine venous return might cause significant harm to both placenta and fetus, but the harm could be magnified if the placenta faces other challenges in addition to obstruction of uterine venous return, such as defective spiral artery remodeling, or other arterial vascular disease such as that from diabetes or chronic hypertension. *CV* chorionic villus, *IVC* inferior vena cava, *IVS* intervillous space, *IVSP* intervillous space pressure, pO_2 partial pressure of oxygen, *UmbArt* umbilical artery, *UmbVein* umbilical vein

Increased external pressure within the intervillous space makes the chorionic arteries behave as if their walls were stiffer, as shown in Fig. 4.10. This externally imposed stiffness constrains arterial expansion during systole, preventing the arteries from storing a large volume of blood for release during diastole, as shown in Figs. 4.11 and 4.12. In this theoretical example, note that—due to the increased stiffness of the chorionic arteries—only 5 arbitrary units of blood are stored in the

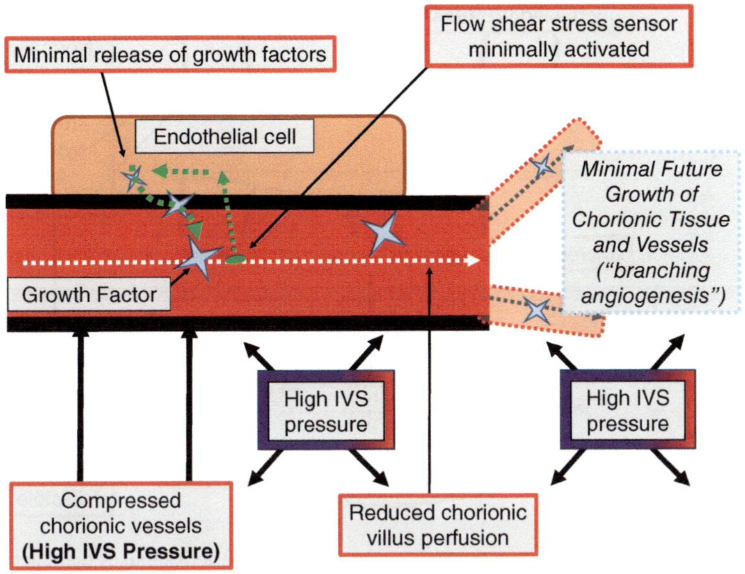

Fig. 4.9 Compression of chorionic villi may reduce the flow shear stress needed for future angiogenesis and chorionic villus growth. Reduction of flow within the compressed chorionic vessels may reduce the release of growth factors from vascular endothelium, resulting in reduced stimulus for angiogenesis and growth. In this fanciful portrayal, intervillous space pressure is high and chorionic villus perfusion and flow shear stress are limited, limiting the release of vascular growth factors and curtailing the growth of this chorionic villus tree. (The chorionic villus stroma located between the intervillous space and the fetal vessel is not shown). *IVS* intervillous space

externally stiffened arterial walls during systole. This lack of blood volume stored during systole leads to low blood flow velocity when that same small amount of blood is released during diastole. So in this example of chorionic arteries stiffened by external intervillous space pressure, the systolic flow would be 95 arbitrary units, whereas the diastolic flow would only be 5 arbitrary units. In this example—which we imagine to be caused by obstruction of uterine venous return—the difference between systolic and diastolic umbilical artery flow velocities—along with the pulsatility index—would be very high—and this is, in fact, the umbilical artery Doppler velocimetry waveform pattern seen in placental insufficiency. *One can therefore theorize that increased intervillous space pressure due to obstruction of uterine venous return may be a cause of placental insufficiency*!

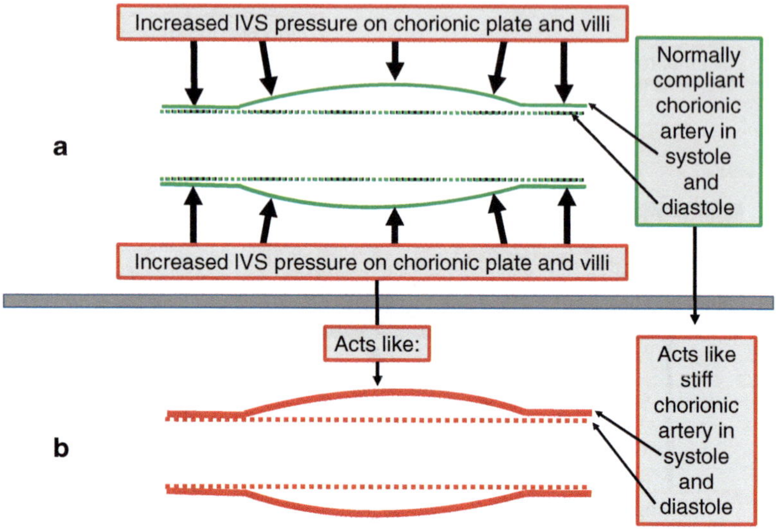

Fig. 4.10 External pressure on normally compliant chorionic arteries makes them act as though they were stiff. This result may occur suddenly with obstruction of uterine venous return and be fully reversible at first. Increased vascular resistance and decreased compliance might produce a rapid positional increase in pulsatility index when a pregnant woman turns into a position which obstructs uterine venous return, but another cause of such an increase in pulsatility index (not shown in the figure) might be the positional triggering of generalized hypoxic fetoplacental vasoconstriction by the reduced intervillous perfusion caused by obstruction of uterine venous return. If this were the mechanism, positional increases in pulsatility index might appear only slowly, since hypoxic fetoplacental vasoconstriction takes time to begin and develops only gradually, as discussed in the text. *IVS* intervillous space

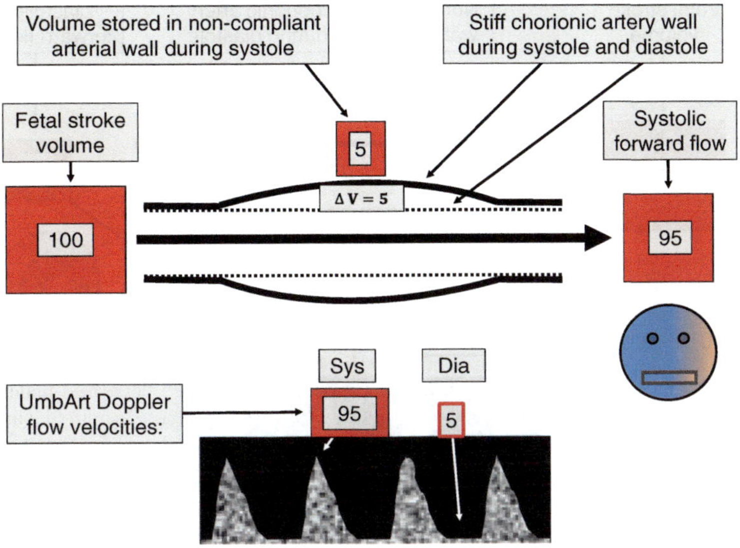

Fig. 4.11 Stiff chorionic arteries with low compliance will produce umbilical artery Doppler waveforms with high pulsatility indices. This figure and the next give numerical examples of how externally imposed and temporary arterial stiffness might show up in the umbilical artery Doppler velocity waveform. In this figure, we see that of the 100 arbitrary units of fetal stroke volume, only 5 units are stored within the stiffened arterial vascular tree during systole and 95 units flow forward. This creates the high systolic flow and low diastolic flow seen in the schematic Doppler velocity waveform at the bottom of the figure. *Dia* diastole, *Sys* systole, *UmbArt* umbilical artery, ΔV change in volume

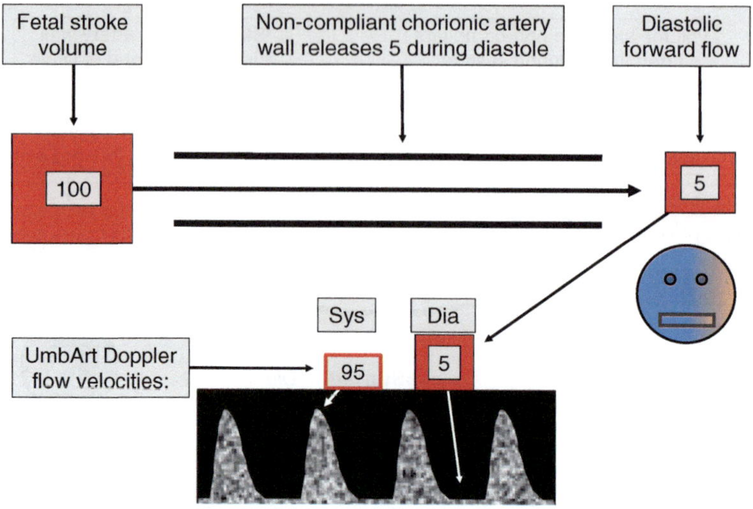

Fig. 4.12 Stiff chorionic arteries have *nothing to give during diastole*. The chorionic arteries, externally compressed due to obstruction of uterine venous return, absorb little volume during systole and therefore have little volume to discharge into the circulation during diastole. This leads to a dramatic reduction in forward flow during diastole—only 5 units! In this way, stiff chorionic arteries lead to a high pulsatility index in the umbilical artery Doppler velocity waveform seen at the bottom of the figure. It is also possible that the arterial walls remodel over time and become stiff permanently, rather than just when they are being compressed by obstruction of uterine venous return. *Dia* diastole, *Sys* systole, *UmbArt* umbilical artery

Possible Remodeling of Chronically Compressed Chorionic Vessels

Figures 4.13 and 4.14 present the theory that gradual remodeling of chorionic vessels subjected to recurrent or prolonged increased intervillous space pressure could convert temporary and reversible vascular *behavior* into *permanent structural change* which would then permanently limit fetal perfusion of the chorionic villus tree. Placentas from cases of fetal growth restriction are characterized by the histologic changes of "fetal vascular malperfusion," which consist of stunted and avascular chorionic villi, as well as chorionic vascular intramural fibrin deposition and stem villus vessel obliteration due to thickening of the vessel walls [9–13]. These vascular changes are portrayed figuratively in Fig. 4.15. It would seem that these histologic changes are consistent with a pathogenesis involving external compression by increased intervillous space pressure—as well as the possible outright destruction of chorionic villi by postulated violent jet flow from unremodeled spiral arteries, which is discussed in the next chapter.

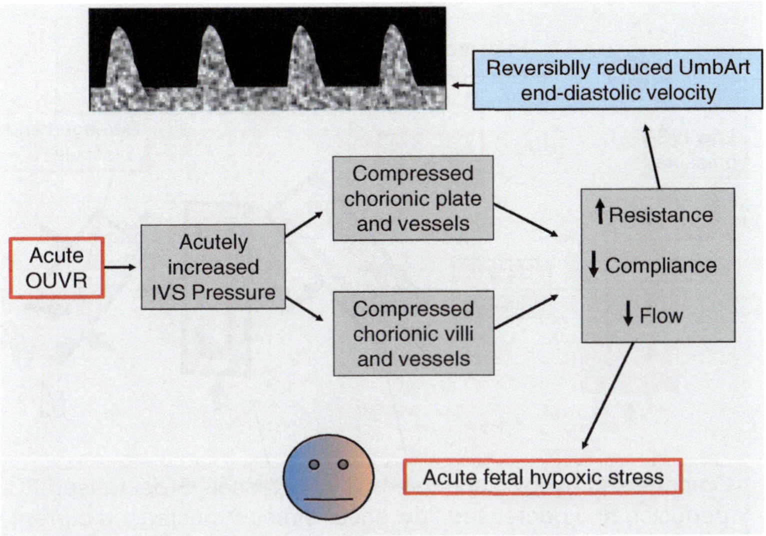

Fig. 4.13 At first, the stiffness of the externally compressed chorionic arteries may be temporary and reversible, entirely due to temporarily increased intervillous space pressure. *IVS* intervillous space, *OUVR* obstruction of uterine venous return, *UmbArt* umbilical artery

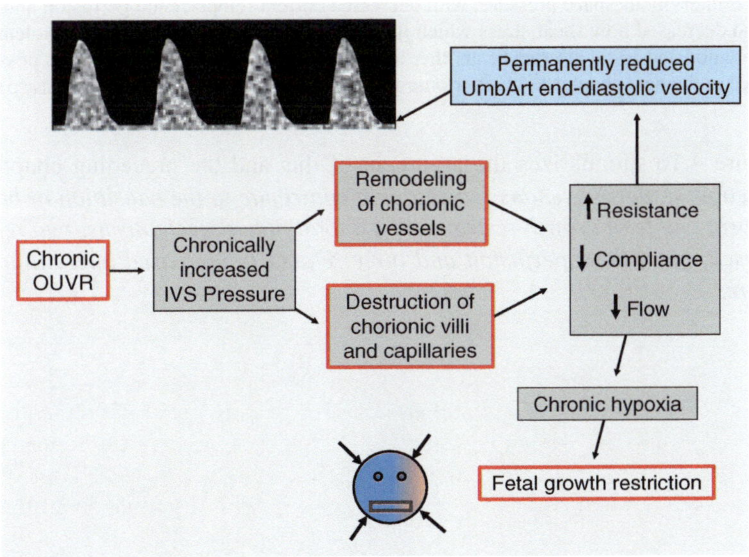

Fig. 4.14 Can the recurrently compressed chorionic arteries *remodel* and become permanently stiff? It is possible that intermittent compression of chorionic arteries causes them to remodel and acquire permanent high resistance and low compliance. If this happens, it might "lock-in" poor fetal perfusion of the placenta and lead to fetal growth restriction and the chorionic villus damage which is seen histologically in cases of placental insufficiency. *IVS* intervillous space, *OUVR* obstruction of uterine venous return, *UmbArt* umbilical artery

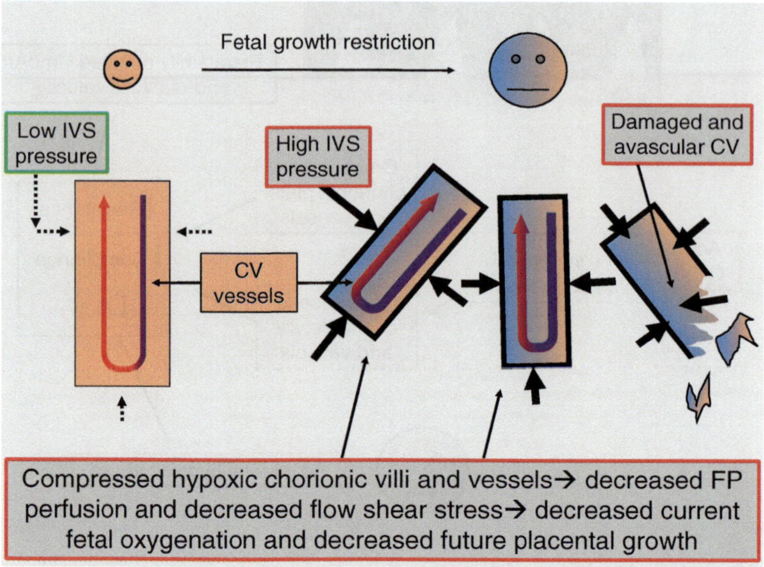

Fig. 4.15 "Locked-in" poor placental growth and destruction of chorionic villi. In fetal growth restriction, avascular and damaged chorionic villi are a prominent feature. Could these pathologic outcomes be set in motion by recurrent episodes of obstruction of uterine venous return and increased intervillous space pressure, with decreased current fetoplacental perfusion and oxygenation and decreased flow shear stress which limits future placental growth? Could violent jet flow from unremodeled spiral arteries be another cause of damage to chorionic villi (this possibility is discussed in the next chapter)? *CV* chorionic villus, *FP* fetoplacental, *IVS* intervillous space

Figure 4.16 summarizes the argument of this and the preceding chapter: *that obstruction of uterine venous return might contribute to the causation of both preeclampsia and fetal growth restriction by a total of five mechanisms: two related to decreased intervillous perfusion and three related to increased intervillous space pressure.*

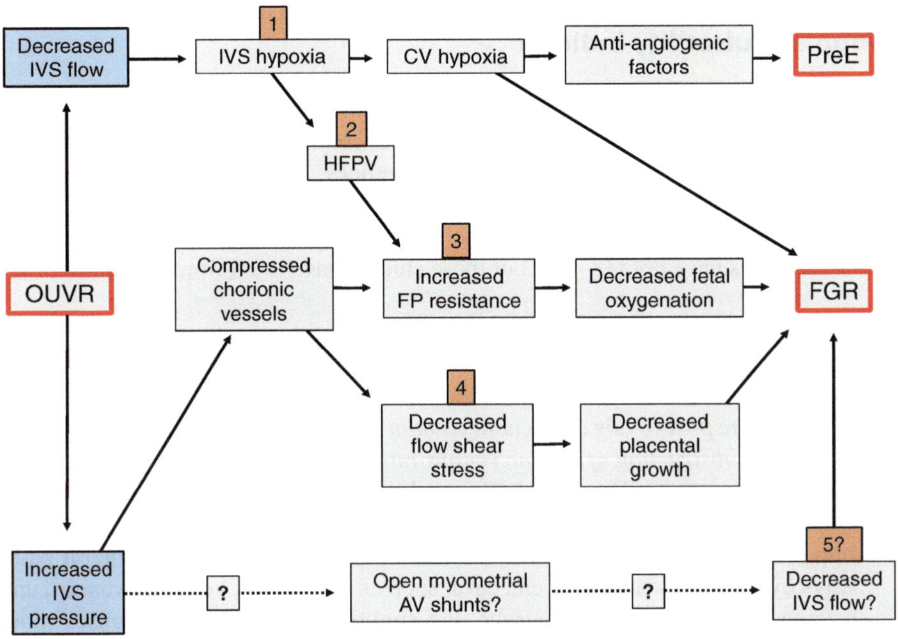

Fig. 4.16 The main message of the last two chapters: how obstruction of uterine venous return may impair placental function. Obstruction of uterine venous return might contribute to the causation of both preeclampsia and fetal growth restriction by a total of five mechanisms: two related to decreased intervillous space perfusion and three related to increased intervillous space pressure. The mechanisms are numbered in the figure and the explanations are as follows: (1) Decreased intervillous space perfusion in the presence of normal chorionic villus oxygen uptake capacity will cause intervillous space and chorionic villus hypoxia. This hypoxia by itself might contribute to both preeclampsia and fetal growth restriction as shown. (2) Intervillous hypoxia—besides being a danger in its own right—can trigger hypoxic fetoplacental vasoconstriction, since the primary stem villus arteries of the chorionic villus tree constrict gradually in response to intervillous hypoxia. This effect of intervillous hypoxia will restrict *fetoplacental* perfusion, with the results shown. (3) Increased intervillous space pressure will directly compress the chorionic villi and the fetal vessels within them, increasing their resistance, reducing their compliance, and—overall—reducing fetoplacental perfusion. This possible effect is the rationale for studies which have sought changes in umbilical artery Doppler waveforms when pregnant women assume the supine position after lying in a lateral position. (4) Increased intervillous space pressure with compression of chorionic vessels may also curtail flow shear stress, which is needed for the release of fetal-blood-borne growth factors which stimulate future chorionic villus growth. This would be an effect taking place over the course of days, weeks, or months. (5) Finally, subplacental arteriovenous shunts are known to exist, but their function is unknown. It may be that they function as a sort of "pressure relief valve" to reduce intervillous space pressure when it becomes excessive [24], and if these shunts open when intervillous space pressure increases due to obstruction of uterine venous return, it could be a cause of decreased perfusion of both the intervillous space and the myometrium (see Chap. 6). *AV* arteriovenous, *CV* chorionic villous, *FGR* fetal growth restriction, *FP* fetoplacental, *HFPV* hypoxic fetoplacental vasoconstriction, *IVS* intervillous space, *OUVR* obstructed uterine venous return, *PreE* preeclampsia

Does the Maternal Supine Position Increase Umbilical Artery Doppler Pulsatility Indices?

If these theories regarding increased intervillous space pressure are correct, one would expect that obstruction of uterine venous return would have been shown to increase umbilical artery Doppler pulsatility indices. Investigators have looked for these increases when pregnant women change from the lateral to the supine position, and some studies have shown the predicted increase in pulsatility indices, whereas others have not [14–20], but these studies have the following limitations:

1. The greatest limitation is that these studies do not demonstrate what is actually happening to venous return, cardiac output, or uterine venous pressure when the study participants adopt the supine and left lateral positions. *The mere adoption of the supine position by a pregnant woman late in gestation does not guarantee significant obstruction of uterine venous return and significant elevation of uterine venous pressure.* The spatial relationships of the inferior vena cava, vertebral column, and uterus vary considerably from person to person and even more important may be the availability—or lack thereof—of venous collateral pathways bypassing the inferior vena cava, such as the lumbar, vertebral venous, and azygos pathway [21]. *On average*, the supine position certainly causes more obstruction of venous return than lateral positions, but this average result says nothing about positional changes in uterine venous return within individual patients. Many patients may not have hemodynamically significant obstruction of uterine venous return in the supine position, whereas a small percentage may have a dangerous degree of obstruction in the supine position which is, in fact, accompanied by the expected umbilical artery Doppler changes. It may only be a relatively small percentage of pregnant women who have significant problems with positional obstruction of uterine venous return—but those patients should be identified as early as possible in gestation so that their propensity for fetal injury based on maternal position can be managed.
   These studies should be repeated but with simultaneous trending of maternal cardiac output, to see if obstruction of uterine venous return as detected by a decrease in maternal cardiac output correlates with umbilical artery Doppler changes. It should not be assumed that the supine position always obstructs uterine venous return or that a lateral position always relieves that obstruction.
2. The studies cited have involved healthy non-obese women without significant co-morbidities and with singleton pregnancies. These women would be expected to have maximal ability to compensate for some degree of obstruction of uterine venous return. Perhaps the studies might be repeated in patients with multiple gestation and with risk factors such as obesity, short stature, diabetes, and chronic hypertension. Furthermore, the studies should be repeated while trending cardiac output, in order to know whether obstruction of uterine venous return is actually occurring or not in a given maternal position.
3. The observation period for umbilical artery Doppler changes has been brief, generally about 5–10 min. It may take time for positional changes in umbilical

artery Doppler waveforms to develop [22, 23], since there may be two distinct mechanisms by which the positional waveform changes might occur. The first mechanism could be that increasing hydrostatic pressure within the intervillous space directly compresses the chorionic villi and the vessels within them, and the time course of this process is not known. The second mechanism might occur via the mediation of hypoxic fetoplacental vasoconstriction. Obstruction of uterine venous return would cause intervillous space hypoxia, which would then trigger generalized hypoxic fetoplacental vasoconstriction. The widespread constriction of the primary stem villus arteries would then be manifest as an increase in placental vascular resistance, a decrease in compliance, and as an increase in the pulsatility index. But hypoxic fetoplacental vasoconstriction appears to take 12–15 min to even *begin* to develop after the experimental imposition of intervillous anoxia [22], and it appears to increase in degree progressively over a period of 30 min or more. Resolution of hypoxic fetoplacental vasoconstriction is similarly slow and gradual [22].

For all these reasons—and despite the studies performed—it still seems unclear under what conditions obstruction of uterine venous return affects the fetoplacental circulation. *More research is required*!

Summary

1. Increased intervillous space pressure caused by obstruction of uterine venous return may impair placental function in three ways: (a) decreasing fetoplacental perfusion by compressing chorionic villi, (b) reducing the beneficial effects of flow shear stress on continued chorionic villus growth, and (c) opening subplacental myometrial arteriovenous shunts which divert maternal blood from either the intervillous space or the myometrium.
2. *Flow shear stress* is an important emerging concept in placental health and processes which impair its beneficial function may impair normal placental growth.
3. Flow shear stress is the force exerted by blood flow on vascular endothelium, and it is detected by flow sensors on the luminal surfaces of vascular endothelial cells. Adequate flow shear stress causes the release of vascular growth factors which support further growth of chorionic villus tissue "downstream."
4. Placental insufficiency is associated with umbilical artery Doppler velocity waveforms with increased pulsatility indices, and it is plausible that increased intervillous space pressure could produce such waveforms. Hence, it is possible that increased intervillous space pressure could be a *cause* of placental insufficiency.
5. Positional increases in pulsatility indices have been sought in women who assume the supine position from a lateral position, and some studies show the expected findings but others do not. These studies have limitations and should be repeated in higher-risk patients and with cardiac output trending in order to confirm whether obstruction of uterine venous return is actually present or not.

References

1. Power GG, Longo LD. Sluice flow in placenta: maternal vascular pressure effects on fetal circulation. Am J Physiol. 1973;225(6):1490–6. https://doi.org/10.1152/ajplegacy.1973.225.6.1490. PMID: 4202497.
2. Karimu AL, Burton GJ. The effects of maternal vascular pressure on the dimensions of the placental capillaries. Br J Obstet Gynaecol. 1994;101(1):57–63. https://doi.org/10.1111/j.1471-0528.1994.tb13011.x. PMID: 8297870.
3. Morley LC, Debant M, Gaunt HJ, Simpson NAB, Beech DJ. Nitric oxide synthase phosphorylation in fetoplacental endothelium is enhanced by agonism of Piezo1 mechanosensor in small for gestational age babies. Reprod Fertil. 2023;4(1):e220100. https://doi.org/10.1530/RAF-22-0100. PMID: 36542598; PMCID: PMC9874955.
4. Morley LC, Debant M, Walker JJ, Beech DJ, Simpson NAB. Placental blood flow sensing and regulation in fetal growth restriction. Placenta. 2021;113:23–8. https://doi.org/10.1016/j.placenta.2021.01.007. Epub 2021 Jan 18. PMID: 33509641; PMCID: PMC8448138.
5. Morley LC, Beech DJ, Walker JJ, Simpson NAB. Emerging concepts of shear stress in placental development and function. Mol Hum Reprod. 2019;25(6):329–39. https://doi.org/10.1093/molehr/gaz018. PMID: 30931481; PMCID: PMC6554190.
6. Morley LC, Shi J, Gaunt HJ, Hyman AJ, Webster PJ, Williams C, Forbes K, Walker JJ, Simpson NAB, Beech DJ. Piezo1 channels are mechanosensors in human fetoplacental endothelial cells. Mol Hum Reprod. 2018;24(10):510–20. https://doi.org/10.1093/molehr/gay033. PMID: 30085186; PMCID: PMC6311101.
7. Scott DB. Inferior vena caval occlusion in late pregnancy and its importance in anaesthesia. Br J Anaesth. 1968;40(2):120–8. https://doi.org/10.1093/bja/40.2.120.
8. Batton B, Li L, Newman NS, Das A, Watterberg KL, Yoder BA, Faix RG, Laughon MM, Stoll BJ, Higgins RD, Walsh MC, Eunice Kennedy Shriver National Institute of Child Health and Human Development Neonatal Research Network. Evolving blood pressure dynamics for extremely preterm infants. J Perinatol. 2014;34(4):301–5. https://doi.org/10.1038/jp.2014.6. Epub 2014 Feb 6. PMID: 24503912; PMCID: PMC3982788.
9. Benirschke's Pathology of the Human Placenta 7th ed., Ch 22, Ed Rebecca N. Baergen, Graham J. Burton, Cynthia G. Kaplan. Springer. ISBN: 978-3-030-84724-1.
10. Benirschke's Pathology of the Human Placenta 7th ed., Ch 9, Ed Rebecca N. Baergen, Graham J. Burton, Cynthia G. Kaplan. Springer. ISBN : 978-3-030-84724-1.
11. Lu L, Kingdom J, Burton GJ, Cindrova-Davies T. Placental stem villus arterial remodeling associated with reduced hydrogen sulfide synthesis contributes to human fetal growth restriction. Am J Pathol. 2017;187(4):908–20. https://doi.org/10.1016/j.ajpath.2016.12.002. Epub 2017 Feb 1. PMID: 28157488; PMCID: PMC5397715.
12. Salafia CM, Pezzullo JC, Minior VK, Divon MY. Placental pathology of absent and reversed end-diastolic flow in growth-restricted fetuses. Obstet Gynecol. 1997;90(5):830–6. https://doi.org/10.1016/S0029-7844(97)00473-0. PMID: 9351773.
13. Las Heras J, Baskerville JC, Harding PG, Haust MD. Morphometric studies of fetal placental stem arteries in hypertensive disorders ('toxaemia') of pregnancy. Placenta. 1985;6(3):217–27. https://doi.org/10.1016/s0143-4004(85)80051-5. PMID: 4022951.
14. Marx GF, Patel S, Berman JA, Farmakides G, Schulman H. Umbilical blood flow velocity waveforms in different maternal positions and with epidural analgesia. Obstet Gynecol. 1986;68(1):61–4. PMID: 3523331.
15. Ryo E, Okai T, Takagi K, Okuno S, Sadatsuki M, Kaneko M, Taketani Y. Comparison of umbilical artery Doppler velocimetry between maternal supine position and complete left lateral position in predicting obstetric complications. Ultrasound Obstet Gynecol. 1998;11(6):415–8. https://doi.org/10.1046/j.1469-0705.1998.11060415.x. PMID: 9674088.
16. Khatib N, Weiner Z, Beloosesky R, Vitner D, Thaler I. The effect of maternal supine position on umbilical and cerebral blood flow indices. Eur J Obstet Gynecol Reprod Biol. 2014;175:112–4. https://doi.org/10.1016/j.ejogrb.2013.12.043. Epub 2014 Jan 9. PMID: 24491277.

17. Silva KP, Hamamoto TENK, Nomura RMY. Transient fetal blood redistribution associated with maternal supine position. J Perinat Med. 2017;45(3):343–7. https://doi.org/10.1515/jpm-2016-0288. PMID: 27831924.
18. Couper S, Clark A, Thompson JMD, Flouri D, Aughwane R, David AL, Melbourne A, Mirjalili A, Stone PR. The effects of maternal position, in late gestation pregnancy, on placental blood flow and oxygenation: an MRI study. J Physiol. 2021;599(6):1901–15. https://doi.org/10.1113/JP280569. Epub 2021 Jan 18. PMID: 33369732; PMCID: PMC7613407.
19. Jani D, Clark A, Couper S, Thompson JMD, David AL, Melbourne A, Mirjalili A, Lydon AM, Stone PR. The effect of maternal position on placental blood flow and fetoplacental oxygenation in late gestation fetal growth restriction: a magnetic resonance imaging study. J Physiol. 2023;601(23):5391–411. https://doi.org/10.1113/JP284269.
20. Wu S, Liao G, Yang J. Effects of right lateral position on changes of fetal hemodynamics in late pregnancy. J Ultrasound Med. 2023;42(10):2341–7. https://doi.org/10.1002/jum.16261.
21. Humphries A, Stone P, Mirjalili SA. The collateral venous system in late pregnancy: a systematic review of the literature. Clin Anat. 2017;30(8):1087–95. https://doi.org/10.1002/ca.22959. Epub 2017 Aug 11. PMID: 28726308.
22. Ramasubramanian R, Johnson RF, Downing JW, Minzter BH, Paschall RL. Hypoxemic fetoplacental vasoconstriction: a graduated response to reduced oxygen conditions in the human placenta. Anesth Analg. 2006;103(2):439–42. https://doi.org/10.1213/01.ane.0000222468.76942.d8. PMID: 16861430.
23. Hampl V, Jakoubek V. Regulation of fetoplacental vascular bed by hypoxia. Physiol Res. 2009;58(Suppl 2):S87–94. https://doi.org/10.33549/physiolres.931922. PMID: 20131940.
24. Schaaps JP, Tsatsaris V, Goffin F, Brichant JF, Delbecque K, Tebache M, Collignon L, Retz MC, Foidart JM. Shunting the intervillous space: new concepts in human uteroplacental vascularization. Am J Obstet Gynecol. 2005;192(1):323–32. https://doi.org/10.1016/j.ajog.2004.06.066. PMID: 15672043.

5 More Perspectives on Preeclampsia and Fetal Growth Restriction

Destruction of Chorionic Villi Within an Unstable and Violent Intervillous Space

In the preceding two chapters, I have suggested that preeclampsia and fetal growth restriction could be due—in part—to decreased intervillous perfusion and increased intervillous pressure, and that obstruction of uterine venous return might cause both of these unfavorable changes. Normal perfusion of the intervillous space in a healthy pregnancy is shown schematically in Fig. 5.1, with the chorionic villus shown only as a rectangular block of tissue. Figure 5.2 shows (in a highly schematic way) the branching structure of a chorionic villous "tree," starting from the umbilical cord, passing through the chorionic plate vessels, the primary stem villus vessels and their many subsequent intermediate villous branches, and finally arriving at the terminal villi filled only with capillaries, where the majority of gas exchange takes place. As shown in Fig. 5.3, the "classical" explanation of preeclampsia suggests that defective spiral artery remodeling causes reduced intervillous flow which causes chorionic villous hypoxia and preeclampsia, on the one hand, and fetal hypoxia and growth restriction on the other [1–4]. But there is another plausible explanation for preeclampsia and fetal growth restriction which involves the destructive power of high-velocity jets of maternal blood emerging from unremodeled and narrow-diameter spiral arteries.

T. L. Archer, *Threats to Fetal, Placental and Myometrial Oxygenation*,
https://doi.org/10.1007/978-3-031-60364-8_5

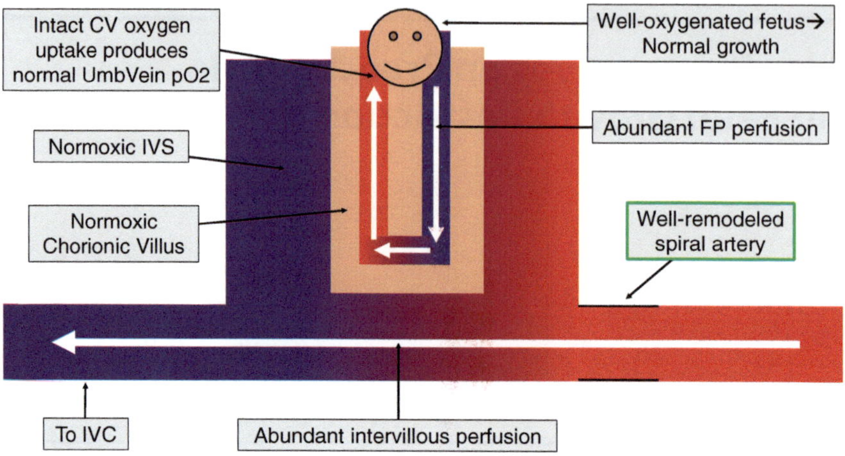

Fig. 5.1 Healthy chorionic villi within a well-perfused and low-pressure intervillous space. The spiral arteries have been remodeled so that they provide an adequate and gentle flow of maternal blood which percolates around the chorionic villi, gives up oxygen to the fetal circulation across the placental barrier, and then exits the intervillous space into a low-pressure uterine venous system which drains into an unobstructed inferior vena cava. The hydrostatic pressure within the intervillous space is low and the chorionic villi are not compressed, so that flow shear stress within the chorionic vessels is adequate to ensure future growth of the chorionic villi in order to keep pace with fetal needs. *CV* chorionic villus, *FP* fetoplacental, *IVC* inferior vena cava, *IVS* intervillous space, pO_2 oxygen partial pressure, *UmbVein* umbilical vein

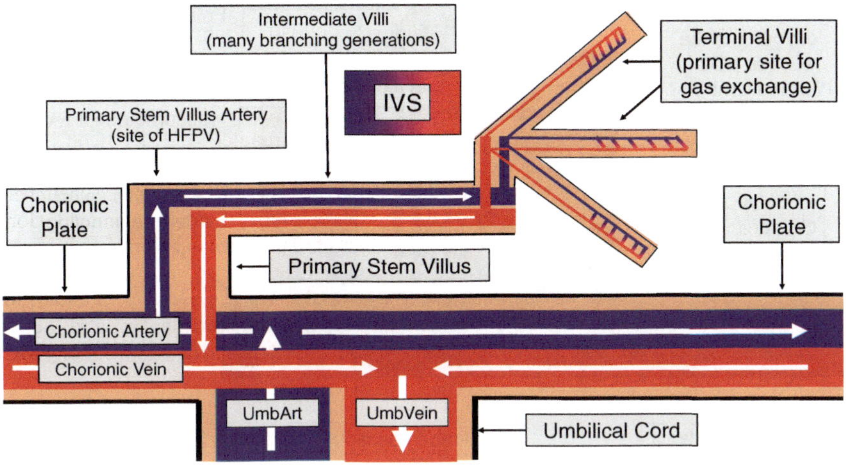

Fig. 5.2 Three levels of chorionic villous branching. This schematic drawing shows the levels of branching of a chorionic villus tree: (1) the umbilical cord containing the umbilical arteries and vein; (2) the chorionic plate containing the chorionic vessels which connect the umbilical vessels to the primary stem villi; (3) the primary stem villus containing the primary stem villus artery and veins, with the artery being thought to be the site of hypoxic fetoplacental vasoconstriction in response to intervillous hypoxia; (4) the many generations (not shown) of branching conducting intermediate villi, which undergo a process of villous maturation which may be affected by variations of the conditions within the intervillous space, such as hydrostatic pressure, oxygen tension, or high-velocity jets of maternal blood; and (5) the terminal villi, where most of the gas and nutrient exchange occurs between mother and fetus, because of the immense total surface area of the terminal villi. *The terminal villi, like the conducting intermediate villi, may be easily damaged by high-velocity jets of maternal blood, and these possible changes can be seen in* Figs. 5.5 and 5.14. *HFPV* hypoxic fetoplacental vasoconstriction, *IVS* intervillous space, *UmbArt* umbilical artery, *UmbVein* umbilical vein

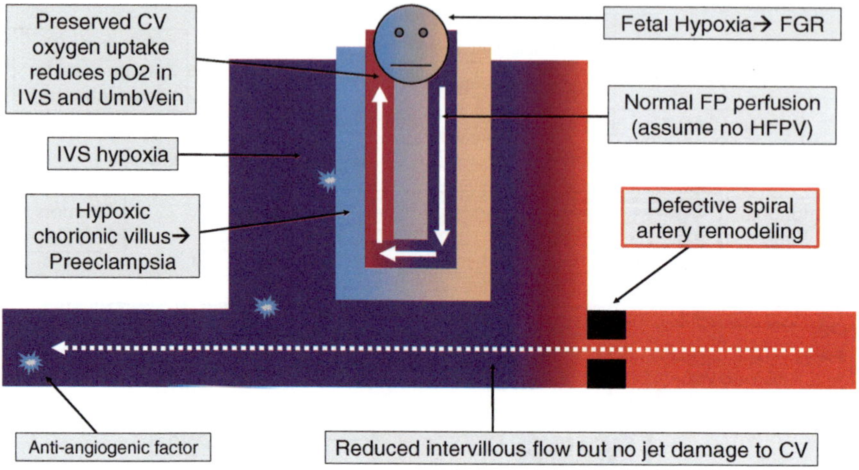

Fig. 5.3 The "classical" theory of preeclampsia. The "classical" theory of preeclampsia is that defective spiral artery remodeling leads to reduced perfusion of intervillous spaces. In the figure, the chorionic villi (shown as a simple rectangle) are intact and avidly take up sufficient oxygen from the intervillous space to barely satisfy the fetus' needs, but the fetus is stressed nevertheless because the oxygen is extracted at a low pO_2. In other words, the fetus may be alive and growing slowly but is growing under hypoxic conditions and perhaps experiencing growth restriction. Intervillous space oxygen tension is low because the usual amount of oxygen has been extracted from a slower flow of maternal blood. The low oxygen tension in the intervillous space stresses the chorionic villi as well, and they are beginning to secrete anti-angiogenic factors into maternal blood, which may eventually cause the preeclampsia syndrome in the mother. Hence, in this "classical" model, the mother may suffer preeclampsia and the fetus may suffer growth restriction, all because of decreased intervillous perfusion due to defective spiral artery remodeling. *CV* chorionic villus, *FGR* fetal growth restriction, *FP* fetoplacental, *IVC* inferior vena cava, *HFPV* hypoxic fetoplacental vasoconstriction, *IVS* intervillous space, *UmbVein* umbilical vein

Violent Jets of Blood from Unremodeled Spiral Arteries Damage Chorionic Villi

Burton and other investigators [5–7] have developed another rheological theory explaining preeclampsia and fetal growth restriction which suggests that defective spiral artery remodeling causes chorionic villus and fetal injury not so much because of reductions in intervillous space blood flow, but rather because the narrow and unremodeled spiral arteries discharge destructive high-velocity jets of maternal blood into the intervillous space which damage or destroy chorionic villi, as shown in Figs. 5.4 and 5.5, and the histologic placental changes seen in fetal growth restriction do appear to be consistent with destruction of chorionic villi [8–10].

This carefully constructed theory, relying on both mathematical modeling and histology, suggests that unremodeled spiral arteries emit a destructive jet of blood into the intervillous space at a velocity approximating 1–2 m/s, whereas blood from

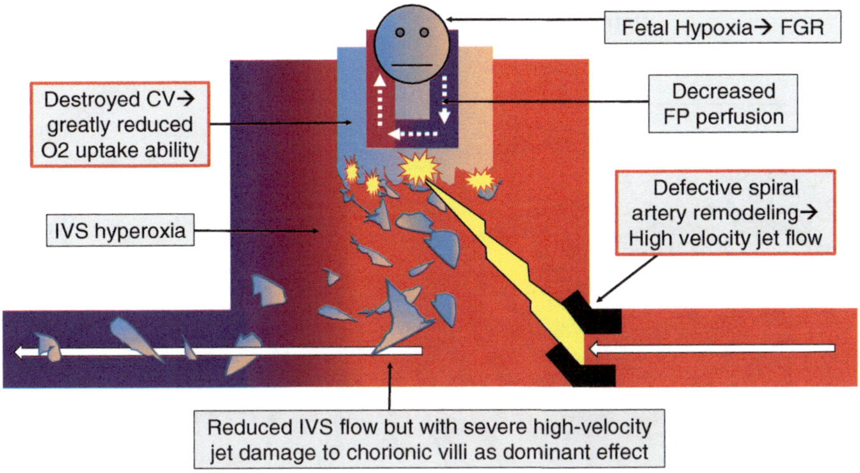

Fig. 5.4 Violent jet flow from unremodeled spiral arteries damages chorionic villi, reducing the surface area available for oxygen absorption by the fetus. This is the rheological theory advanced by Burton, which maintains that the most important effect of defective spiral artery remodeling is that it allows high-velocity jets of maternal blood to enter the intervillous space and damage the chorionic villi. This destruction of chorionic villus tissue decreases the ability of the chorionic villi to take up oxygen from the intervillous space. This fact—combined with the speed with which the maternal blood may traverse the space—may cause the pO_2 in the intervillous space to be high—and not low—despite the fact that the fetus is hypoxic! The Burton model predicts that defective spiral artery remodeling will reduce intervillous perfusion by 27% [5], as well as creating high-velocity jets of blood, but it is the contention of the theory that the reduction of intervillous blood flow does not impair **fetal oxygenation nearly as much as the damage to chorionic villi by the high-velocity jets** [5]. The combined result of the effects shown in this figure and in Fig. 5.3 would be that a preeclamptic placenta would show a wider distribution of oxygen tensions than a normal placenta, and this result has been found in a recent in vivo MRI study of placental oxygenation in preeclamptic patients [15]. See also Fig. 5.13. *CV* chorionic villus, *FGR* fetal growth restriction, *FP* fetoplacental, *IVS* intervillous space, O_2 oxygen

properly remodeled spiral arteries gently flows into the intervillous space at an approximate velocity of only 10 cm/s. As shown on the left side of Fig. 5.5, the much slower stream of blood in the healthy placenta percolates gently through the chorionic villi, allowing adequate time for gas exchange, and does not physically damage the villi, whereas the momentum of the high-velocity jet of blood destroys chorionic villi as shown in Fig. 5.4 and on the right side of Fig. 5.5. Furthermore, the blood from this violent and destructive jet may pass through the intervillous space quickly, without allowing adequate time for gas exchange with those chorionic villi which are still intact. The theory maintains that the value of spiral artery remodeling to the pregnancy is not so much to increase intervillous space flow as it is to decrease the velocity and destructive force with which maternal blood enters the intervillous space.

It must be added, however, that Burton's model does predict a decrease in intervillous space *flow volume* (in mL/s) when spiral artery remodeling is defective—but

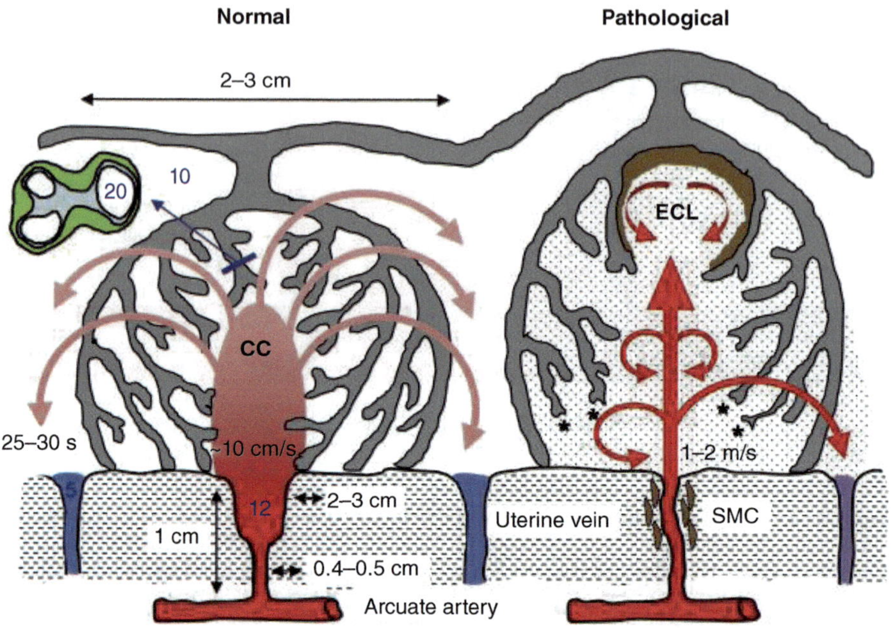

Fig. 5.5 Jet flow damage to chorionic villi in a more anatomically accurate representation. This diagram comes from the original paper of Burton et al. regarding their rheological theory of preeclampsia [5]. Notable features are: (1) high-velocity jet blood flow from the defectively remodeled spiral arteries (on the right side of the figure) is estimated to enter the intervillous space at a velocity of 1–2 m/s, whereas blood from normally remodeled vessels (on the left side of the figure) enters at a velocity approximating 10 cm/s. The jet flow is estimated to be 10–20 times faster than the normal flow, and the momentum of this jet is theorized to cause extensive destruction of terminal and intermediate villi, with a consequent loss of surface area for gas exchange. The physiology of this situation is similar to that of pulmonary emphysema, in which many alveoli are simply destroyed by the disease process, limiting the amount of alveolar capillary membrane available for gas exchange between alveolar gas and alveolar capillary blood. The ability of the chorionic villi to take up oxygen is severely impaired because much of the chorionic villus tree no longer exists! The "tree" appears to have been severely "pruned," as shown on the right side of Fig. 5.14 in the process of "accelerated villous maturation," which is characteristic of "maternal vascular malperfusion." Perhaps the anatomy shown would better be described as "accelerated villous *destruction*." *ECL* echogenic cystic lesion, *CC* central cavity, *SMC* smooth muscle cells. Tightly looped arrows on the right show turbulent high velocity flow. Note the wide mouth of normally remodeled spiral artery on the left, which greatly slows the velocity of blood flow into the intervillous space in m/s while at the same time modestly increasing the volume flow rate in mL/s. Figure from reference [5]. This is an open access article distributed under the terms of the Creative Commons CC BY license. Publisher is Elsevier. Caption has been modified

it is a decreased flow *volume* with a 10- to 20-fold increase in jet flow *velocity* (in m/s)! Hence, Burton's theory, while adding the suggestion of chorionic villus damage due to high-velocity jet flow, preserves the assumption of the "classical" preeclampsia model that defective spiral artery remodeling decreases intervillous flow, perhaps by 27% [5]. In short, Burton's model seems to suggest that with defective spiral artery remodeling, intervillous space flow *volume* will be reduced, but that the blood flow which does occur will have a much higher—and more destructive—*velocity*. The theory essentially proposes that defective spiral artery remodeling offers the "worst of both worlds"—*less intervillous oxygen being supplied, but in a more destructive manner!*

Figure 5.3 shows how reduced intervillous space flow volume—without violent jet flow and with preserved chorionic villous structure and oxygen uptake—will produce low intervillous oxygen tensions, whereas high velocity perfusion of intervillous spaces in which the chorionic villi have been severely damaged and are unable to take up normal amounts of oxygen will have relatively "high" oxygen tensions (but never greater than that of maternal arterial blood), as shown in Fig. 5.4.

"V/Q Mismatch" Within the Placenta

Another useful way of conceptualizing and summarizing this complicated situation with multiple processes at work is that variations in spiral artery remodeling and intervillous pressure will create a *mismatch* of maternal and fetal perfusion within the placenta. This concept of a "mismatch" between oxygen supply and demand in the placenta is analogous to "*V*/*Q* mismatch" in the lung [11], where "*V*" is alveolar ventilation and "*Q*" is pulmonary blood flow, as shown in Fig. 5.6. In this analogy with the lung, the "*V*" within the placenta corresponds to *maternal perfusion of the* intervillous spaces, while the "*Q*" corresponds to *fetal perfusion of the chorionic villi* [12–14], as shown in Fig. 5.7. In both placenta and lung, the mismatching of oxygen supply and demand leads to hypoxia of the organism. Episodic obstruction of uterine venous return would further reduce both uteroplacental and fetoplacental perfusion, making both chorionic villous and fetal oxygenation even worse.

Figures 5.8, 5.9, 5.10, and 5.11 portray four different scenarios in which defective spiral artery remodeling—with or without the destructive effects of high-velocity jet flow—might interact with obstruction of uterine venous return to produce fetal and chorionic villous hypoxia. In varying combinations, the four scenarios would probably produce a placenta with some regions having low oxygen tension and other regions having high oxygen tension, and in a recent in vivo MRI study of placentas in preeclamptic patients compared to those in healthy controls [15], Gowland et al. found regions of increased blood flow velocity (as shown in Fig. 5.12) as well as increased regional heterogeneity of placental oxygenation, with some regions being highly oxygenated and other regions being very hypoxic (as shown in Fig. 5.13).

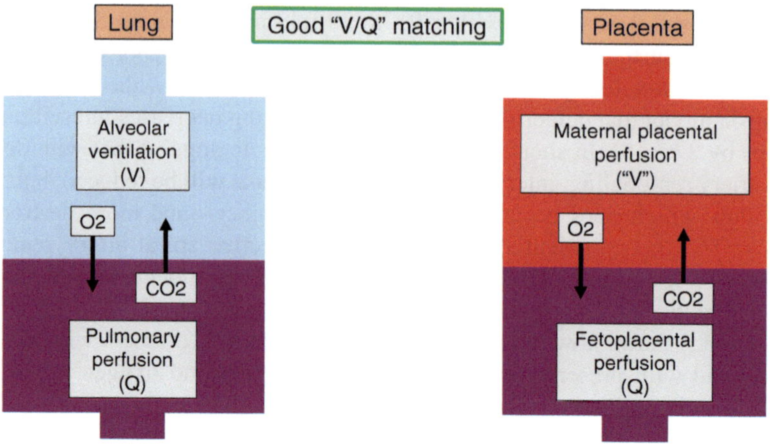

Fig. 5.6 "*V/Q* matching" in lung and placenta. The concept of the successful *bringing together*—or "matching"—of alveolar ventilation with pulmonary perfusion in the lung was introduced by John West in the late 1960s [11], and the concept was later applied to the placenta, in which the "*V*" is actually the *maternal perfusion of the placenta* and the "*Q*" is *the fetal perfusion of the placenta.* In both organs, it is essential that the *supply* of oxygen be brought together—or "matched" with the *demand* for oxygen. If the two flows are not successfully matched up so that gas transfer can occur, the entire function of both lung and placenta is undermined. Imagine a pair of lungs in which one lung receives all the blood flow and the other lung receives all of the ventilation—the organism would die! CO_2 carbon dioxide, O_2 oxygen, *V/Q* ratio of ventilation to perfusion in the lung

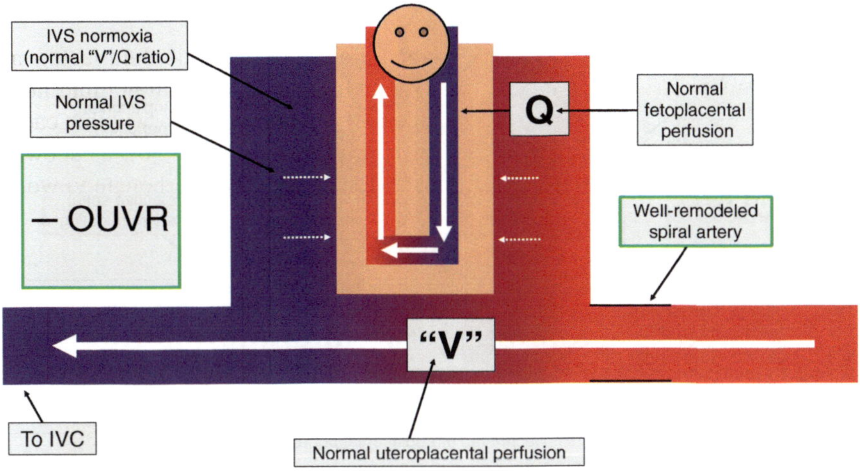

Fig. 5.7 Healthy "*V*/*Q* matching" in the placenta. This figure shows that in the analogy with the lung, the "ventilation" ("*V*")—or *supply* of oxygen—is *maternal placental perfusion* (or "uteroplacental perfusion"), whereas the *demand* for oxygen is fetal perfusion of the chorionic villi (*Q*, or "fetoplacental perfusion"). When "*V*" and *Q* are well matched, the fetus receives oxygen and eliminates carbon dioxide easily. The use of a "*V*" to describe a flow of blood is confusing at first, but the analogy with the lung is very useful conceptually. *IVC* inferior vena cava, *IVS* intervillous space, *–OUVR* absence of obstruction of uterine venous return, *Q* fetoplacental perfusion of chorionic villi, *"V"/Q* the ratio of uteroplacental (maternal) to fetoplacental perfusion. In the placenta, the "ventilation"—or source of oxygen—is the flow of maternal blood through the intervillous space and is denoted as "*V*"

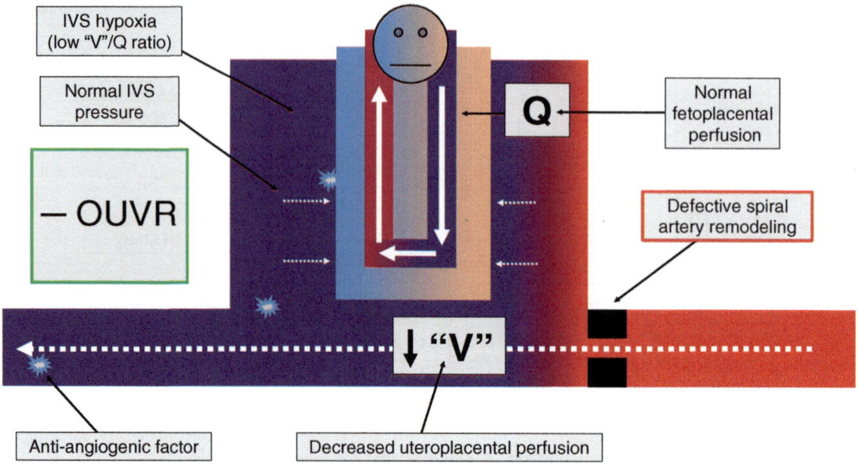

Fig. 5.8 The decreased "*V*"/*Q* ratio of the classical preeclampsia model. In the "classical" preeclampsia model of decreased uteroplacental (maternal) perfusion of the intervillous space due to defective spiral artery remodeling, only the "*V*" component—the uteroplacental perfusion—is decreased. The chorionic villi, their fetal blood vessels and their oxygen uptake capacity are intact, and therefore more oxygen is extracted by the chorionic villi from a decreased maternal blood flow, driving down the intervillous space pO_2. Intervillous space pressure is normal, since there is no obstruction of uterine venous return. The "*V*"/*Q* ratio is decreased and this decreases the intervillous space oxygen tension. *IVS* intervillous space, *−OUVR* absence of obstruction of uterine venous return, *Q* fetoplacental perfusion of chorionic villi, *"V"/Q* the ratio of uteroplacental (maternal) to fetoplacental perfusion. In the placenta, the "ventilation"—or source of oxygen—is the flow of maternal blood through the intervillous space and is denoted as "*V*"

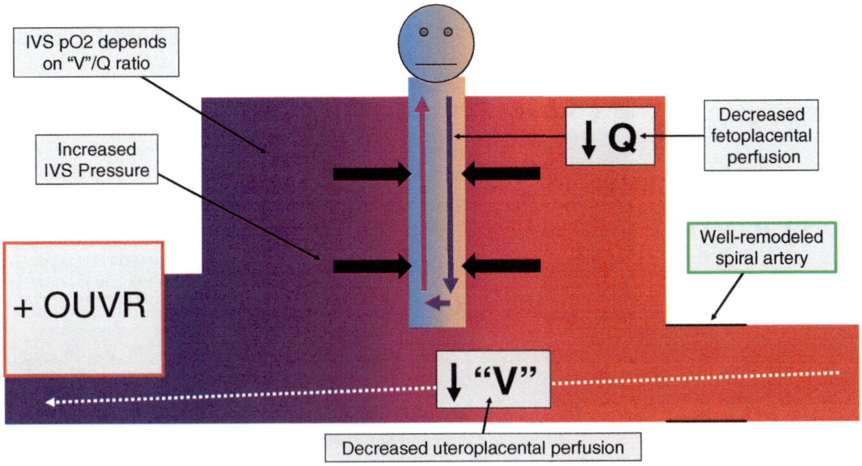

Fig. 5.9 Obstruction of uterine venous return reduces "*V*" but may also reduce *Q*. Obstruction of uterine venous return may disturb placental function in two ways: decreased intervillous space perfusion and increased intervillous space pressure. The decreased perfusion will decrease intervillous space oxygen tension—*assuming that the chorionic villi take up normal amounts of oxygen.* But what if the chorionic villi do not take up normal amounts of oxygen? Decreased oxygen uptake could be caused by two processes: (1) reduced fetal perfusion of intact chorionic villi (as shown in this figure) or (2) destruction of chorionic villi along with their fetal blood vessels (as shown in Fig. 5.10). In this figure, obstruction of uterine venous return increases intervillous space pressure which compresses intact chorionic villi and the fetal blood vessels within them, reducing fetal oxygen uptake capacity (as well as increasing afterload on the fetal right ventricle which perfuses the placenta). These effects will almost certainly reduce oxygen uptake by the fetus, but the final effect on intervillous space pO_2 will depend on the comparative *degree* of reduction in uteroplacental and fetoplacental perfusion (the "*V*" and the *Q*). In other words, the intervillous space pO_2 could be normal due to an equal reduction in "*V*" and *Q*. *The fetus would still suffer, however, because it is taking up less oxygen—despite the "normal" oxygen tension within the intervillous space! IVS* intervillous space, *+OUVR* obstruction of uterine venous return is present, *pO_2* oxygen partial pressure, *"V"/Q* the ratio of uteroplacental (maternal) to fetoplacental perfusion. In the placenta, the "ventilation"—or source of oxygen—is the flow of maternal blood through the intervillous space and is denoted as "*V*"

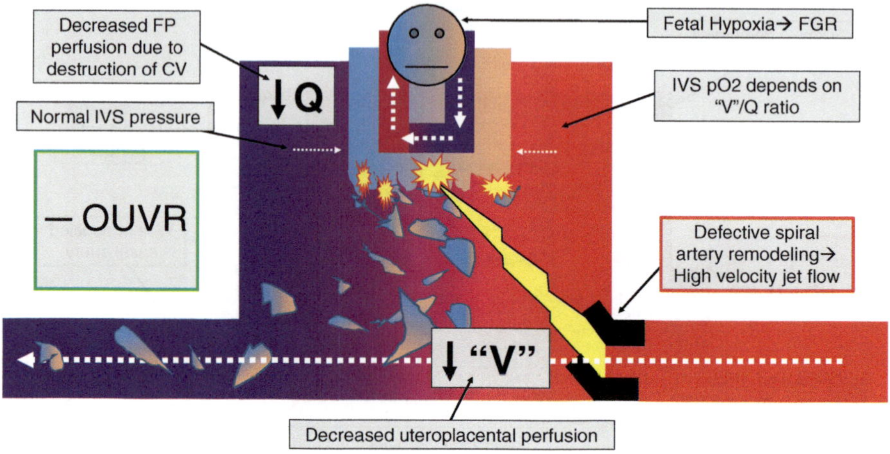

Fig. 5.10 Destruction of chorionic villi will reduce fetoplacental perfusion (*Q*). If chorionic villi have been destroyed by jets of high velocity blood emerging from defectively remodeled spiral arteries, they can no longer take up oxygen. Therefore, even if intervillous space pressure is normal, the oxygen uptake capacity of the chorionic villi will be reduced because chorionic villus perfusion has been forcibly reduced by outright destruction. Therefore, in this scenario, *Q* is reduced. But even Burton's model suggests that defective spiral artery remodeling reduces intervillous space perfusion, perhaps by 27%. So "*V*" is reduced as well, and the final pO_2 of the intervillous space will depend on the comparative reductions of uteroplacental and fetoplacental perfusion ("*V*" and *Q*), as in Fig. 5.9. *Also, as in* Fig. 5.9, *total fetal oxygen uptake will certainly be reduced, despite the fact that the oxygen tension within the intervillous space* pO_2 *may be normal. CV* chorionic villi, *FGR* fetal growth restriction, *FP* fetoplacental, *IVS* intervillous space, *−OUVR* absence of obstruction of uterine venous return, pO_2 oxygen tension in mmHg, *"V"/Q* ratio the ratio of uteroplacental (maternal) to fetoplacental perfusion. In the placenta, the "ventilation"—or source of oxygen—is the flow of maternal blood through the intervillous space and is denoted as "*V*"

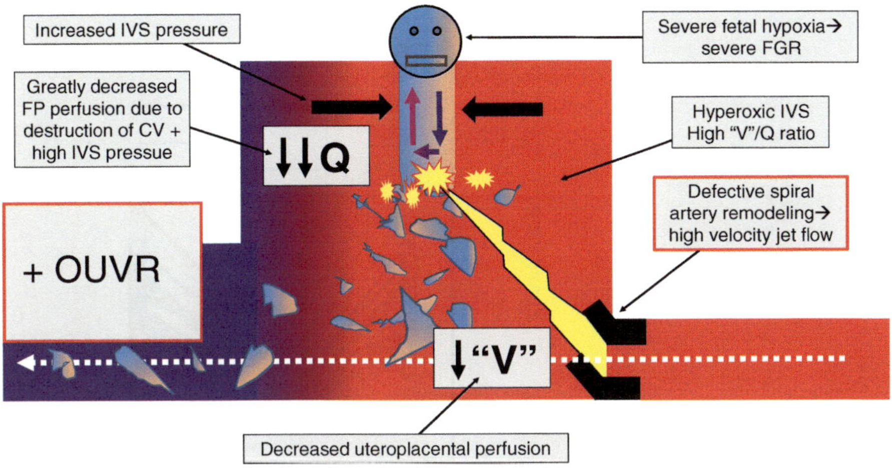

Fig. 5.11 Destruction of chorionic villi combined with obstruction of uterine venous return will greatly reduce Q and may cause hyperoxia in intervillous spaces. This placenta is in terrible shape. It has multiple bad things happening within it: (1) uteroplacental perfusion is reduced by (a) defective spiral artery remodeling and (b) obstruction of uterine venous return; (2) additionally, fetal oxygen uptake is impaired by two separate processes: (c) destruction of chorionic tissue and their fetal blood vessels by high-velocity jets of maternal blood, and (d) compression of surviving chorionic villi and their fetal vessels by increased intervillous space pressure due to obstruction of uterine venous return. *In this example, again, the final intervillous space* pO_2 *will depend on the comparative degree of impairment of uteroplacental and fetoplacental perfusion, but the net result will be greatly impaired fetal oxygen uptake, no matter what the intervillous space* pO_2 *is.* Hyperoxic intervillous spaces may be the result when chorionic villus destruction and impairment outweigh the effects of decreased uteroplacental perfusion. *CV* chorionic villi, *FGR* fetal growth restriction, *FP* fetoplacental, *IVS* intervillous space, + *OUVR* obstruction of uterine venous return is present, pO_2 oxygen partial pressure, *"V"/Q* ratio the ratio of uteroplacental (maternal) to fetoplacental perfusion. In the placenta, the "ventilation"—or source of oxygen—is the flow of maternal blood through the intervillous space and is denoted as "*V*"

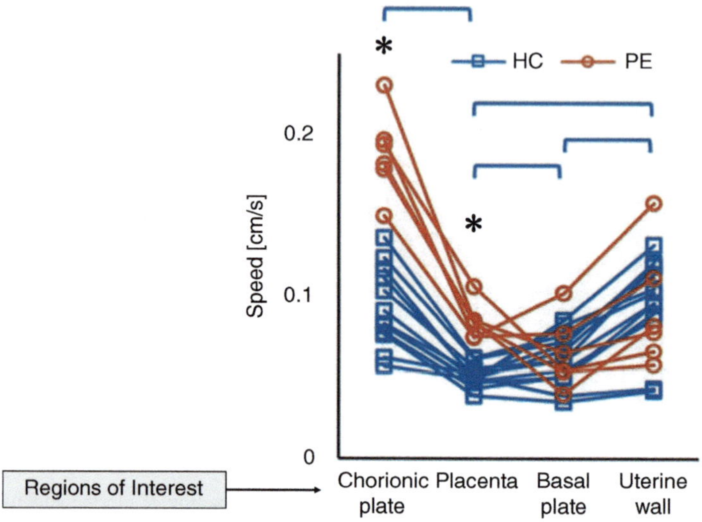

Fig. 5.12 Chorionic and placental blood flow is faster in preeclamptic than in healthy placentas. This figure, modified from [15], contains a lot of information and requires explanation. The information with asterisks over the data points are the only ones we are interested in at this time, and they show that blood velocities in the chorionic plate and placenta are higher in preeclamptic than in healthy pregnant women. These findings are consistent with the hypothesis that preeclampsia involves high velocity blood flow emerging from unremodeled spiral arteries [5]. *HC* healthy control placentas, *PE* preeclamptic placentas. Figure from reference [15]. Copyright: © 2020 Dellschaft et al. This is an open access article distributed under the terms of the Creative Commons Attribution License, which permits unrestricted use, distribution, and reproduction in any medium, provided the original author and source are credited

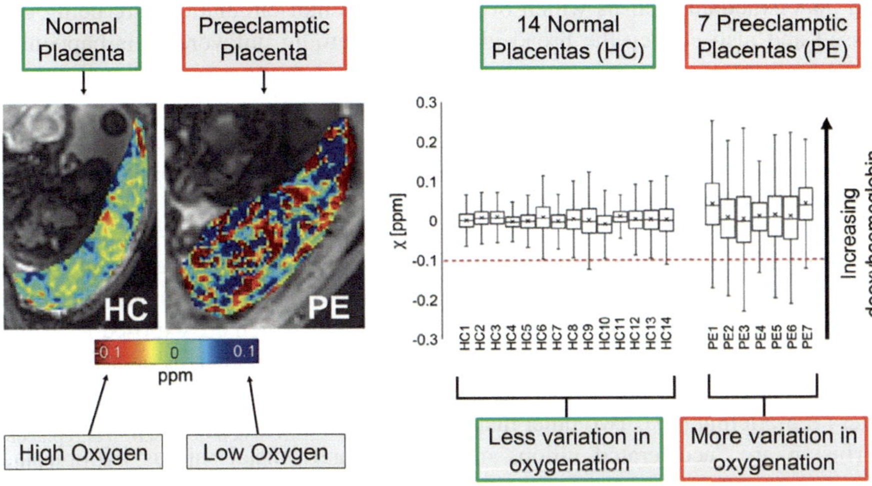

Fig. 5.13 By MRI examination, there is more heterogeneity of oxygenation in vivo in preeclamptic placentas than in normal ones. This figure shows more regional variation in oxygenation in the preeclamptic placenta than in the healthy one. This increased regional variability in preeclampsia is consistent with a combination of the "classical" theory of preeclampsia involving underperfusion of some intervillous spaces which have normal oxygen uptake by intact chorionic villi (as shown in Fig. 5.8), together with the "Burton modification" of the "classical" theory, which predicts spiral artery jet flow which destroys chorionic villi and thereby drastically reduces chorionic villous oxygen uptake capacity, as shown in Fig. 5.10. The classical theory predicts hypoxic regions in the preeclamptic placenta, and the "Burton modification" of the theory provides an elegant mechanism for explaining hyperoxic regions of the placenta. I am proposing that intermittent obstruction of uterine venous return would further decrease both uteroplacental and fetoplacental perfusion and make the fetal hypoxia already caused by preeclamptic "*V*"/*Q* mismatch even worse. Prevention of obstruction of uterine venous return might do nothing to prevent the fundamental pathology of preeclampsia and FGR, but it might mitigate the damage or delay the onset of both fetal and maternal disease and allow delivery at a later date. *HC* healthy control placentas, *PE* preeclamptic placentas, *X* (ppm) chi, an index of the amount of deoxyhemoglobin present, with high oxygen showing as red at −0.1 and low oxygen as blue at +0.1—as shown in the color scale. Figure from [15]. Copyright: © 2020 Dellschaft et al. This is an open access article distributed under the terms of the Creative Commons Attribution License

Placental Histology in Preeclampsia and Fetal Growth Restriction

A conference held in Amsterdam in 2015 appears to have brought some useful changes to what had been a confusing system of terminology in placental pathology. The conference introduced the terms "maternal vascular malperfusion" and "fetal vascular malperfusion" to the lexicon of the field, and as a non-specialist I find these terms refreshing both for their specificity and their modesty [16]. The terms openly and understandably tell us which of the two placental circulations are being discussed and also convey the broad idea that something unfavorable is happening which prevents the placenta from properly bringing the two circulations into the close contact needed for adequate gas exchange and fetal growth.

Maternal Vascular Malperfusion

This term tells us that something bad is happening with the maternal circulation of the placenta, that is, with the spiral arteries, intervillous space, or the chorionic villi—which of course contain fetal blood vessels but which are exposed to maternal blood within the intervillous space. Maternal vascular malperfusion can be characterized by low placental weight, chorionic villous infarction, and abnormal spiral artery remodeling [17]. Two other histological hallmarks of maternal vascular malperfusion are "accelerated villous maturation" and "distal villous hypoplasia." These two "villous maturation disorders" are morphological changes of the chorionic villi which are found in fetal growth restriction and which could be expected to make oxygen uptake by the fetus less efficient [17]. Figure 5.14 is my attempt to

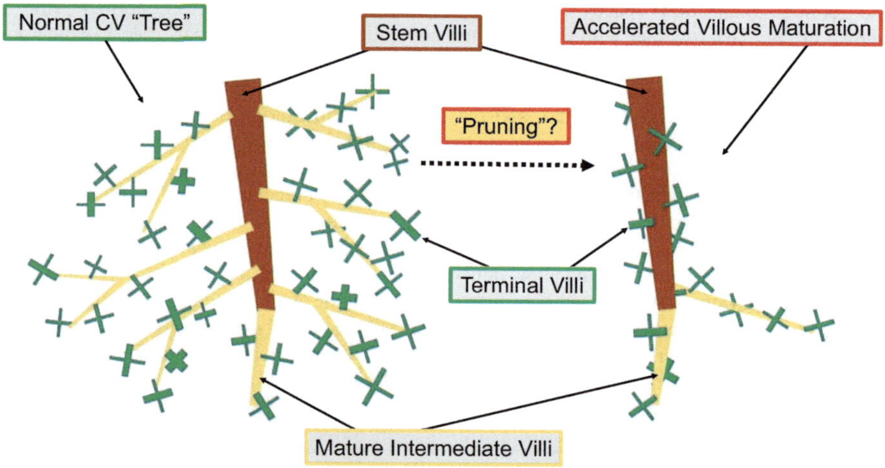

Fig. 5.14 Disorders of villous maturation. The structural hallmarks of maternal vascular malperfusion are *accelerated villous maturation* as shown on the right side of this figure and *distal villous hypoplasia,* which has a similar appearance but is not shown. These disorders of villous maturation are often found in the placentas of growth-restricted newborns. To my non-pathologist's eye, the structure of accelerated villous maturation appears like an upside-down tree that has been pruned aggressively, when compared to the normal "branches" of the normal villous tree on the left. This "pruning" or destruction of the mature intermediate villi might be due to (1) decreased intervillous perfusion, (2) increased intervillous pressure, or (3) high-velocity jet flow due to defective spiral artery remodeling. I would pose the following question: are these changes a disorder of villous *maturation* or are they the result of a process of *creation followed by destruction?* Perhaps it amounts to the same thing. Figure was drawn by the author based on Figure 19.11 on page 527 of [17]

show that the abnormal chorionic villus "trees" found in accelerated villous maturation appear to contain fewer "mature intermediate villi" than are found in normal villus trees, and the authors of [17] speculate that this absence of intermediate villi could be due to violent jet flow and chorionic villus destruction as proposed by Burton et al. [5]. The three classes of *functional* uteroplacental perfusion disorders we have been discussing—decreased intervillous perfusion, increased intervillous space pressure, and violent, high-velocity intervillous jet blood flow—might all contribute to what appears *structurally* to be a "pruning" process involving the absence or destruction of mature intermediate and terminal villi, which is portrayed in various ways in Figs. 5.5, 5.10, 5.11, and 5.14. Since obstruction of uterine venous return could cause both decreased intervillous perfusion and increased intervillous pressure, it is possible that such obstruction could help explain the pathological changes of the two "villous maturation disorders" seen in fetal growth restriction. In short, it appears possible that the pathological changes seen in fetal growth restriction may not be due to abnormal villous *maturation*, but rather to abnormal villous *destruction*, and that some of this destruction might be mediated by obstruction of uterine venous return, as well as by high-velocity jets of blood emerging from unremodeled spiral arteries.

In a recent review of the placental pathology seen in cases of intrauterine death of fetuses without birth defects, 92% of the placentas were histologically abnormal, with a very high incidence of villous maturation disorders and histological evidence of fetal hypoxia [18], both of which might be due to decreased IVS flow, increased IVS pressure, or high spiral artery jet flow velocity.

Fetal Vascular Malperfusion

This term simply tells us that something bad is happening with the fetal side of the placental circulation. The hallmarks of fetal vascular malperfusion are disorders of the fetal blood vessels within the umbilical cord and chorionic plate and villi, such as thrombosis of vessels, thickened vessel walls with or without vessel obliteration, and completely avascular villi [19, 20]. It seems that decreased maternal intervillous perfusion, increased intervillous pressure, and violent intervillous jet flow might all contribute to these pathological changes in chorionic vessels. It would seem, however, that increased intervillous pressure might have special weight in causing fetal vascular malperfusion since increased intervillous space pressure will directly compress the fetal vasculature within the chorionic villi and may cause thickening and remodeling of those vessels. Disorders of the umbilical cord causing venous obstruction are cited as prominent causes of fetal vascular malperfusion, and I would propose that increased intervillous space pressure due to obstruction of uterine venous return may be another cause of chorionic vessel remodeling and thickening, thrombosis, obliteration, and chorionic villus avascularity. This picture would be consistent with the high pulsatility index umbilical artery Doppler changes seen in fetal growth restriction—involving high fetoplacental resistance and low compliance, as discussed in Chap. 4.

Chorionic Villi May Need a Stable Environment for Optimal Growth

For healthy chorionic villus growth, three aspects of the intervillous space—hydrostatic pressure, oxygen tension, and maternal blood flow velocity—may all need to be maintained within acceptable ranges, and variations outside those ranges may cause problems for both maternal and fetal circulations. Figure 5.15 shows how this concept might apply to the flow shear stress experienced by the external surface of chorionic villi: on the left side of Fig. 5.15 we see that flow shear stress is inadequate to support optimal chorionic villus growth, whereas on the right side of the figure, high flow shear stress—perhaps caused by violent jets of blood emerging from unremodeled spiral arteries—causes gross physical damage to chorionic villi.

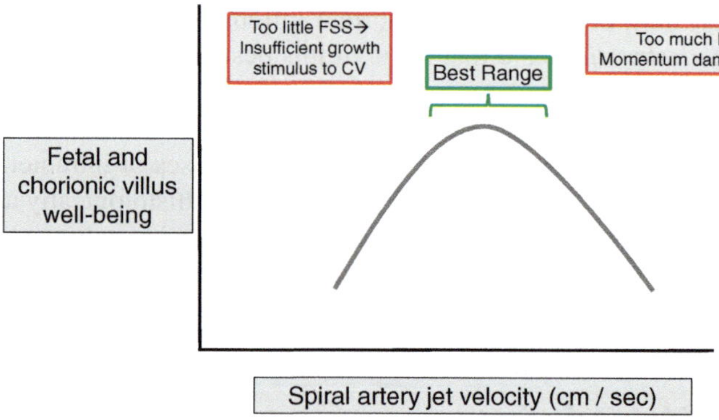

Fig. 5.15 Optimum spiral artery jet flow velocity (in cm/s, not mL/min). Flow shear stress is a stimulus to chorionic villus growth functions on the *outside* of chorionic villi, as well as *within* chorionic fetal vessels. Insufficient velocity of maternal blood flow within the intervillous space may not provide optimal stimulation of chorionic villus growth from the *outside surface of the villi*, just as insufficient fetal perfusion of the chorionic villi may not provide optimal stimulation of chorionic villus growth *from inside the chorionic villus*. Excessive velocity, however, may cause direct momentum damage to the chorionic villi. Hence, there is probably an optimal intervillous space perfusion velocity, and intermittent obstruction of uterine venous return may reduce this velocity in a way which compromises chorionic villus growth. *CV* chorionic villus, *FSS* flow shear stress, *IVS* intervillous space

Intermittent Obstruction of Uterine Venous Return May Cause Ischemia and Reperfusion Injury to Chorionic Villi

As suggested schematically in Fig. 5.16, *wide variations* in intervillous oxygen tension may cause more chorionic villous injury than *lower oxygen tension* per se [21–26], and intermittent obstruction of uterine venous return could be a cause of that wide variation. In other words, the chorionic villi and fetus may be able to adapt to a relatively wide range of oxygen tension *as long as that specific oxygen tension is held reasonably stable over time.* A corollary of this insight is that it may be misleading to characterize one intervillous space as "hypoxic" just because its oxygen tension is lower than that of another intervillous space, since the term "hypoxic" is often used to describe a level of oxygenation that is injurious in and of itself. The finding by Thuring et al. that discontinuous uterine *venous* blood flow is associated with preeclampsia and fetal growth restriction is also consistent with this hypothesis [27]. There may be nothing that can be done at present about defective spiral artery

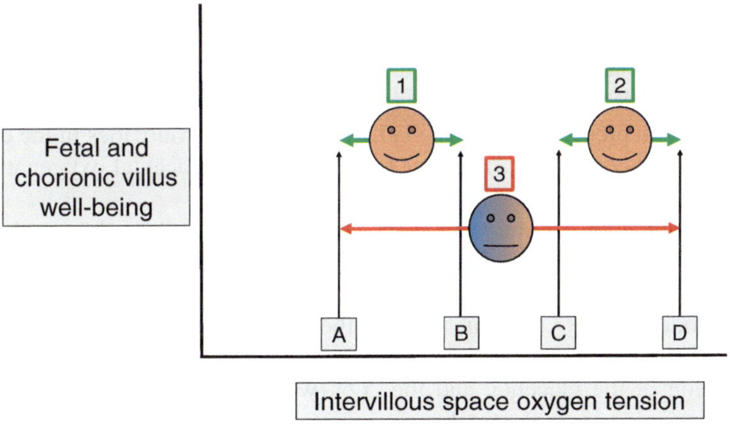

Fig. 5.16 Wide variations in intervillous oxygen tension may be more injurious to chorionic villi than lower oxygen tensions per se. Lower oxygen tensions per se (within limits) may not injure chorionic villi and the fetus as much as wide *variations* in intervillous space oxygen tension. In other words, the chorionic villi and fetus may be able to adapt to a relatively wide range of oxygen tension *as long as that specific oxygen tension is held reasonably stable over time.* This figure is an attempt to convey that idea schematically: Both Fetus #1 and Fetus #2 are thriving, despite the fact that the average intervillous oxygen tension to which Fetus #1 is exposed is lower than that for Fetus #2. A corollary of this insight is that it might well be misleading to characterize the intervillous space of Fetus #1 as "hypoxic" compared to that of Fetus #2, since the word "hypoxia" often implies a level of oxygenation which is harmful by itself if maintained. The key to the probable good outcomes for both Fetus #1 and Fetus #2 is that the *variation* of intervillous oxygenation to which they are exposed during intrauterine life is minimal (the green double arrows are short). By contrast, Fetus #3 is not doing well because its exposure to oxygen varies widely throughout the day—perhaps as a result of intermittent obstruction of uterine venous return (the double red arrow is long) [26]

remodeling, but prevention of obstruction of uterine venous return might mitigate its harmful influence by stabilizing intervillous oxygen tension and hydrostatic pressure within narrower ranges. In this way, elimination of obstruction of uterine venous return might help the chorionic villi to grow optimally and the fetus to achieve its full potential during its life ahead.

Summary

1. The "classical" theory of preeclampsia is that decreased intervillous perfusion from defectively remodeled spiral arteries causes intervillous hypoxia, which damages both chorionic villi and the fetus, causing either preeclampsia, fetal growth restriction, or both syndromes together.
2. Graham Burton and his colleagues have advanced a competing—or perhaps complementary—theory, which is that defective spiral artery remodeling is indeed a cause of preeclampsia, but that it causes its damage not so much by reducing intervillous perfusion, as by allowing high-velocity jets of maternal blood to enter the intervillous space and cause direct momentum-related structural damage to the chorionic villi.
3. Recent MRI work by Gowland et al. has presented evidence which supports Burton's model. She and her colleagues have found that, in vivo, the placentas of women with preeclampsia have (1) higher blood flow velocities in the chorionic plate and placenta and (2) greater heterogeneity of placental oxygenation, than the placentas of healthy control pregnant women.
4. The combination of the "classical" and the "Burton" model would predict exactly these findings—high velocity flow and a wider variation of placental oxygenation than in normal placentas.
5. The model of "*V*/*Q* mismatching" in the lung can be fruitfully adapted to the placenta, in which the "*V*" or ventilation in the lung is analogous to the maternal perfusion of the placenta, and the "*Q*" (which is pulmonary perfusion in the lung) is analogous to the fetal perfusion of the chorionic villi.
6. Intermittent obstruction of uterine venous return adds another "layer" of instability and variation to the picture, and the net result of obstruction of uterine venous return in a placenta at risk for causing preeclampsia or fetal growth restriction may be to further decrease fetal and chorionic villus oxygenation and accelerate the onset of clinical injury to both chorionic villi and the fetus. Even in the presence of poor spiral artery remodeling or other risk factors, avoidance of obstruction of uterine venous return might therefore allow prolongation of intrauterine fetal growth with delivery at a later date and might thereby improve the ability of the fetus to achieve its full potential in its life to come.

References

1. Erez O, Romero R, Jung E, Chaemsaithong P, Bosco M, Suksai M, Gallo DM, Gotsch F. Preeclampsia and eclampsia: the conceptual evolution of a syndrome. Am J Obstet Gynecol. 2022;226(2S):S786–803. https://doi.org/10.1016/j.ajog.2021.12.001. PMID: 35177220; PMCID: PMC8941666.
2. Redman CWG, Staff AC, Roberts JM. Syncytiotrophoblast stress in preeclampsia: the convergence point for multiple pathways. Am J Obstet Gynecol. 2022;226(2S):S907–27. https://doi.org/10.1016/j.ajog.2020.09.047. Epub 2021 Feb 2. PMID: 33546842.
3. Burton GJ, Jauniaux E. Pathophysiology of placental-derived fetal growth restriction. Am J Obstet Gynecol. 2018;218(2S):S745–61. https://doi.org/10.1016/j.ajog.2017.11.577. PMID: 29422210.
4. Schoots MH, Gordijn SJ, Scherjon SA, van Goor H, Hillebrands JL. Oxidative stress in placental pathology. Placenta. 2018;69:153–61. https://doi.org/10.1016/j.placenta.2018.03.003. Epub 2018 Mar 16. PMID: 29622278.
5. Burton GJ, Woods AW, Jauniaux E, Kingdom JC. Rheological and physiological consequences of conversion of the maternal spiral arteries for uteroplacental blood flow during human pregnancy. Placenta. 2009;30(6):473–82. https://doi.org/10.1016/j.placenta.2009.02.009. Epub 2009 Apr 17. PMID: 19375795; PMCID: PMC2697319.
6. Roth CJ, Haeussner E, Ruebelmann T, Koch FV, Schmitz C, Frank HG, Wall WA. Dynamic modeling of uteroplacental blood flow in IUGR indicates vortices and elevated pressure in the intervillous space - a pilot study. Sci Rep. 2017;7:40771. https://doi.org/10.1038/srep40771. PMID: 28102332; PMCID: PMC5244422.
7. Saghian R, James JL, Tawhai MH, Collins SL, Clark AR. Association of placental jets and mega-jets with reduced villous density. J Biomech Eng. 2017;139(5):0510011–05100110. https://doi.org/10.1115/1.4036145. PMID: 28267189; PMCID: PMC7104759.
8. Biagiotti R, Sgambati E, Brizzi E. Placental morphometry in pregnancies complicated by intrauterine growth retardation with absent or reversed end diastolic flow in the umbilical artery. Ital J Anat Embryol. 1999;104(4):201–7. PMID: 10684184.
9. Spinillo A, Gardella B, Adamo L, Muscettola G, Fiandrino G, Cesari S. Pathologic placental lesions in early and late fetal growth restriction. Acta Obstet Gynecol Scand. 2019;98(12):1585–94. https://doi.org/10.1111/aogs.13699. Epub 2019 Sep 18. PMID: 31370094.
10. Junaid TO, Brownbill P, Chalmers N, Johnstone ED, Aplin JD. Fetoplacental vascular alterations associated with fetal growth restriction. Placenta. 2014;35(10):808–15. https://doi.org/10.1016/j.placenta.2014.07.013. Epub 2014 Aug 6. PMID: 25145956.
11. West JB. A lifetime of pulmonary gas exchange. Physiol Rep. 2018;6(20):e13903. https://doi.org/10.14814/phy2.13903. PMID: 30350350; PMCID: PMC6198137.
12. Downing JW, Brock-Utne JG, Mankowitz M. Aspects of intra-uterine fetal resuscitation. S Afr Med J. 1980;58(9):373–5. PMID: 7404259.
13. Sebire NJ, Talbert D. 'Cor placentale': placental intervillus/intravillus blood flow mismatch is the pathophysiological mechanism in severe intrauterine growth restriction due to uteroplacental disease. Med Hypotheses. 2001;57(3):354–7. https://doi.org/10.1054/mehy.2001.1347. PMID: 11516228.
14. Sebire NJ, Talbert D. The role of intraplacental vascular smooth muscle in the dynamic placenta: a conceptual framework for understanding uteroplacental disease. Med Hypotheses. 2002;58(4):347–51. https://doi.org/10.1054/mehy.2001.1538.
15. Dellschaft NS, Hutchinson G, Shah S, Jones NW, Bradley C, Leach L, Platt C, Bowtell R, Gowland PA. The haemodynamics of the human placenta in utero. PLoS Biol. 2020;18(5):e3000676. https://doi.org/10.1371/journal.pbio.3000676. PMID: 32463837; PMCID: PMC7255609.

16. Redline RW, Ravishankar S, Bagby CM, Saab ST, Zarei S. Four major patterns of placental injury: a stepwise guide for understanding and implementing the 2016 Amsterdam consensus. Mod Pathol. 2021;34(6):1074–92. https://doi.org/10.1038/s41379-021-00747-4. Epub 2021 Feb 8. PMID: 33558658.
17. Benirschke's Pathology of the Human Placenta 7th ed., Ch 19, Ed Rebecca N. Baergen, Graham J. Burton, Cynthia G. Kaplan. Springer. ISBN : 978-3-030-84724-1.
18. Jaiman S, Romero R, Pacora P, Jung E, Bhatti G, Yeo L, Kim YM, Kim B, Kim CJ, Kim JS, Qureshi F, Jacques SM, Erez O, Gomez-Lopez N, Hsu CD. Disorders of placental villous maturation in fetal death. J Perinat Med. 2020 Apr 1:/j/jpme.ahead-of-print/jpm-2020-0030/jpm-2020-0030.xml. https://doi.org/10.1515/jpm-2020-0030. Epub ahead of print. PMID: 32238609; PMCID: PMC8262362.
19. Benirschke's Pathology of the Human Placenta 7th ed., Ch 22, Ed Rebecca N. Baergen, Graham J. Burton, Cynthia G. Kaplan. Springer. ISBN : 978-3-030-84724-1.
20. Khong TY, Mooney EE, Ariel I, Balmus NC, Boyd TK, Brundler MAT, Derricott H, Evans MJ, Faye-Petersen OM, Gillan JE, Heazell AEP, Heller DS, Jacques SM, Keating S, Kelehan P, Maes A, McKay EM, Morgan TK, Nikkels PGJ, Parks WT, Redline RW, Scheimberg I, Schoots MH, Sebire NJ, Timmer T, Turowski G, van der Voorn JP, van Lijnschoten I, Gordijn SJ. Sampling and definitions of placental lesions: Amsterdam placental workshop group consensus statement. Arch Pathol Lab Med. 2016;140:698–713.
21. Baker BC, Heazell AEP, Sibley C, Wright R, Bischof H, Beards F, Guevara T, Girard S, Jones RL. Hypoxia and oxidative stress induce sterile placental inflammation in vitro. Sci Rep. 2021;11(1):7281. https://doi.org/10.1038/s41598-021-86268-1. PMID: 33790316; PMCID: PMC8012380.
22. Sultana Z, Qiao Y, Maiti K, Smith R. Involvement of oxidative stress in placental dysfunction, the pathophysiology of fetal death and pregnancy disorders. Reproduction. 2023;166(2):R25–38. https://doi.org/10.1530/REP-22-0278. PMID: 37318094.
23. Hung TH, Skepper JN, Burton GJ. In vitro ischemia-reperfusion injury in term human placenta as a model for oxidative stress in pathological pregnancies. Am J Pathol. 2001;159(3):1031–43. https://doi.org/10.1016/S0002-9440(10)61778-6. PMID: 11549595; PMCID: PMC1850466.
24. Cindrova-Davies T, Yung HW, Johns J, Spasic-Boskovic O, Korolchuk S, Jauniaux E, Burton GJ, Charnock-Jones DS. Oxidative stress, gene expression, and protein changes induced in the human placenta during labor. Am J Pathol. 2007;171(4):1168–79. https://doi.org/10.2353/ajpath.2007.070528. Epub 2007 Sep 6. PMID: 17823277; PMCID: PMC1988867.
25. Burton GJ, Cindrova-Davies T, Yung HW, Jauniaux E. Hypoxia and reproductive health: oxygen and development of the human placenta. Reproduction. 2021;161(1):F53–65. https://doi.org/10.1530/REP-20-0153. PMID:32438347.
26. Graham J. Burton, personal communication. I am greatly indebted to Dr. Burton for his discussion and clarification of these issues.
27. Thuring A, Laurini R, Marsál K. Uterine venous blood flow in normal and complicated pregnancies: a methodological study. Ultrasound Obstet Gynecol. 2010;35(4):462–7. https://doi.org/10.1002/uog.7572. PMID: 20127752.

Dysfunctional Labor and Uterine Atony

6

Personal Note
Because one of the members of the Reproductive Medicine faculty at the University of California San Diego had started a Maternal Weight and Wellness Program, we anesthesiologists had the opportunity to help care for a large number of very obese women. I was using ultrasound to facilitate the placement of epidurals and spinals, and the residents and I had found it particularly helpful in obese patients. But in very obese patients, a common scenario was that a woman would arrive at Labor and Delivery in early labor and we would place a well-functioning epidural before the contractions got very intense, often at 3–4 cm of cervical dilation. The practice was well-established that maternal request for pain relief was sufficient indication for epidural placement, since—it was said—labor could always be augmented with oxytocin if uterine contractions seemed to diminish after the epidural had relieved the patient's pain. Years before, many obstetricians had insisted that anesthesiologists delay epidural placement until the patient's cervix had dilated to a certain number of centimeters (usually 5 or 6 cm), because they thought that earlier epidural placement might impair the progress of labor. This practice often led to dissatisfaction on the part of the patient, the nursing staff and not a few anesthesiologists who were eager to relieve a woman's labor pain, which—in many cases—was excruciating long before her cervix had dilated to the required degree. Gradually, it seemed, obstetricians had come to agree with the argument that labor could always be augmented with an oxytocin infusion if necessary, and the practice of placing an epidural upon maternal request had become widespread. Another rationale for early epidural placement in obese patients—besides pain relief—was that epidural placement might be difficult and there was a high probability that the obese patient would need full epidural anesthesia for a cesarean delivery.

Frequently with obese patients, it seemed, labor would progress to a certain point, with or without oxytocin augmentation, but would then slow down or stop entirely, resulting in the diagnosis of "dysfunctional labor" and a cesarean delivery. Of course it was satisfying for us anesthesiologists that the patient's epidural which

T. L. Archer, *Threats to Fetal, Placental and Myometrial Oxygenation*,
https://doi.org/10.1007/978-3-031-60364-8_6

had worked well for labor also worked well for the cesarean surgery, but why did obese women so often end up with dysfunctional labor followed by cesarean delivery?

Dysfunctional Labor and Postpartum Uterine Atony: Two Sequelae of Myometrial Hypoxia?

"Failure to progress," "dystocia," or "dysfunctional labor" have traditionally been described as being caused by problems with the "powers, passage, or passenger," as shown in Figs. 6.1 and 6.2. In this chapter, we only consider dysfunctional labor due to inadequate myometrial contractions—that is, to a failure of the Powers.

Figure 6.3 shows the many ways in which obesity and multiple gestation can contribute to poor myometrial perfusion and resulting myometrial hypoxia and acidosis. With the patient in the supine position, the inferior vena cava is compressed not only by the uterus itself but also by the weight of the obese abdominal wall—which also contributes to generally increased intra-abdominal pressure. Besides compressing the inferior vena cava by its weight, the obese abdominal wall also directly compresses the myometrial tissue beneath it, increasing local myometrial

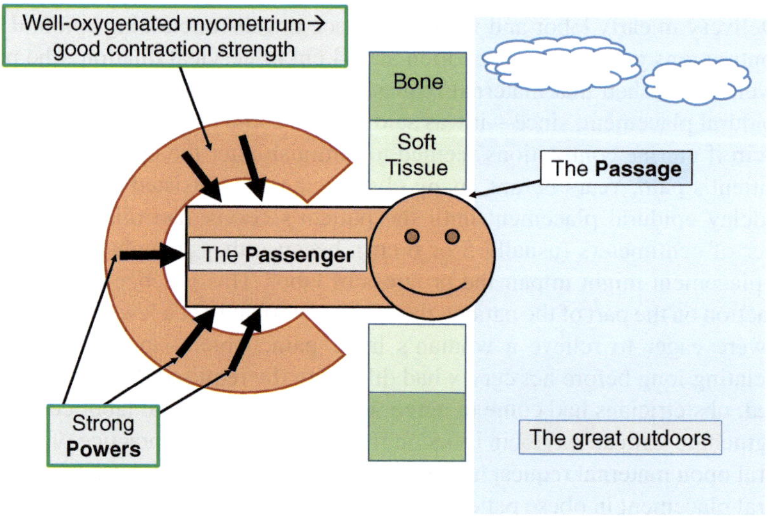

Fig. 6.1 Optimal myometrial oxygenation optimizes the chance for a vaginal delivery. The causes of dysfunctional labor are traditionally classified as The Three P's: The Powers, the Passage, and the Passenger. The terminology for dysfunctional labor is vague and confusing since the words used do not usually specify which of The Three P's is causing the problem—and it is often not clear to providers why the baby is not progressing down the birth canal! This chapter considers only problems with the Powers of labor—that is, how hard and well the myometrium contracts. Intrauterine pressure catheters can be placed to monitor the strength of uterine contractions and this puts the diagnosis of a problem with The Powers on an objective basis, but it does not tell us *why* the contractions are weak

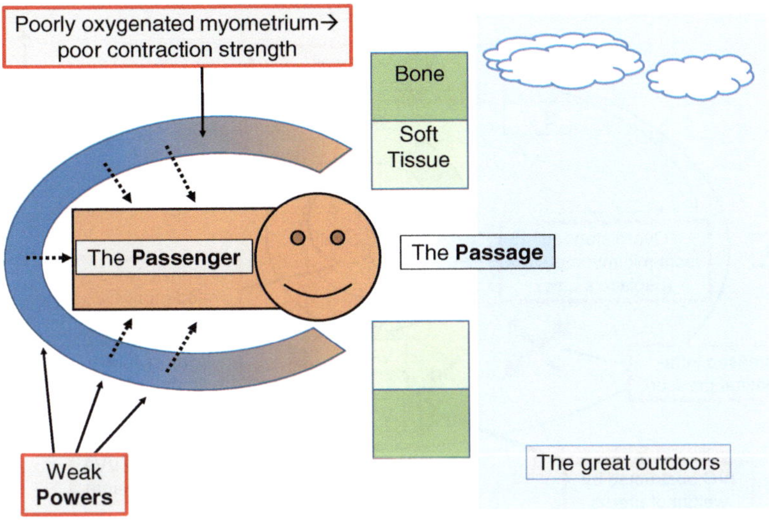

Fig. 6.2 Poor myometrial oxygenation may reduce the "Powers" and force a cesarean delivery. Myometrial hypoxia might be an under-recognized cause of dysfunctional labor. It is often implicitly assumed during labor that if the fetus is doing well—as judged by fetal heart rate and variability—there is no oxygenation problem with the hard-working myometrium. But this assumption may not be correct since the myometrium has its own oxygen needs, separate from those of the fetus. This is especially true during labor when the myometrium is working hard and interrupting its own oxygen supply—as well as that of the fetus—with each contraction

tissue pressure and obstructing uterine veins *within the myometrium itself.* The presence of a twin gestation increases the overall oxygen demand of the uterus, not only because of the oxygen needs of the twins but also because of the increased oxygen needs of the increased amount of myometrial tissue. Also—as if that were not enough—the larger uterus will have an increased opportunity of obstructing its own venous return by virtue of its very size!

Only one of the factors shown in Fig. 6.3 is reversible, and that is *patient position*. Figure 6.4 shows that even though we cannot change the patient's obesity or multiple gestation, we can improve myometrial perfusion by turning the patient onto her side! Even with the patient positioned on her side, her myometrium and fetus may still experience some limitation of myometrial and fetal oxygenation, due to the multiple gestation and the increased myometrial wall tension and tissue pressure due to Laplace's law, but much of the weight burden is removed from the uterus and the inferior vena cava. Both the compression of the inferior vena cava and the myometrium itself—as well as the intra-abdominal pressure—have a positional component which will be relieved when the patient lies turned all the way onto her side [1]. One would expect that this favorable change in positioning would be heralded by an increase in maternal cardiac output and a decrease in uterine venous pressure, and if this were the case, then this maneuver would represent a successful application of cardiac output-guided maternal positioning.

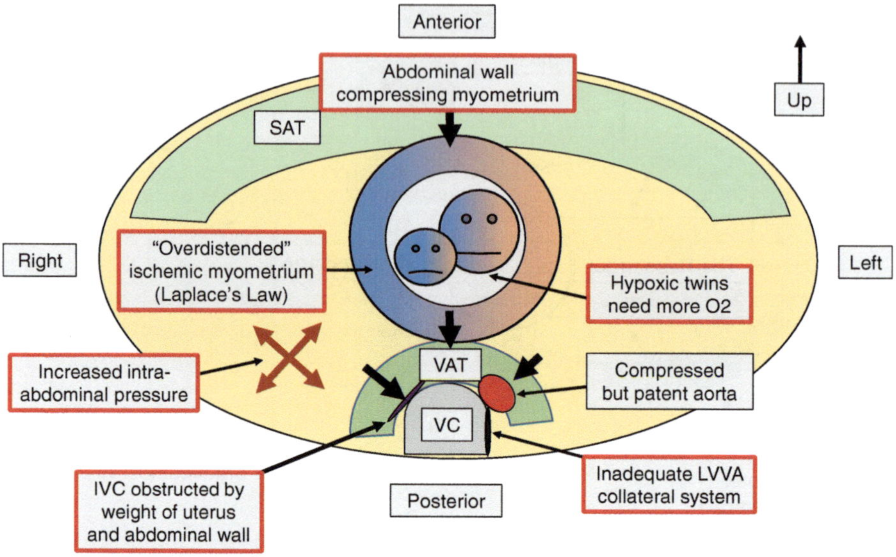

Fig. 6.3 Multiple stresses to myometrial oxygenation in the supine position. This figure shows six stresses on myometrial oxygenation in a short and obese woman carrying twins and lying in the supine position: (1) Obstruction of uterine venous return by the combined weight of the uterus and the obese abdominal wall, (2) generally increased intra-abdominal pressure, (3) an "overdistended" (large) uterus with increased wall tension and tissue pressure due to Laplace's law, (4) an obese abdominal wall applying direct pressure to the myometrium and thereby increasing local tissue pressure, (5) a twin gestation and an increased amount of myometrial tissue, increasing the oxygen demands of the uterus as a whole, and (6) an inadequate lumbar, vertebral venous, and azygos collateral venous system. *IVC* inferior vena cava, *LVVA* lumbar vertebral venous and azygos collateral venous system, O_2 oxygen, *SAT* subcutaneous adipose tissue, *VAT* visceral adipose tissue, *VC* vertebral column

Figure 6.5 shows how maternal short stature would make all of these obstructive tendencies even worse: there is simply not enough room within the abdomen of a woman with short stature to avoid unwanted compression of the inferior vena cava or of the myometrium itself.

Myometrial biopsies taken at cesarean deliveries performed for dysfunctional labor show a significantly lower pH and pO_2 than biopsies taken at cesarean deliveries performed electively or for fetal indications during normal labor with adequate contractions [2]. This association suggests that dysfunctional labor may be caused by myometrial hypoxia and lactic acidosis [3], and the suggestion has been made that obstruction of uterine venous return might be a cause of the myometrial hypoxia causing dysfunctional labor [4].

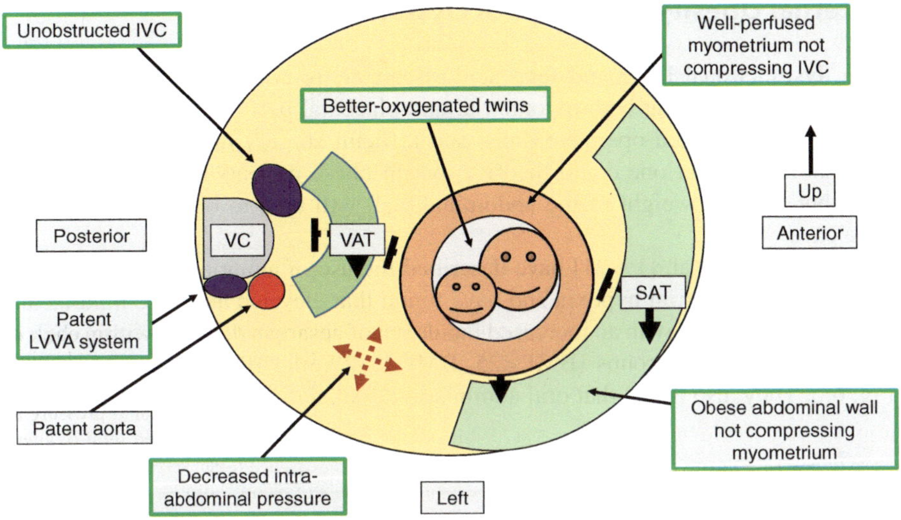

Fig. 6.4 The left lateral decubitus position greatly improves myometrial perfusion. The obese and short woman with twins has turned into the left lateral decubitus position and myometrial perfusion has improved, despite the fact that the woman is still carrying twins and is still short and obese. The point is that the relief of obstruction of uterine venous return may be very helpful, despite the persistence of underlying and unchangeable stressors. Another way of saying this is that there may be a positional component to the impairment of myometrial perfusion, despite the persistence of other risk factors. *IVC* inferior vena cava, *LVVA* lumbar vertebral venous and azygos collateral venous system, *SAT* subcutaneous adipose tissue, *VAT* visceral adipose tissue, *VC* vertebral column

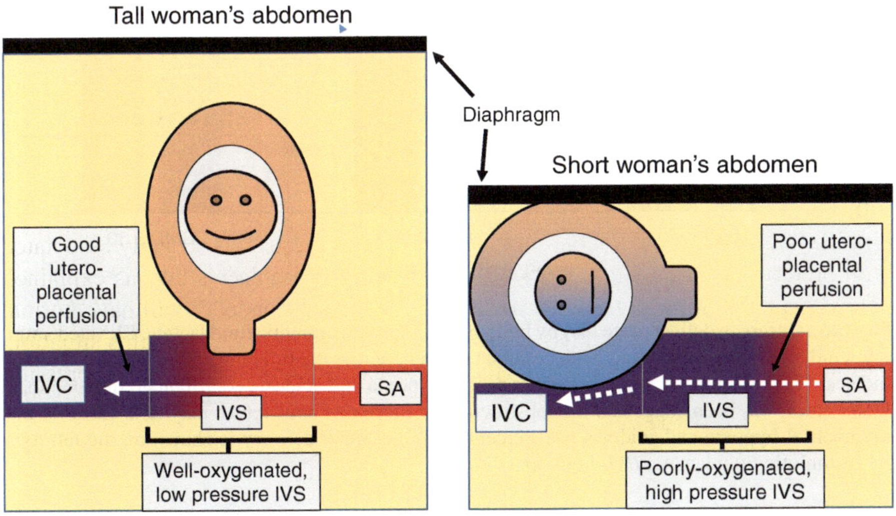

Fig. 6.5 A short woman has less volume within the abdomen than a taller woman. This simple fact will favor uterine venous obstruction both at the inferior vena cava and within the myometrium. Pressure will increase throughout the abdomen, threatening to create an "abdominal compartment syndrome." *IVC* inferior vena cava, *IVS* intervillous space, *SA* spiral artery

Maternal Obesity as a Cause of Dysfunctional Labor

Both dysfunctional labor and fetal acidosis are more common in obese patients [5–18], suggesting that both myometrial and placental perfusion may be impaired by obesity. Prolonged operative times and difficult surgery may explain the fetal acidosis in part, but one could theorize that in obese patients not only the uterus itself but also the weight of the abdominal wall will tend to obstruct the inferior vena cava.

Wiberg-Itzel et al. [19–21] have described the use of amniotic fluid lactate as a marker for myometrial hypoxia and have found that elevated amniotic fluid lactate levels are associated with an increased incidence of cesarean delivery within each of three different BMI groups (BMI <25, BMI 25–29, and BMI ≥30), as shown in Fig. 6.6. They also found that oral administration of sodium bicarbonate to women

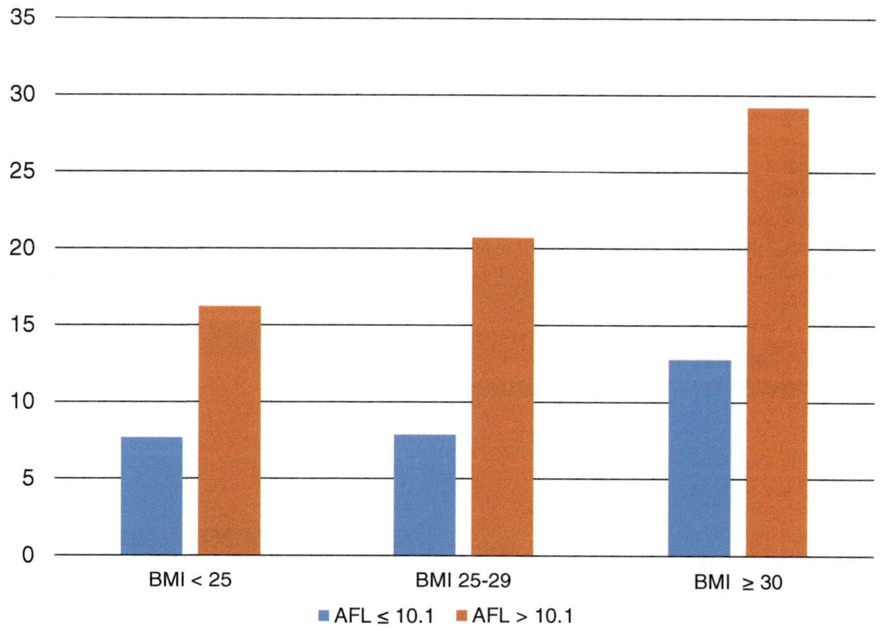

Fig. 6.6 Cesarean delivery rate (%) by body mass index and amniotic fluid lactate. Elevated amniotic fluid lactate levels correlate with cesarean delivery across the full range of maternal body mass indices. This research [2, 3, 20, 21] suggests that hypoxia and acidosis contribute to dysfunctional labor, and it has been suggested that obstruction of uterine venous return may be a cause of that myometrial hypoxia and acidosis [4]. Percentage of cesarean delivery is shown on the left axis. *AFL* amniotic fluid lactate, *BMI* body mass index

Table 6.1 Mechanisms by which obesity and short stature may decrease myometrial perfusion

1. Positional obstruction of uterine venous return by the uterus
2. Positional obstruction of uterine venous return by the obese abdominal wall
3. Positional direct pressure by the obese abdominal wall on myometrial tissue
4. Position-independent increased intra-abdominal pressure with generalized obstruction to abdominal venous return

with high amniotic fluid lactate improves myometrial function and increases the rate of vaginal delivery [21]. These authors discuss the need to "flush out" lactate from myometrium between uterine contractions but do not mention the possibility that obstruction of uterine venous return could be a cause of increased myometrial hypoxia and lactic acid accumulation during labor. Prevention of obstruction of uterine venous return during labor by cardiac output-guided maternal positioning might reduce the incidence of both dysfunctional labor and postpartum uterine atony [4].

Table 6.1 shows four mechanisms by which obesity and short stature may reduce myometrial perfusion, causing hypoxia and acidosis and contributing to dysfunctional labor and/or postpartum uterine atony and hemorrhage.

Maternal Hypotension as a Cause of Poor Myometrial Perfusion and Tissue Hypoxia and Acidosis

Prolonged maternal hypotension is known to cause poor myometrial perfusion which then leads to tissue hypoxia and acidosis—which in turn causes poor uterine tone. Perfusion pressure determines tissue perfusion and is defined as arterial inflow pressure minus venous outflow pressure—unless tissue pressure exceeds venous pressure, in which case perfusion pressure is arterial pressure minus tissue pressure. In Fig. 6.7, we see that maternal arterial hypotension—perhaps from hemorrhage or neuraxial anesthesia—can reduce the mean arterial pressure and cause myometrial hypoxia and acidosis, even though uterine venous pressure and myometrial tissue pressures are normal.

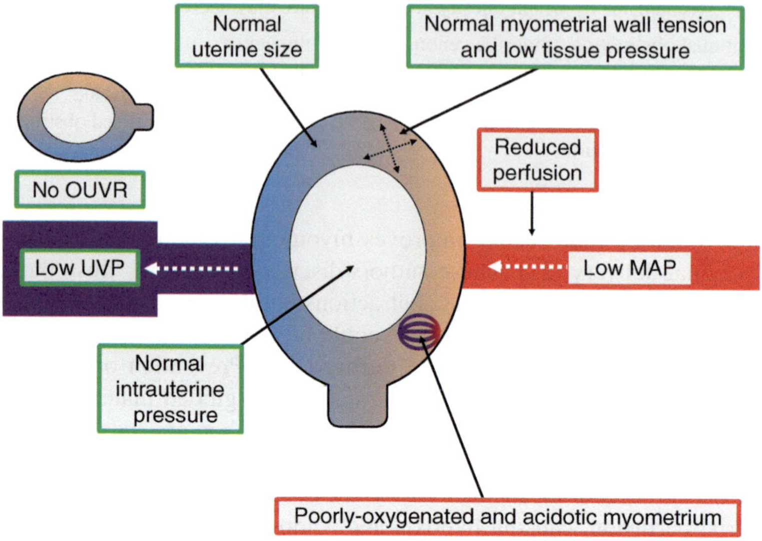

Fig. 6.7 Maternal arterial hypotension as a cause of poor myometrial perfusion. Hemorrhage or neuraxial anesthesia can reduce the arterial blood pressure perfusing the myometrium. Hence, patients who are hypotensive, or who have recently been hypotensive, may be at special risk of poor myometrial contractility and in need of "myometrial resuscitation" via restoration of arterial pressure and proper positioning to minimize uterine venous pressure. This renewed perfusion will wash lactic acid out of the myometrium, restore oxidative metabolism, and eventually restore full function, but that process takes time. *MAP* mean arterial pressure, *OUVR* obstruction of uterine venous return, *UVP* uterine venous pressure

Increased Uterine Venous Pressure Decreases Myometrial Perfusion Pressure

Figure 6.8 shows healthy myometrial perfusion, with adequate arterial pressure and normal venous and myometrial tissue pressures. Figure 6.9, in contrast, shows how obstruction of uterine venous return will increase uterine venous pressure and reduce myometrial perfusion pressure, causing myometrial hypoxia, acidosis, and

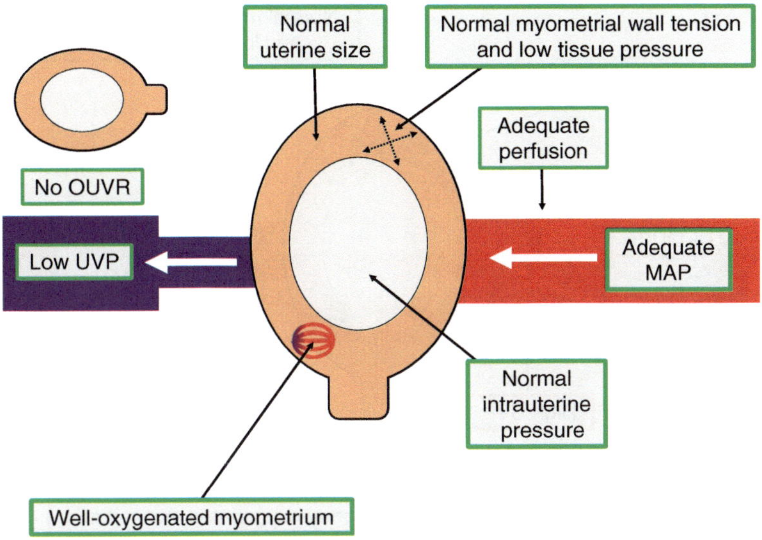

Fig. 6.8 Healthy myometrial perfusion. Three major determinants of myometrial perfusion are: (1) maternal arterial pressure, (2) uterine venous pressure, and (3) myometrial tissue pressure. In all tissues—myometrium included—perfusion pressure (a key indicator of future tissue viability) is defined as arterial inflow pressure minus venous outflow pressure—*unless the pressure inside the tissue—the tissue pressure—exceeds the venous pressure*. If this latter condition exists, then perfusion pressure is defined as arterial pressure minus tissue pressure. In the well-perfused myometrium shown in this figure, the arterial pressure is adequate and the venous and myometrial tissue pressures are low—perfect for optimal myometrial perfusion! *MAP* mean arterial pressure, *OUVR* obstruction of uterine venous return, *UVP* uterine venous pressure

dysfunction. This would seem to be a simple explanation for some cases of dysfunctional labor, and this possibility needs to be investigated since the solution might be simple: cardiac output-guided maternal positioning. Obstruction of uterine venous return might also contribute to myometrial edema, thereby increasing tissue pressure and increasing the distance that oxygen has to diffuse from capillaries to myometrial muscle cells, which would further impair myometrial function during labor.

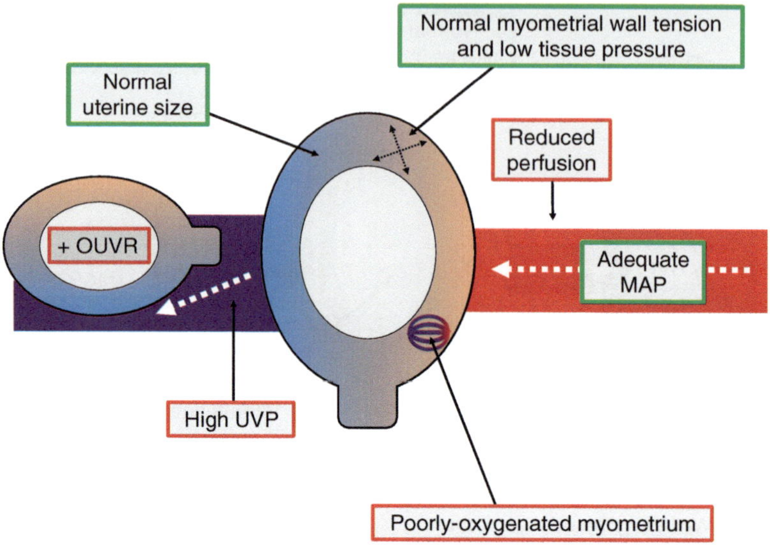

Fig. 6.9 Obstruction of uterine venous return increases uterine venous pressure and reduces myometrial perfusion. Obstruction of uterine venous return—by the uterus itself or an obese abdominal wall—will increase uterine venous pressure and decrease uterine perfusion. Increased uterine venous pressure will also promote congestion and edema formation within the myometrium, which would raise tissue pressure and increase the distance that oxygen has to diffuse from capillaries to myometrial smooth muscle cells. *MAP* mean arterial pressure, *OUVR* obstruction of uterine venous return, *UVP* uterine venous pressure

Uterine "Overdistention" as a Cause of Poor Myometrial Perfusion and Tissue Hypoxia and Acidosis

With maternal arterial hypotension due to blood loss or neuraxial anesthesia, the cause of poor myometrial perfusion is simply low arterial pressure—a global failure of the cardiovascular system. But with the so-called uterine overdistention (which is really just another way of saying "a large uterus"), an impediment to myometrial perfusion may reside within the myometrium itself [22], due to Laplace's Law, as shown in Fig. 6.10. Laplace's law states (in effect) that a larger uterus will have greater wall tension and tissue pressure than a smaller uterus, for a given intrauterine pressure and myometrial wall thickness. The myometrial wall thickness in twin gestation is not significantly different from that found in a singleton gestation [23], and intrauterine pressure inside a large uterus probably tends to be greater than that within a small one, due to the finite size of the abdominal cavity and the limited distensibility of the abdominal wall. For these two reasons, myometrial tissue pressure may well exceed uterine venous pressure in a large uterus and therefore become the limiting factor for myometrial perfusion. Thus, increased myometrial tissue pressure in a large uterus may make myometrial perfusion more precarious than it

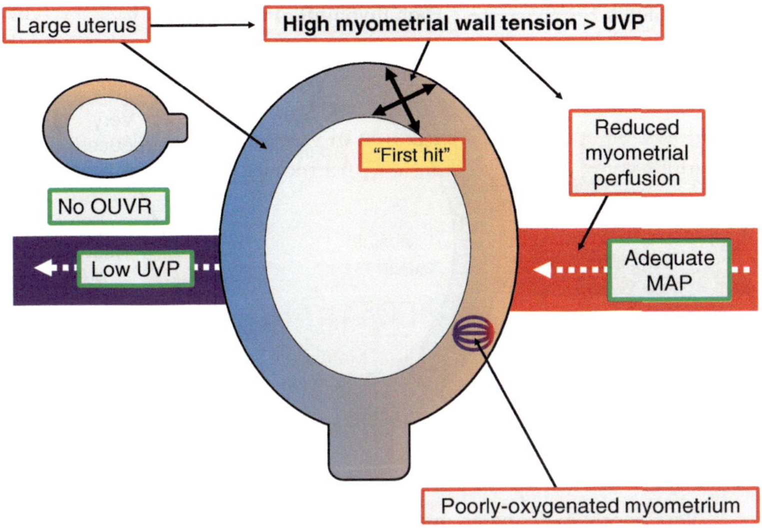

Fig. 6.10 Increased uterine size ("uterine overdistention") is a cause of increased myometrial wall tension and tissue pressure, due to Laplace's law. Laplace's law states that for a given intracavitary pressure and wall thickness, a larger elastic chamber will have higher wall tension than a smaller one. The myometrial wall thickness in twin gestation is the same as that in a singleton gestation, which supports the idea that wall tension and tissue pressure are increased in the larger uterus of a multiple gestation. Because the myometrial tissue pressure exceeds the uterine venous pressure in this example, the myometrial perfusion pressure is the mean arterial pressure minus the tissue pressure. *The increased tissue pressure in the large uterus will reduce perfusion of both the myometrium itself and the placenta, since the arteries and veins serving the placenta traverse the myometrium, even though they do not supply the myometrium with oxygen.* In this Figure, increased myometrial wall tension is delivering a "first hit" to myometrial and placental perfusion, but there is no obstruction of perfusion at the inferior vena cava external to the uterus, and so perfusion is only blocked at one location—there is no "second hit." *This is a key insight—that myometrial and placental perfusion can both be obstructed at two points: (1) the inferior vena cava and (2) within the myometrial wall itself. MAP* mean arterial pressure, *OUVR* obstruction of uterine venous return, *UVP* uterine venous pressure

would be in a smaller uterus. Obstruction of uterine venous return will reduce myometrial perfusion in a uterus of any size, but it may be particularly dangerous when myometrial perfusion pressure has already been reduced due to the working of Laplace's law within the wall of an "overdistended uterus," as shown in Fig. 6.11. In this situation, two distinct obstructive processes are at work in series, as shown schematically in Fig. 6.12. Increased myometrial tissue pressure (the "first hit") and obstruction of uterine venous return external to the uterus (the "second hit") reinforce each other in reducing myometrial oxygenation.

In summary, the oxygenation of the myometrium is more precarious in a large uterus than in a small one—with or without the additional stress caused by obstruction of uterine venous return—and it may be especially important to avoid obstruction of uterine venous return in patients with "uterine overdistention" due to multiple gestation or polyhydramnios.

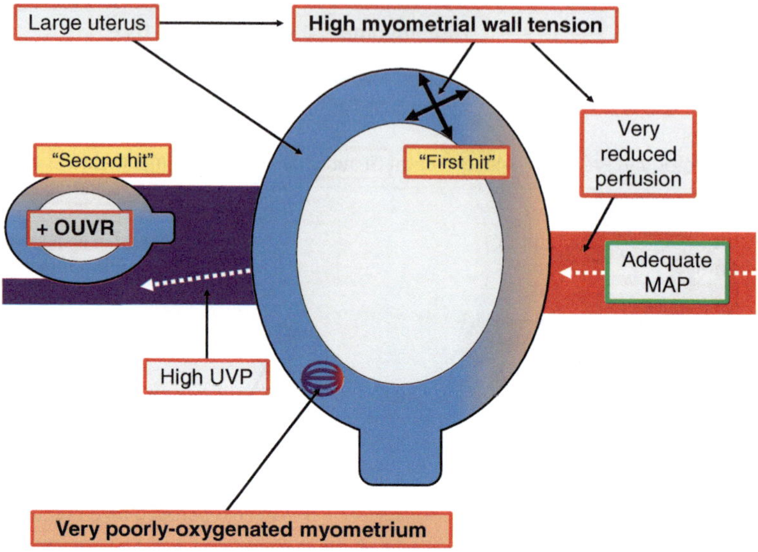

Fig. 6.11 Risk factors for decreased myometrial oxygenation can work in combination, further increasing risk. This Figure shows how obstruction of uterine venous return (a "second hit") can further impair myometrial and fetal oxygenation in a large uterus in which myometrial and placental perfusion are already precarious due to Laplace's law (the "first hit"). *MAP* mean arterial pressure, *OUVR* obstruction of uterine venous return, *UVP* uterine venous pressure

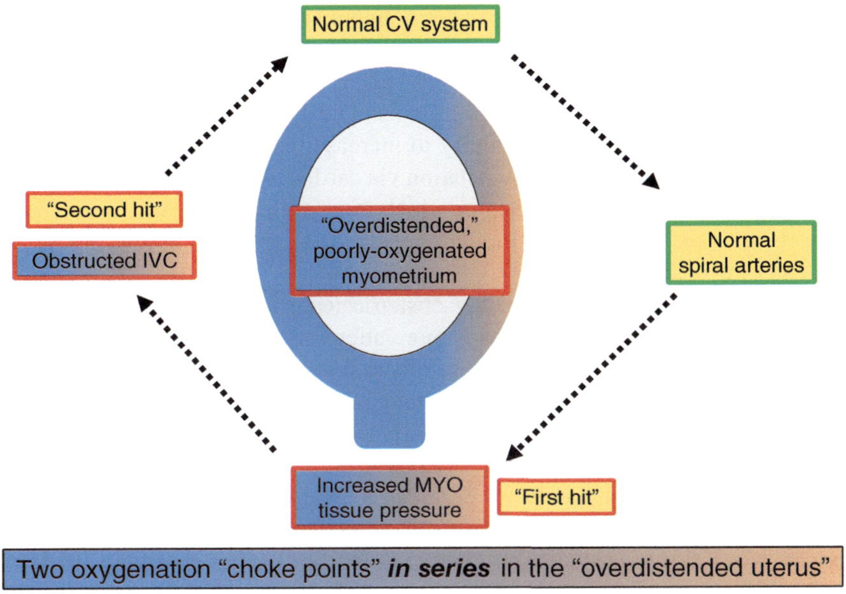

Fig. 6.12 Increased myometrial tissue pressure due to an "overdistended uterus" combines with obstruction of uterine venous return external to the uterus to cause profound myometrial hypoxia and acidosis. This situation could easily cause dysfunctional labor requiring a cesarean delivery. Nothing could have been done about the large uterus, but the obstruction of uterine venous return might have been prevented via "cardiac output-guided maternal positioning." In the Figure, high myometrial wall tension and tissue pressure are considered to be the "first hit," and obstruction of uterine veins external to the uterus is considered to be the "second hit." *CV* cardiovascular, *IVC* inferior vena cava, *MYO* myometrial

Nulliparity, Short Stature, and Decreased Mobility as Causes of Poor Myometrial Perfusion During Labor

Nulliparity [24], maternal short stature [25, 26], and limited maternal mobility [27–29] appear to be associated with dysfunctional labor, and those conditions are also associated with possible limitations on myometrial perfusion during labor. Nulliparity may be associated with the lack of development of lumbar, vertebral venous, and azygos collaterals to the inferior vena cava; short stature may be associated with generally increased intra-abdominal pressure and decreased abdominal volume; and lack of movement and position change during labor may allow prolonged obstruction of uterine venous return.

Of course it is possible that the Powers of the myometrium in obese pregnant women—and in women with an "overdistended" uterus—are weakened by metabolic or structural changes which have nothing to do with myometrial hypoxia and acidosis [30, 31]. But since positional obstruction of uterine venous return is a known and easily correctable cause of *fetal* hypoxia in labor, it would seem that this same positional mechanism should be investigated as a possible cause of *myometrial* hypoxia during labor. Once labor has begun, we cannot change the presentation (or size!) of the baby, and certainly nothing can be done about the size of the pelvis, so it may be that our best opportunity to increase the Powers of the myometrium during labor is to improve its oxygenation via cardiac output-guided maternal positioning. At present, the myometrium which does not contract well during normal labor receives oxytocin, but no thought appears to be given to improving its perfusion and oxygenation.

During labor, the attention of the obstetric team is intensely focused on fetal heart rate and variability, but perhaps more attention should be paid to myometrial oxygen needs independent from those of the fetus [4]. I have speculated that the hypoxic myometrium could be "resuscitated" within the mother, just as the fetus can be resuscitated within the uterus [32]. Intrauterine resuscitation of the fetus consists of a constellation of interventions to improve fetal oxygenation without resorting (at least immediately) to cesarean delivery—such as empirical maternal position change and oxygen administration, together with fluids, vasopressors, and perhaps tocolytics to stop uterine contractions from further depriving the fetus of oxygen. Even if the fetus is not showing signs of hypoxia, these same interventions might resuscitate a hypoxic myometrium which is causing dysfunctional labor. *But rather than having to resuscitate a myometrium after it had become hypoxic and acidotic, it would be better to prevent myometrial hypoxia in the first place—perhaps by means of cardiac output-guided maternal positioning provided continuously from the very onset of labor!*

Uterine Atony and Postpartum Hemorrhage Caused by Myometrial Hypoxia and Acidosis

After delivery, uterine atony leading to postpartum hemorrhage may be another instance of "hypoxic uterine contraction failure." Uterine atony is the most common cause of postpartum hemorrhage and continues to be a significant cause of maternal death worldwide. The following risk factors are associated with postpartum uterine atony and hemorrhage: nulliparity, grand multiparity, hypotension, obesity, polyhydramnios, multiple gestation, labor augmentation with oxytocin, and prolonged first or second stage of labor, and all of these associations (except perhaps grand multiparity) are consistent with the theory that uterine atony—like dysfunctional labor—may be caused in part by myometrial hypoxia caused by decreased myometrial perfusion during labor.

One more possible source of myometrial ischemia and hypoxia leading to dysfunctional labor is shown in Figs. 6.13 and 6.14: subplacental myometrial arteriovenous (AV) shunts [33]. These shunts might provide an alternate pathway for uterine blood flow to bypass both the placenta and myometrial capillaries—especially when intervillous pressure has been elevated by obstruction of uterine venous return, as shown in Fig. 6.14. The actual role for these subplacental myometrial shunts is unclear, but it has been proposed that they may function as a "pressure relief valve" to decompress the intervillous space when its pressure is excessive and threatens to block fetoplacental perfusion by compressing the chorionic villi.

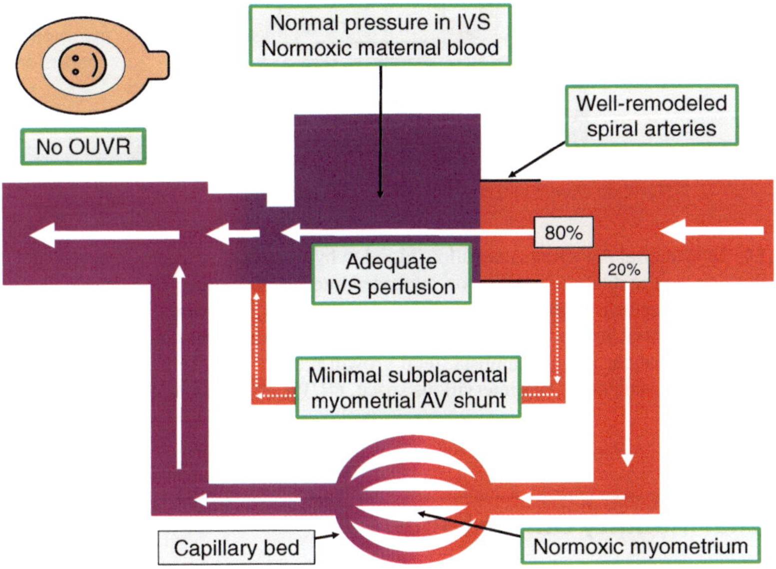

Fig. 6.13 Subplacental myometrial arteriovenous shunts—what do they do? The figure shows that uterine perfusion—far from being in series (with all uterine perfusion flowing through intervillous spaces)—is actually in parallel, with three alternative pathways for blood flow through the uterus: (1) the intervillous spaces of the placenta, (2) myometrial muscle tissue, and (3) subplacental myometrial arteriovenous shunts. The function of the shunts is unknown, but it has been proposed that they serve as a sort of "pressure relief valve" which opens if intervillous space pressure increases sufficiently to threaten the complete suppression of fetoplacental perfusion by compression of the chorionic villi. Their existence may explain the fact that *uterine* artery (not *umbilical* artery) Doppler velocity waveforms maintain their low-resistance characteristics even postpartum, when the myometrium has contracted tightly. In this Figure, intervillous space pressure is low, most perfusion occurs through those spaces and the shunts are not forced open by increased intervillous space pressure. *AV* arteriovenous, *IVS* intervillous space, *OUVR* obstruction of uterine venous return

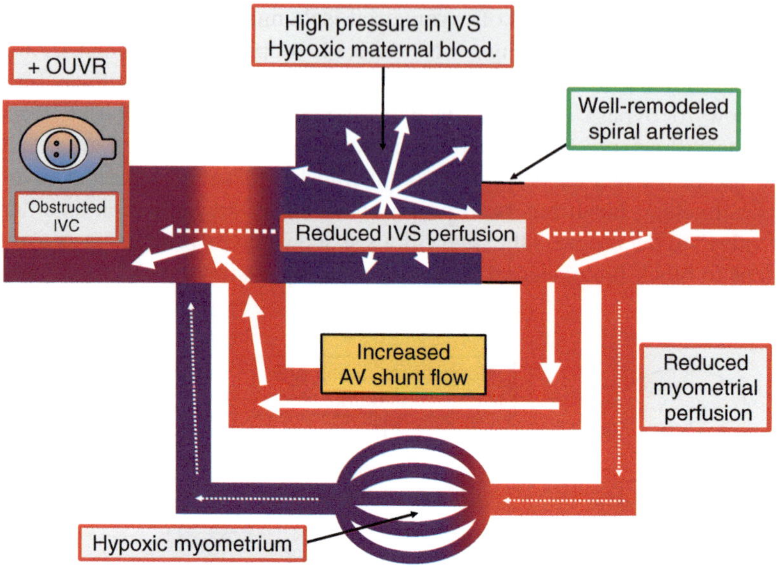

Fig. 6.14 Myometrial AV shunts may allow blood to bypass both intervillous spaces and myometrium. With respect to dysfunctional labor, increased intervillous space pressure due to obstruction of uterine venous return might open the shunt pathways and steal blood from the myometrium, increasing myometrial hypoxia, acidosis, and dysfunction. Shunting could also occur earlier in gestation and contribute to preeclampsia, fetal growth restriction, or preterm birth. *AV* arteriovenous, *IVC* inferior vena cava, *IVS* intervillous space, *OUVR* obstruction of uterine venous return

Maternal Mobility During Labor

Maternal mobility during labor may be more beneficial than some of us have thought. Midwifery practice encourages maternal mobility and physical activity during labor. Patients use birthing balls, hydrotherapy, and bending and stretching exercises to cope with labor discomfort. Contrast this activity—most of which is performed in the standing or sitting position—with a common scenario in patients who receive epidurals. Once the epidural has been placed and the patient has been relieved of her pain, she is usually content to rest quietly and comfortably in bed as her labor progresses. Sometimes her "lateral tilt" is minimal, since the quasi-supine position facilitates nursing care, obstetric exams, and procedures such as the placement of a bladder or intrauterine pressure catheter. In the author's experience, it is common practice to consider that the fetal heart rate and variability serve as valid proxies for the adequacy of overall fetal and myometrial perfusion. As long as the fetal heart rate and variability are adequate, no one seems to consider that the myometrium may have needs for oxygen that are separate from those of the fetus. If the myometrium begins to contract poorly, an oxytocin infusion is begun, and if myometrial performance does not improve, a cesarean delivery is performed for dysfunctional labor. It may be that—in some cases of dysfunctional labor—what the myometrium needs is more oxygen and not more oxytocin, and that its separate needs for oxygen may not be reflected in unfavorable fetal heart rate changes. In other words, the fetus is saying that it is doing well, but the myometrium is not doing well—but has no way of telling us!

Studies have emerged recently [27–29] endorsing the value of increased maternal activity, both during both labor and much earlier in gestation. The onset of the "active phase" of labor also appears to be in the process of re-definition from 4 cm of cervical dilation to 6 cm, and some authors recommend delaying routine admission to the hospital until the cervix has dilated to 6 cm [29]. This practice would appear to implicitly endorse the value of maternal movement and voluntary position change for longer than may be the norm currently. Other authors recommend closer collaboration between midwives and obstetricians. It may be that a little-recognized benefit of increased activity during labor is to optimize uterine perfusion and minimize uterine venous pressure. In this case, an early epidural combined with cardiac output-guided maternal positioning might provide the best of both worlds—excellent and early pain relief, along with optimal placental and myometrial perfusion and oxygenation.

Summary

1. Myometrial hypoxia and acidosis may contribute to both dysfunctional labor and postpartum uterine atony.
2. Myometrial hypoxia and acidosis might be caused by obstruction of uterine venous return and prevented by the use of cardiac output-guided maternal positioning.
3. Known risk factors for dysfunctional labor are: obesity, short stature, hypotension, a large uterus ("uterine overdistention"), nulliparity, grand multiparity, and decreased maternal mobility in labor, and all of these conditions (except for grand multiparity) are also associated with inherent limitation of myometrial perfusion. In other words, dysfunctional labor is associated with conditions in which uterine perfusion is precarious to begin with, even without the added stress of obstruction of uterine venous return.
4. Obstruction of uterine venous return may have an additive or synergistic effect with the above-mentioned conditions involving pre-existing limitations of myometrial perfusion.
5. Epidural analgesia is wonderful for relieving labor pain, but it is possible that the hemodynamics associated with its administration could be improved by cardiac output-guided maternal positioning. This practice might give patients the "best of both worlds"—a pain-free labor and delivery and a lower incidence of dysfunctional labor, cesarean delivery and postpartum uterine atony.

References

1. Garg D, Tyagi A, Kumar M. Intraabdominal pressure and its relation with organ dysfunction in patients scheduled for elective cesarean section: effect of supine vs left lateral tilt position. Acta Obstet Gynecol Scand. 2021;100(1):101–8. https://doi.org/10.1111/aogs.13965. Epub 2020 Aug 19. PMID: 32726457.
2. Quenby S, Pierce SJ, Brigham S, Wray S. Dysfunctional labor and myometrial lactic acidosis. Obstet Gynecol. 2004;103(4):718–23. https://doi.org/10.1097/01.AOG.0000118306.82556.43. Erratum in: Obstet Gynecol. 2004;103(6):1344. PMID: 15051564.
3. Wray S, Alruwaili M, Prendergast C. Hypoxia and reproductive health: hypoxia and labour. Reproduction. 2021;161(1):F67–80. https://doi.org/10.1530/REP-20-0327. PMID: 33112773.
4. Archer TL. Obstructed uterine venous return: a preventable cause of dysfunctional labor? Reproduction. 2021;161(4):V15–7. https://doi.org/10.1530/REP-21-0002. PMID: 33617462.
5. Zhang J, Bricker L, Wray S, Quenby S. Poor uterine contractility in obese women. BJOG. 2007;114(3):343–8. https://doi.org/10.1111/j.1471-0528.2006.01233.x. Epub 2007 Jan 22. PMID: 17261121.
6. Vince K, Brkić M, Poljičanin T, Matijević R. Prevalence and impact of pre-pregnancy body mass index on pregnancy outcome: a cross-sectional study in Croatia. J Obstet Gynaecol. 2021;41(1):55–9. https://doi.org/10.1080/01443615.2019.1706157. Epub 2020 Feb 6.
7. DeBolt CA, Sarker M, Trejo FE, Feldman K, Kaplowitz E, Rattner P, Paul K, Jagannatham S, Ferrara L, Doulaveris G, Bernstein PS, Brustman L, Glazer KB, Stone J, Bianco A. Association between obesity and fetal acidosis at scheduled cesarean delivery. Obstet Gynecol. 2022;140(6):950–7. https://doi.org/10.1097/AOG.0000000000004968. Epub 2022 Nov 2. PMID: 36357997.
8. Bligard KH, Cameo T, McCallum KN, Rubin A, Rimsza RR, Cahill AG, Palanisamy A, Odibo AO, Raghuraman N. The association of fetal acidemia with adverse neonatal outcomes at time of scheduled cesarean delivery. Am J Obstet Gynecol. 2022;227(2):265.e1–8. https://doi.org/10.1016/j.ajog.2022.04.037. Epub 2022 Apr 27.
9. Edwards RK, Cantu J, Cliver S, Biggio JR Jr, Owen J, Tita ATN. The association of maternal obesity with fetal pH and base deficit at cesarean delivery. Obstet Gynecol. 2013;122(2 Pt 1):262–7. https://doi.org/10.1097/AOG.0b013e31829b1e62.
10. Kominiarek MA, Vanveldhuisen P, Hibbard J, Landy H, Haberman S, Learman L, Wilkins I, Bailit J, Branch W, Burkman R, Gonzalez-Quintero VH, Gregory K, Hatjis C, Hoffman M, Ramirez M, Reddy UM, Troendle J, Zhang J, Consortium on Safe Labor. The maternal body mass index: a strong association with delivery route. Am J Obstet Gynecol. 2010;203(3):264.e1–7. https://doi.org/10.1016/j.ajog.2010.06.024. Epub 2010 Jul 31. PMID: 20673867; PMCID: PMC2933947.
11. Barau G, Robillard PY, Hulsey TC, Dedecker F, Laffite A, Gérardin P, Kauffmann E. Linear association between maternal pre-pregnancy body mass index and risk of caesarean section in term deliveries. BJOG. 2006;113(10):1173–7. https://doi.org/10.1111/j.1471-0528.2006.01038.x. PMID: 16972860.
12. Ehrenberg HM, Durnwald CP, Catalano P, Mercer BM. The influence of obesity and diabetes on the risk of cesarean delivery. Am J Obstet Gynecol. 2004;191(3):969–74. https://doi.org/10.1016/j.ajog.2004.06.057. PMID: 15467574.
13. Sarkar RK, Cooley SM, Donnelly JC, Walsh T, Collins C, Geary MP. The incidence and impact of increased body mass index on maternal and fetal morbidity in the low-risk primigravid population. J Matern Fetal Neonatal Med. 2007;20(12):879–83. https://doi.org/10.1080/14767050701713090.
14. Walsh J, Foley M, O'Herlihy C. Dystocia correlates with body mass index in both spontaneous and induced nulliparous labors. J Matern Fetal Neonatal Med. 2011;24(6):817–21. https://doi.org/10.3109/14767058.2010.531313. Epub 2010 Dec 15. PMID: 21158492.
15. Lynch CM, Sexton DJ, Hession M, Morrison JJ. Obesity and mode of delivery in primigravid and multigravid women. Am J Perinatol. 2008;25(3):163–7. https://doi.org/10.1055/s-2008-1061496. Epub 2008 Feb 25. PMID: 18300188.

16. Poston L, Caleyachetty R, Cnattingius S, et al. Preconceptional and maternal obesity: epidemiology and health consequences. Lancet Diabetes Endocrinol. 2016;4(12):1025–36. https://doi.org/10.1016/S2213-8587(16)30217-0.
17. Kyozuka H, Hiraiwa T, Murata T, Sugeno M, Jin T, Ito F, Suzuki D, Nomura Y, Fukuda T, Yasuda S, Fujimori K. Gestational weight gain as a risk factor for dystocia during first delivery: a multicenter retrospective cohort study in Japan. BMC Pregnancy Childbirth. 2022;22(1):728. https://doi.org/10.1186/s12884-022-05055-6. PMID: 36151536; PMCID: PMC9503209.
18. Verdiales M, Pacheco C, Cohen WR. The effect of maternal obesity on the course of labor. J Perinat Med. 2009;37(6):651–5. https://doi.org/10.1515/JPM.2009.110. PMID: 19591559.
19. Karlsson S, Patavoukas E, Sterpu I, Wallstrom T, Wiberg-Itzel E. Body mass index and labor outcome associated with the level of amniotic fluid lactate. A cross-sectional study of women with labor dystocia. J Matern Fetal Neonatal Med. 2022;35(25):8521–9. https://doi.org/10.1080/14767058.2021.1986811. Epub 2021 Oct 25. PMID: 34696678.
20. Wiberg-Itzel E. Amniotic fluid lactate (AFL): a new predictor of labor outcome in dystocic deliveries. J Matern Fetal Neonatal Med. 2022;35(25):7306–11. https://doi.org/10.1080/14767058.2021.1946790. Epub 2021 Nov 10. PMID: 34758684.
21. Wiberg-Itzel E, Wray S, Åkerud H. A randomized controlled trial of a new treatment for labor dystocia. J Matern Fetal Neonatal Med. 2018;31(17):2237–44. https://doi.org/10.1080/14767058.2017.1339268. Epub 2017 Jun 22. PMID: 28587493.
22. Dike NO, Ibine R. Hypotonic labor. [Updated 2022 Oct 24]. In: StatPearls [Internet]. Treasure Island (FL): StatPearls Publishing; 2023 Jan-. Available from: https://www.ncbi.nlm.nih.gov/books/NBK564403/.
23. Sfakianaki AK, Buhimschi IA, Pettker CM, Magloire LK, Turan OM, Hamar BD, Buhimschi CS. Ultrasonographic evaluation of myometrial thickness in twin pregnancies. Am J Obstet Gynecol. 2008;198(5):530.e1–10. https://doi.org/10.1016/j.ajog.2007.11.022. Epub 2008 Feb 15. PMID: 18279826.
24. LeFevre NM, Krumm E, Cobb WJ. Labor dystocia in nulliparous women. Am Fam Physician. 2021;103(2):90–6. PMID: 33448772.
25. Mehraban SS, Pessolano JC, Ponterio JM, et al. The vertical dimension of obesity: adverse pregnancy outcomes in the short obese versus tall obese parturient. J Obstet Gynaecol. 2022;42(1):43–8. https://doi.org/10.1080/01443615.2021.1871887.
26. Leybovitz-Haleluya N, Sheiner E, Wainstock T. Obstetric and perinatal outcome in short-stature patients. Int J Gynaecol Obstet. 2023;163(3):978–82. https://doi.org/10.1002/ijgo.14907.
27. Zwelling E. Overcoming the challenges: maternal movement and positioning to facilitate labor progress. MCN Am J Matern Child Nurs. 2010;35(2):72–80. https://doi.org/10.1097/NMC.0b013e3181caeab3.
28. Souter V, Nethery E, Kopas ML, Wurz H, Sitcov K, Caughey AB. Comparison of midwifery and obstetric care in low-risk hospital births. Obstet Gynecol. 2019;134(5):1056–65. https://doi.org/10.1097/AOG.0000000000003521. PMID: 31599830.
29. Thuillier C, Roy S, Peyronnet V, Quibel T, Nlandu A, Rozenberg P. Impact of recommended changes in labor management for prevention of the primary cesarean delivery. Am J Obstet Gynecol. 2018;218(3):341.e1–9. https://doi.org/10.1016/j.ajog.2017.12.228. Epub 2017 Dec 29. PMID: 29291413.
30. Carvajal JA, Oporto JI. The myometrium in pregnant women with obesity. Curr Vasc Pharmacol. 2021;19(2):193–200. https://doi.org/10.2174/1570161118666200525133530.
31. Chin JR, Henry E, Holmgren CM, Varner MW, Branch DW. Maternal obesity and contraction strength in the first stage of labor. Am J Obstet Gynecol. 2012;207(2):129.e1–1296. https://doi.org/10.1016/j.ajog.2012.06.044.
32. Archer TL. Obstetric anesthesia: a case-based and visual approach. Chapter 32. Archer TL ed. Springer Nature Switzerland AG.
33. Schaaps JP, Tsatsaris V, Goffin F, Brichant JF, Delbecque K, Tebache M, Collignon L, Retz MC, Foidart JM. Shunting the intervillous space: new concepts in human uteroplacental vascularization. Am J Obstet Gynecol. 2005;192(1):323–32. https://doi.org/10.1016/j.ajog.2004.06.066. PMID: 15672043.

Preterm Birth

7

Personal Note

Labor and Delivery was quiet, and I decided to see if I could consent some more pregnant patients for our hemodynamic studies. We were starting to ask ourselves whether obstruction of uterine venous return might cause problems in pregnancy long before term, so we decided to take positional cardiac output measurements in hospitalized pregnant patients who were not in active labor, just to see if any patterns emerged. I entered the room of a patient who had been hospitalized for preterm labor at 26 + 3/7 weeks estimated gestation age. She was on bed rest with bathroom privileges and was lying supine with the head of the bed raised about 45°, in a position that I thought might be associated with obstruction of uterine venous return and increased intra-abdominal pressure. After she consented to our study, I lowered the head of the bed and obtained the hemodynamic measurements shown in Fig. 1.25. Her cardiac output varied markedly depending on her position and this surprised me greatly. I thought that perhaps I had stumbled across something significant. Despite what I expected her to say—based on the measurements I had just taken—the patient said that she felt equally comfortable in all positions, but that the doctors had told her to spend as much time as possible lying on one side or the other—but to avoid lying supine.

As I was taking off the patches and wires used for the electrical cardiometry measurements, a perinatologist I knew came into the room to see the same patient, and I showed him the results I had just obtained: the patient's cardiac output was lowest in the full right lateral position, slightly higher in the supine position, and highest by far in the left lateral position—and these changes were reproducible.

His first response was to ask if the effect could be some sort of artifact and I said that while that was possible, most pregnant patients at similar gestational ages did not show such pronounced changes—at least in my very limited experience.

The patient was short in stature and we noted that her abdomen was very tense. We explained to the patient that we were investigating whether different body

T. L. Archer, *Threats to Fetal, Placental and Myometrial Oxygenation*,
https://doi.org/10.1007/978-3-031-60364-8_7

positions might cause different degrees of obstruction to blood flow into and out of the uterus and how that might affect the baby. Later on, the perinatologist said that it seemed to him that many of the preterm labor patients he saw were short in stature and had tight abdomens, and he went on to suggest that perhaps his clinical impression should be studied formally. As we parted company he added with a smile, "Yes, it seems like all that pressure within the abdomen can't be good for uterine perfusion. Maybe that pressure has something to do with causing preterm labor. Hopefully your research will tell us." The year was 2010. Was the perinatologist correct in thinking that patients with preterm labor often had tense abdomens? Now, in 2024, I think he was correct—and this chapter explains why.

Preterm Birth and Obstruction of Uterine Venous Return

Known and suspected risk factors and mechanisms for preterm birth include: (1) obesity, (2) maternal short stature, (3) uterine "overdistention," (4) placental abruption (decidual hemorrhage), (5) fetal hypoxic stress-induced premature activation of the fetal hypothalamic-pituitary-adrenal axis, (6) sterile myometrial inflammation, (7) infectious chorioamnionitis, (8) vaginal microbiome changes, and (9) ethnicity. Table 7.1 presents these risk factors.

At first glance, these risk factors and mechanisms appear to have little in common, but three of them—obesity, maternal short stature, and "uterine overdistention"—may involve an intrinsic vulnerability of tissue oxygenation—a "first hit"—which obstruction of uterine venous return—as a "second hit"—converts into actual injury. Other risk factors and mechanisms—placental abruption, sterile myometrial inflammation, vaginal microbiome changes, and infectious chorioamnionitis—might be caused solely or largely by obstruction of uterine venous return, by both oxygenation and pressure mechanisms. We now examine these risk factors and mechanisms for preterm birth in greater detail and start by exploring the perinatologist's observation that a tense abdomen might be a cause of preterm birth:

Table 7.1 Known and suspected risk factors and mechanisms for preterm birth

Obesity
Maternal short stature
Uterine "overdistention" (a large uterus)
Placental abruption (decidual hemorrhage)
Fetal hypoxic stress-induced activation of the fetal hypothalamic-pituitary-adrenal axis
Sterile myometrial inflammation
Vaginal microbiome changes
Infectious chorioamnionitis
Ethnicity

Both Obesity and Maternal Short Stature Can Block Abdominal Venous Return, in What Resembles an Early Abdominal Compartment Syndrome

Maternal short stature [1–4] and obesity [5–8] are both associated with preterm birth, and a simple explanation for that association could be that both conditions make venous obstruction more likely. Several authors have discussed the abdominal compartment syndrome in pregnancy [9–14], and—as shown in Figs. 7.1 and 7.2—both maternal short stature and obesity will tend to make the following three conditions more frequent and severe: a) obstruction of uterine venous return external to the uterus, b) direct compression of myometrium causing intra-myometrial venous obstruction, and c) generally increased intra-abdominal pressure. These three conditions may cause fetal, placental, myometrial, and vaginal hypoxia, along with increased abdominal, pelvic, and lower extremity venous pressure and edema. This

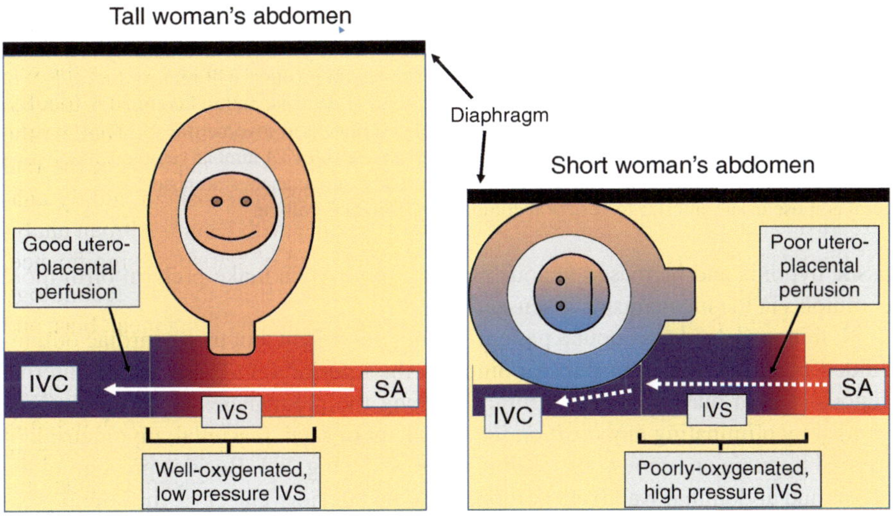

Fig. 7.1 Maternal short stature provides less space for the gravid uterus, facilitating an incipient abdominal compartment syndrome. Maternal short stature is a risk factor for premature birth, independent of BMI. The figure shows a theory as to why this might be the case: a short woman simply has less room within her abdomen for the uterus than a taller woman. This lack of available volume in the abdomen may cause (1) more frequent and more severe obstruction of the inferior vena cava by the uterus and (2) increased myometrial tissue pressure due to external compression of the uterus by the diaphragm, abdominal wall, and other organs. Both of these sources of decreased perfusion and increased pressure will decrease fetal and myometrial oxygenation. This situation could, in fact, be described as an incipient "abdominal compartment syndrome," as has been suggested [9–14], and may explain the high incidence of preterm birth in short women. Although some of the detrimental effects of short stature are probably not related to maternal position, other effects may have a positional component, in which case cardiac output-guided maternal positioning might prevent preterm birth or delay it sufficiently to improve neonatal outcomes. *IVC* inferior vena cava, *IVS* intervillous space, *SA* spiral artery (from uterine arteries)

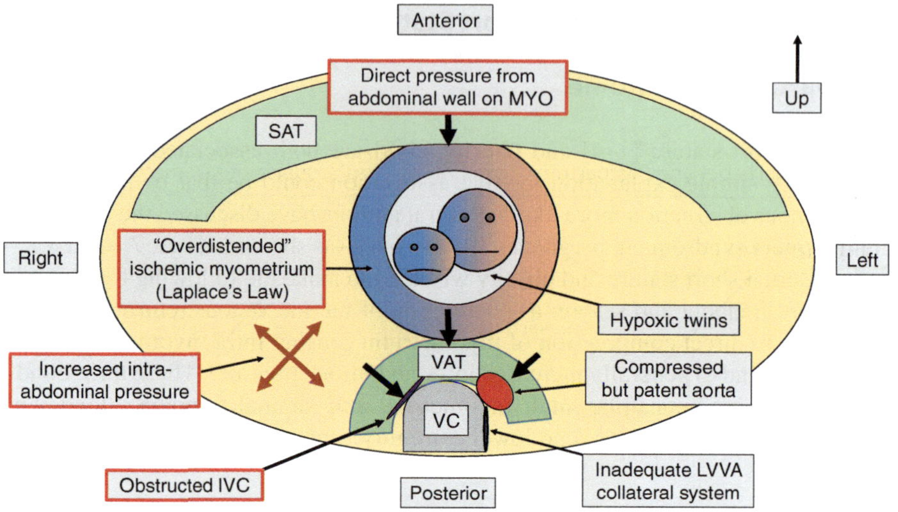

Fig. 7.2 The supine position may be particularly dangerous in pregnant women who are obese or short. In an obese pregnant woman who is lying supine, both the uterus and a heavy abdominal wall will tend to compress the inferior vena cava. The lateral position will remove the weight of both structures from the inferior vena cava and will tend to decrease intra-abdominal pressure as well (see Fig. 7.3), so there is probably a positional component to myometrial and fetal oxygenation in women who are obese or short. *IVC* inferior vena cava, *LVVA* lumbar vertebral venous and azygos collateral venous system, *MYO* myometrium, *SAT* subcutaneous adipose tissue, *VAT* visceral adipose tissue anterior to vertebral column, *VC* vertebral column

tissue hypoxia and increased venous pressure might then make preterm birth more common via the mechanisms discussed below.

Nothing can be done about a patient's height or weight, but using cardiac output-guided maternal positioning to decompress the inferior vena cava and the uterine venous system during gestation might prolong the pregnancies of short or obese women by eliminating any *positional* component of fetal, placental, myometrial, or vaginal hypoxia or venous obstruction as shown in Fig. 7.3. Besides preventing the uterus and abdominal wall from compressing the inferior vena cava, the lateral position has been shown to decrease intra-abdominal pressure in pregnant women [15].

Uterine "Overdistention" Increases Myometrial Wall Tension and Tissue Pressure, Threatening Fetal, Placental, and Myometrial Oxygenation

Uterine "overdistention" (another name for a "large uterus") is strongly associated with preterm birth, perhaps due to the functioning of Laplace's law, as explained below. A uterus of average size (one that is not "overdistended") will have normal myometrial wall tension and tissue pressure, as shown in Fig. 7.4. In this situation, uterine venous pressure external to the uterus exceeds myometrial tissue pressure

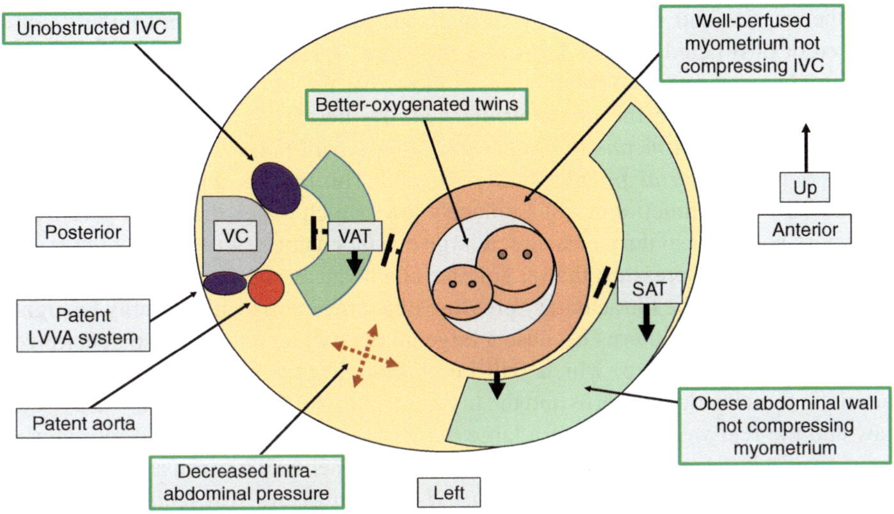

Fig. 7.3 Resolution of myometrial and fetal hypoxia with lateral position. The lateral position may be particularly beneficial in short or obese pregnant women, since their abdomens may be very tense and have low compliance. Lying in a lateral position will prevent the weight of the uterus and the abdominal wall from pressing on the inferior vena cava and the uterus itself. *IVC* inferior vena cava, *LVVA* lumbar vertebral venous and azygos collateral venous system, *SAT* subcutaneous adipose tissue, *VAT* visceral adipose tissue anterior to vertebral column, *VC* vertebral column

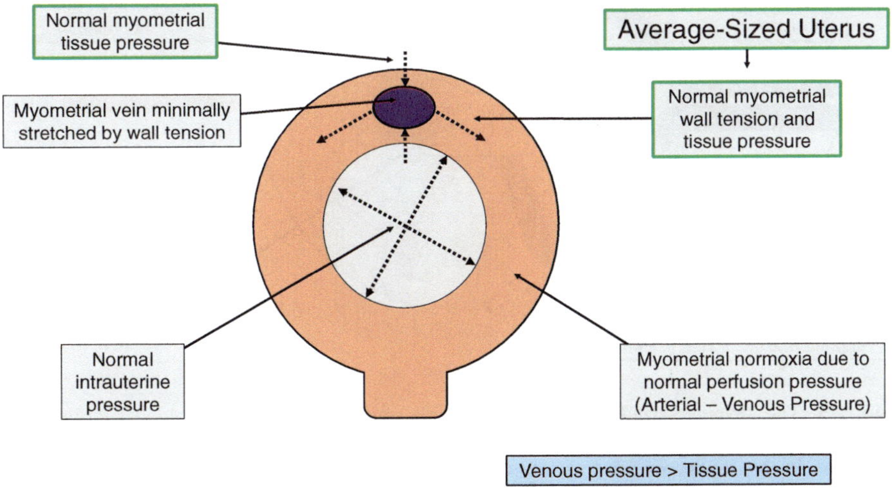

Fig. 7.4 The "average-sized" uterus: due to Laplace's law, for a given intrauterine pressure, a smaller uterus will have lower wall tension and tissue pressure than a larger uterus. A "normal-sized" uterus (one that is not "overdistended") will have normal myometrial wall tension and tissue pressure. Normally, uterine venous pressure probably exceeds myometrial tissue pressure and the arteries and veins traversing the myometrium are not unduly compressed or obstructed. Both the myometrium and placenta receive adequate perfusion, since perfusion pressure (arterial–venous) is normal

and the arteries and veins passing through the myometrium are not unduly compressed or obstructed. Figure 7.5 shows the same "average-sized" uterus but brings the fetoplacental unit into the picture to show that the blood vessels perfusing the placenta pass through the myometrium and are therefore exposed to myometrial tissue pressure. *This means that increased myometrial tissue pressure will tend to reduce both myometrial and placental perfusion.* This increased tissue pressure may be caused by the functioning of Laplace's law, which states that for a given wall thickness and intracavitary pressure, a large elastic chamber will have a higher wall tension and tissue pressure than a smaller chamber, as shown in Fig. 7.6. In real patients, however, the intracavitary pressure of a large uterus will probably be higher than that of a smaller uterus because a large uterus will tend to increase generalized intra-abdominal pressure, which will be communicated—at least in part—to the amniotic fluid inside the uterus and the myometrium. So, for two reasons—Laplace's law and the real-world effect of a large uterus on intra-abdominal and intrauterine pressure—a large uterus will tend to have much higher wall tension and tissue pressure than a smaller uterus. *This increased tissue pressure will tend to limit both myometrial and placental perfusion—even in the absence of obstruction of uterine venous return external to the uterus, as shown in* Fig. 7.7. Figure 7.8 shows how

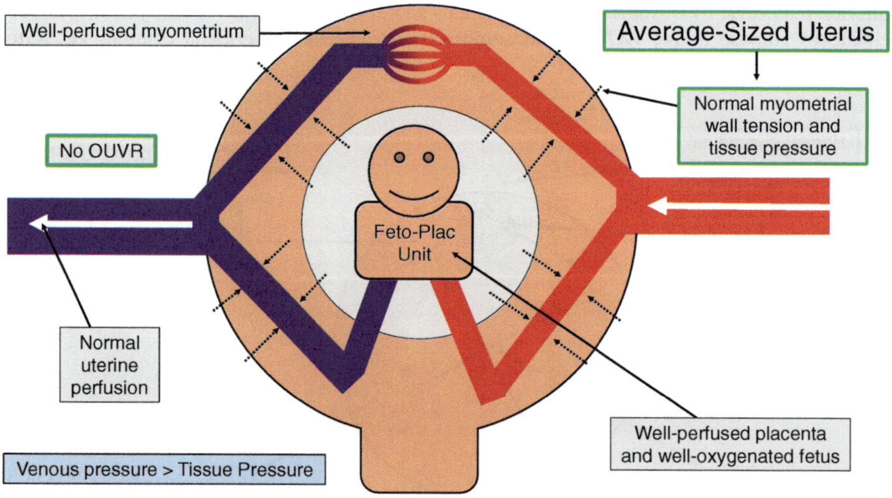

Fig. 7.5 The "average-sized" uterus: both the placental and myometrial blood supplies pass through the myometrium, making both vulnerable to restriction by increased myometrial tissue pressure. In this figure, we are focusing on the blood supply of the fetoplacental unit (which is good in this figure). The key message of this figure is that *increases in myometrial tissue pressure—from whatever cause—will reduce the perfusion pressure for both the myometrium itself and for the placenta.* Myometrial tissue pressure can be increased by (1) a large uterus (by Laplace's law), (2) external pressure due to obesity or maternal short stature, or (3) generally increased intra-abdominal pressure—none of which is present in this figure. *Feto-Plac* unit fetoplacental unit, *OUVR* obstruction of uterine venous return

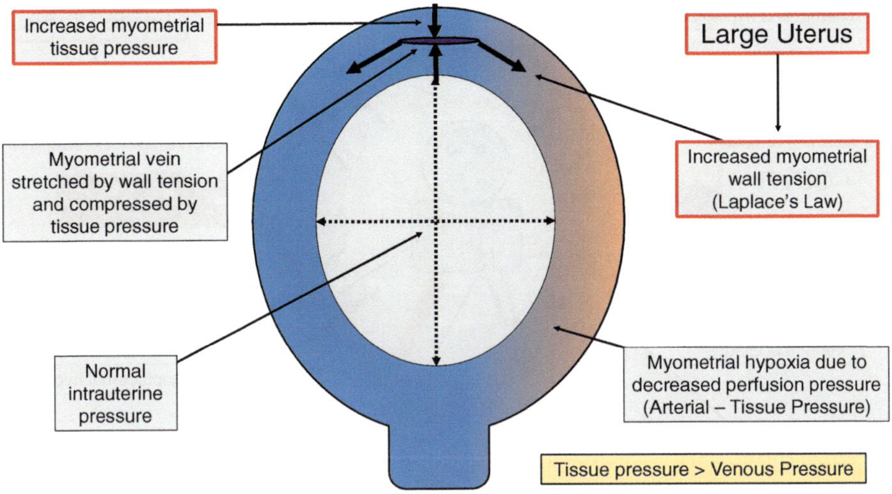

Fig. 7.6 The large uterus: due to Laplace's law, for a given intrauterine pressure, a larger uterus will have higher wall tension and tissue pressure than a smaller uterus. This implies that *by its very size* a larger uterus will tend to have a lower perfusion pressure for both myometrium and placenta than a smaller uterus—at least when tissue pressure exceeds venous pressure. This would imply that myometrial and fetal oxygenation are often more *precarious* in a larger uterus than in a smaller one

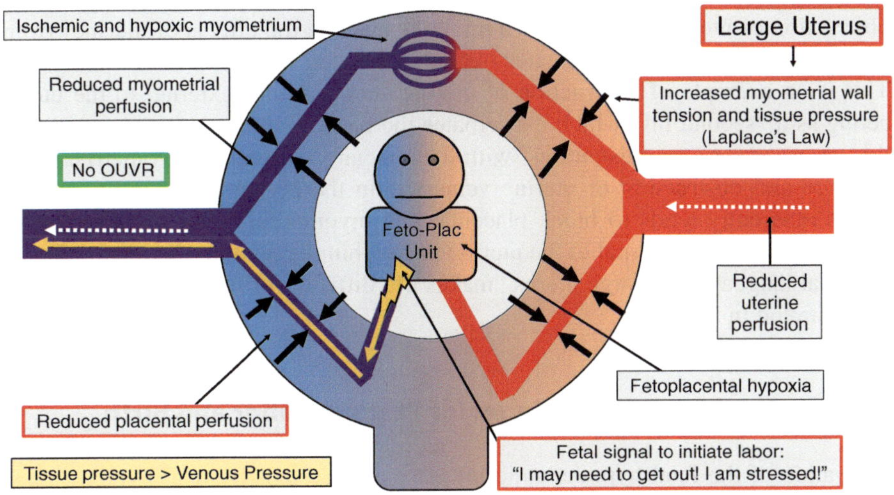

Fig. 7.7 Increased myometrial tissue pressure threatens the oxygenation of both the fetus and the myometrium. The arteries and veins serving the placenta and myometrium pass through the myometrium, and therefore increased myometrial tissue pressure associated with a large uterus may reduce perfusion of both placenta and myometrium. In this figure, the fetus is experiencing hypoxic stress and is sending a signal of some sort to the mother to initiate premature labor [16]—even without the additional stress of obstruction of uterine venous return. Such a signal may arise because of activation of the fetal hypothalamic-pituitary-adrenal axis. *Feto-Plac* unit fetoplacental unit, *OUVR* obstruction of uterine venous return

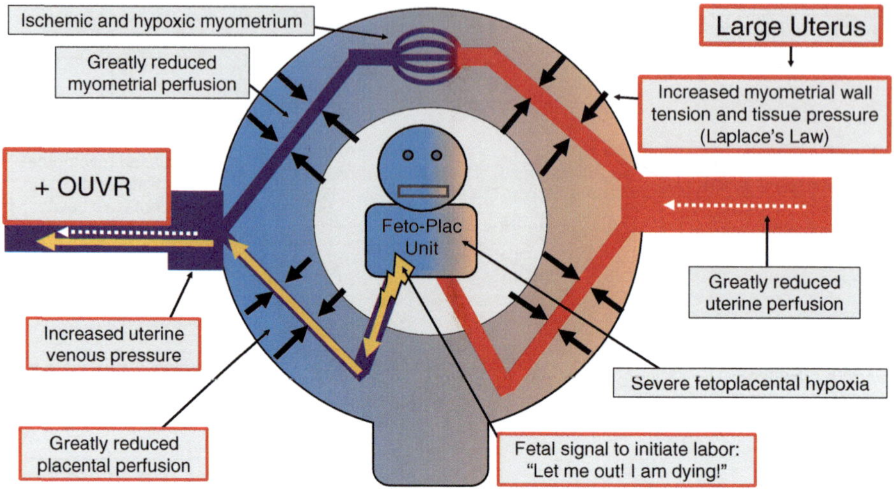

Fig. 7.8 Obstruction of uterine venous return may exacerbate pre-existing placental and myometrial hypoxia caused by "uterine overdistention". Obstruction of uterine venous return might exacerbate the pre-existing effects of uterine "overdistention" in producing fetal hypoxic stress. This would be an excellent example of obstruction of uterine venous return acting as a "second hit" which exacerbates the harmful effects of a "first hit"—in this case, uterine "overdistention." The "first hit" could also be obesity, maternal short stature, or uterine arterial disease. *Feto-Plac Unit* fetoplacental unit, *OUVR* obstruction of uterine venous return

obstruction of uterine venous return might exacerbate the effects of uterine "overdistention," producing even greater hypoxic stress on the myometrium and fetus. This is an example of obstruction of uterine venous return external to the uterus acting as a "second hit" which exacerbates the harmful effects of a "first hit"—in this case, uterine "overdistention" with its associated increased myometrial tissue pressure and obstruction of uterine veins within the myometrium itself. A large uterus inherently tends to block placental and myometrial perfusion, both at the inferior vena cava (external to the uterus) and within the myometrium itself. To use informal language, the large uterus "makes life difficult for itself" in several ways, as illustrated in Fig. 7.9.

Hypoxic Fetal Stress as a Trigger for Preterm Labor and Birth

Activation of the fetal hypothalamic-pituitary-adrenal axis by fetal hypoxic stress due to an "overdistended" uterus and its elevated tissue pressure—with or without superimposed obstruction of uterine venous return—may send a signal to the mother and her myometrium to begin labor [16], as shown in Figs. 7.7 and 7.8. But Fig. 7.10 shows that a large uterus is only one of the three potential causes of increased myometrial tissue pressure and increased fetal and myometrial vulnerability to obstruction of uterine venous return. The other two causes are obesity and maternal short stature—both of which are known risk factors for preterm birth!

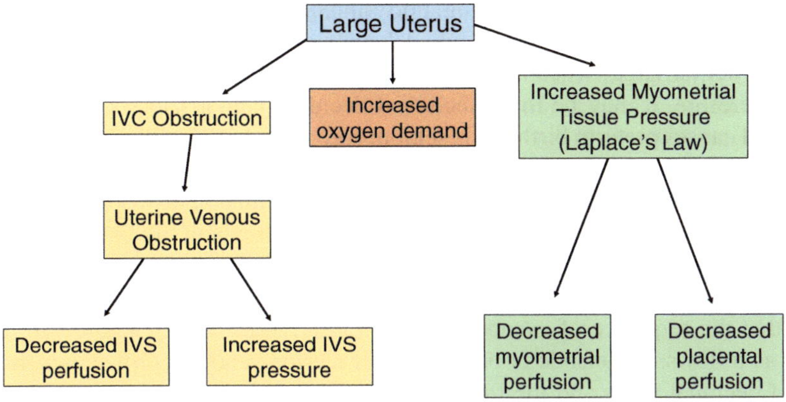

Fig. 7.9 In multiple ways, a large uterus can make life hard for itself and the fetus inside. *IVC* inferior vena cava, *IVS* intervillous space

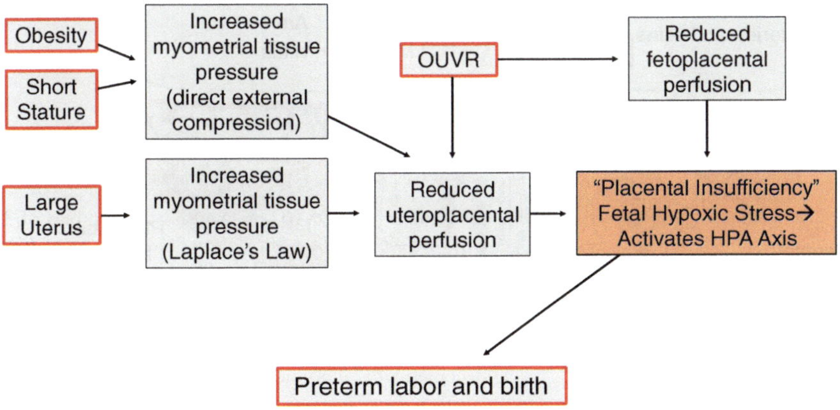

Fig. 7.10 Obesity and maternal short stature will also tend to increase myometrial tissue pressure, thereby possibly contributing to preterm birth. A large uterus is only one of the three potential "first hit" causes of increased myometrial tissue pressure. The other two causes are obesity and maternal short stature—both of which are known risk factors for preterm birth! If obstruction of uterine venous return is also present (as a "second hit"), it may powerfully potentiate the pre-existing hypoxic stress associated with increased myometrial tissue pressure due to maternal obesity or short stature. *HPA* hypothalamic pituitary adrenal, *OUVR* obstruction of uterine venous return

Placental Abruption Creates Thrombin Which Makes the Myometrium Contract

The incidence of clinically apparent placental abruption (or "decidual hemorrhage") during pregnancy is about 1%, whereas the incidence of preterm birth is about 10.2% [17]. How could placental abruption be a significant cause of preterm birth? The answer may be that only a fraction of decidual hemorrhages become clinically apparent by causing vaginal bleeding. Forty-three percent (43%) of preterm placentas show histologic evidence (decidual hemosiderin) of clinically unrecognized decidual hemorrhage, whereas only 0.8% of term placentas show such evidence [18]. Therefore, it may be that subclinical decidual hemorrhage occurs relatively often and causes preterm birth but is seldom recognized clinically due to the lack of vaginal bleeding. By increasing uterine venous pressure, obstruction of uterine venous return may increase the risk of rupture of decidual veins with the formation of a decidual hematoma next to the myometrium, as shown in Fig. 7.11. The coagulation of the decidual hemorrhage involves the formation of thrombin, and thrombin is a potent stimulant to myometrial contractility [19–23]. Therefore, it seems possible that the sequence of events shown in Figs. 7.12, 7.13, 7.14, and 7.15 could occur as follows: an episode of obstruction of uterine venous return causes the rupture of decidual veins and the formation of a blood clot next to the myometrium.

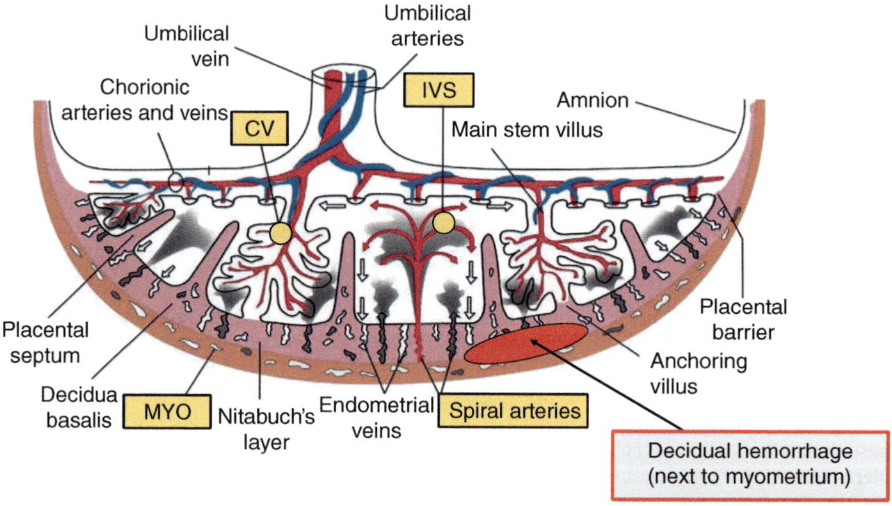

Fig. 7.11 Decidual hemorrhage makes the myometrium contract. This is an anatomic view of a placenta showing that decidual hemorrhage occurs adjacent to myometrium. Obstruction of uterine venous return increases the hydrostatic pressure within decidual veins and this could cause them to rupture, forming a hematoma. In a small abruption, the loss of gas exchange capacity between mother and fetus may not be significant. What causes preterm labor after a small abruption may be that the thrombin generated in the process of blood coagulation stimulates the myometrium to contract. Hence, it is possible that subclinical decidual hemorrhage which does not manifest either as vaginal bleeding or as changes in the fetal heart rate could nevertheless cause preterm labor days or weeks after the hemorrhage. Figure reference: [32]. Caption has been changed and Figure has been modified by addition of labels, yellow marking dots and a red "decidual hemorrhage oval". © 2020 The Authors. Acta Obstetricia et Gynecologica Scandinavica published by John Wiley & Sons Ltd on behalf of Nordic Federation of Societies of Obstetrics and Gynecology (NFOG). This is an open access article distributed under the terms of the Creative Commons CC BY license

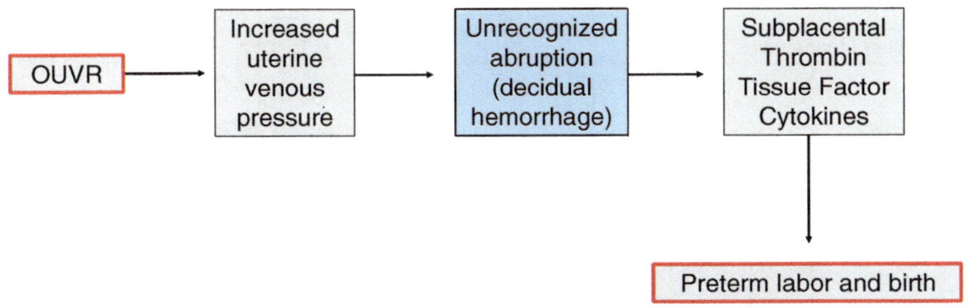

Fig. 7.12 Unrecognized placental abruption as a cause of preterm labor and birth. Increased uterine venous pressure from obstruction of uterine venous return may increase the risk of decidual hemorrhage—which can also be termed a small placental abruption. The resulting hematoma can provoke preterm labor via the formation of thrombin, a known stimulant of myometrial contractility. A high percentage of preterm placentas show histologic evidence of clinically unrecognized decidual hemorrhage. Thus, a small and unrecognized placental abruption not resulting in vaginal bleeding might cause preterm labor days or weeks after the decidual hemorrhage takes place. *OUVR* obstruction of uterine venous return

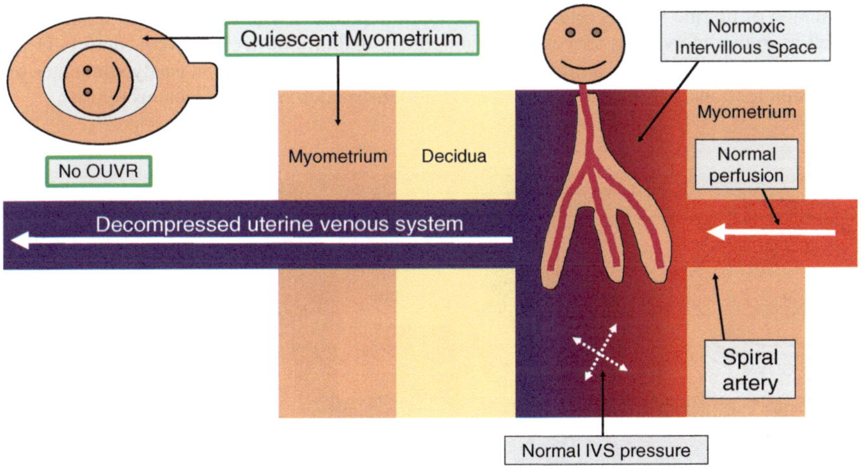

Fig. 7.13 A healthy uterine wall with low venous pressure and a quiescent myometrium. This figure shows a normal intervillous space, decidua, and myometrium without obstruction of uterine venous return. Low hydrostatic pressure within intervillous spaces and decidual veins reduces the risk of decidual hemorrhage. The figure is anatomically misleading since it shows myometrium on both sides of the intervillous space, but it was drawn this way to emphasize the fact that the maternal arteries and veins serving the placenta (and the myometrium itself) pass through the myometrium and are subject to compression by myometrial tissue pressure. *OUVR* obstruction of uterine venous return

The thrombin involved in forming the clot then triggers myometrial contractions, perhaps days or weeks after the unrecognized abruption occurs.

The supine position with obstruction of uterine venous return is mentioned as a cause of clinically apparent placental abruption in a few articles and case reports [24–26], and care-givers are routinely cautioned not to transport pregnant patients

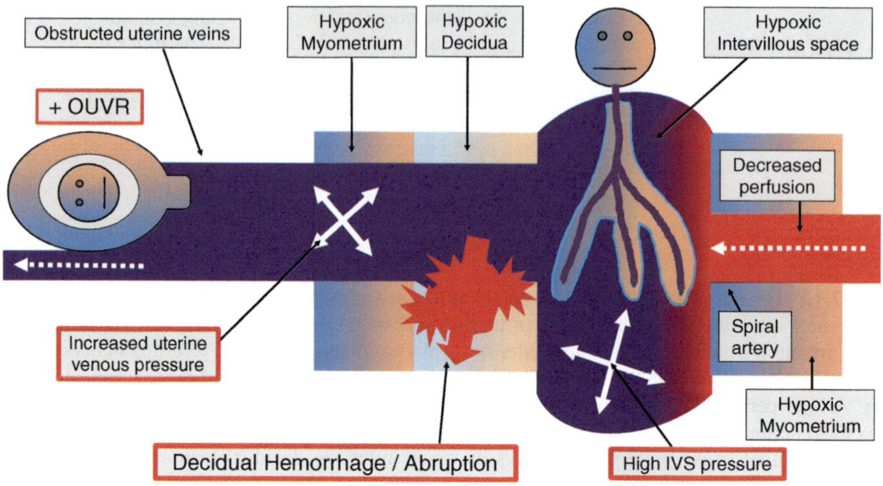

Fig. 7.14 Rupture of decidual veins due to increased uterine venous pressure. In this figure, obstruction of uterine venous return has increased the pressure within uterine and decidual veins as well as in the intervillous spaces, increasing the probability of decidual vein rupture. Decidua lies just inside myometrium, so thrombin generated during clot formation easily stimulates myometrial contractions. *IVS* intervillous space, *OUVR* obstruction of uterine venous return

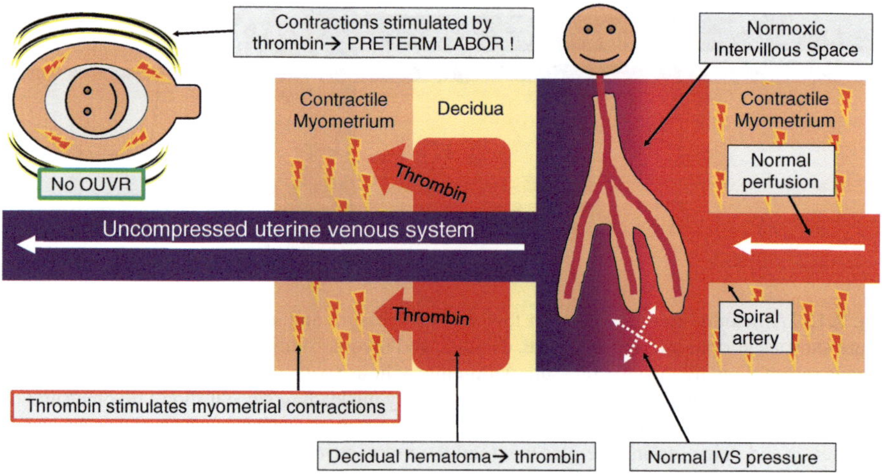

Fig. 7.15 Thrombin stimulates myometrium to contract after decidual hemorrhage. Thrombin produced in the process of decidual clot formation provokes myometrial contractions, which might start days or weeks after the original hemorrhage. The elevated uterine venous pressure which may have provoked the hemorrhage may have been the result of heavy physical effort by the mother and/or the result of an episode of obstruction of uterine venous return. Decidual cells are rich in tissue factor which triggers the coagulation sequence, resulting in the formation of thrombin and the conversion of fibrinogen to the fibrin clot. *IVS* intervillous space, *OUVR* obstruction of uterine venous return

in the supine position to avoid causing placental abruption as well as the supine hypotensive syndrome of pregnancy. But no one appears to have suggested previously that positional obstruction of uterine venous return could be a cause of unrecognized decidual hemorrhage and *delayed* preterm birth.

Myometrial Ischemia and Reperfusion May Cause Sterile Myometrial Inflammation and Preterm Labor

We have argued that *fetal* hypoxic stress due to obstruction of uterine venous return—with or without uterine "overdistention"—might trigger preterm labor. Figure 7.16 presents a variation on this argument by suggesting that repetitive cycles of *myometrial* ischemia followed by reperfusion might create sterile myometrial inflammation which prematurely activates the inflammatory pathways involved in the normal onset of labor at term [27, 28]. Figures 7.17 and 7.18 portray the two extremes of this cyclical process, with Fig. 7.17 showing the "ischemia" phase and Fig. 7.18 showing the "reperfusion" phase. The end result is shown in Fig. 7.19: a myometrium that has been transformed by ischemia and reperfusion into the contractile phenotype—and which then starts to contract prematurely. This sequence of events could occur in an average-sized uterus with a singleton gestation, but it might be more likely to occur in an "overdistended" uterus in which the myometrium

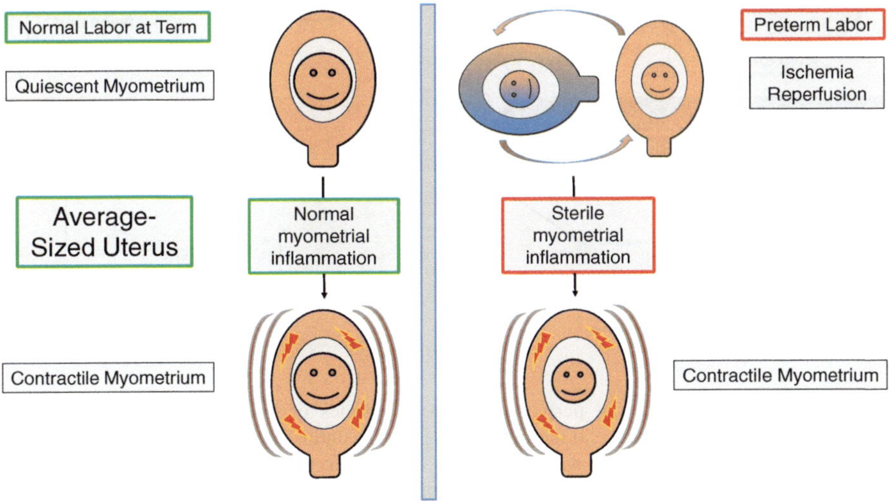

Fig. 7.16 Could ischemia and reperfusion of the myometrium cause sterile myometrial inflammation and preterm labor? The "contractile phenotype" present in normal labor is the result of a normal inflammatory process in the myometrium, which converts it from the quiescent to the contractile phenotype. Preterm birth is also associated with myometrial inflammation, but of a different character than that associated with term labor. It is possible that repeated cycles of myometrial ischemia and reperfusion due to intermittent obstruction of uterine venous return create sterile inflammation which prematurely triggers the onset of labor

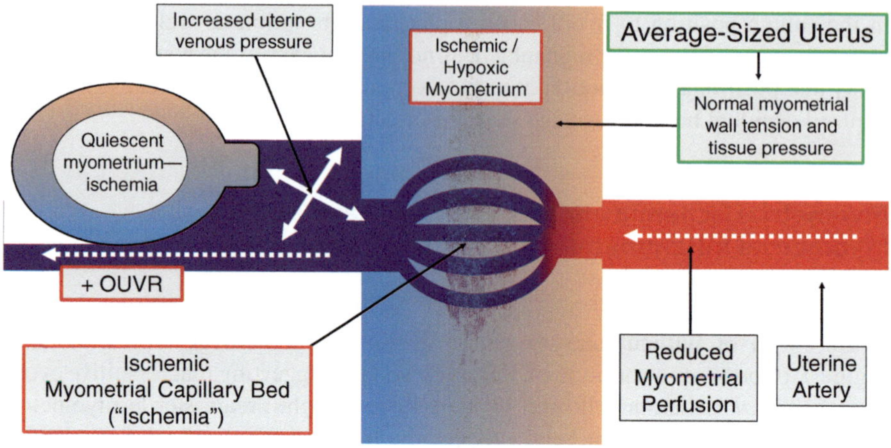

Fig. 7.17 The ischemia phase of myometrial ischemia and reperfusion. If obstruction of uterine venous return does occur from time to time—as shown in this figure—this state of venous congestion and poor myometrial perfusion would constitute the "ischemia" phase within the paradigm of "ischemia and reperfusion injury." *OUVR* obstruction of uterine venous return

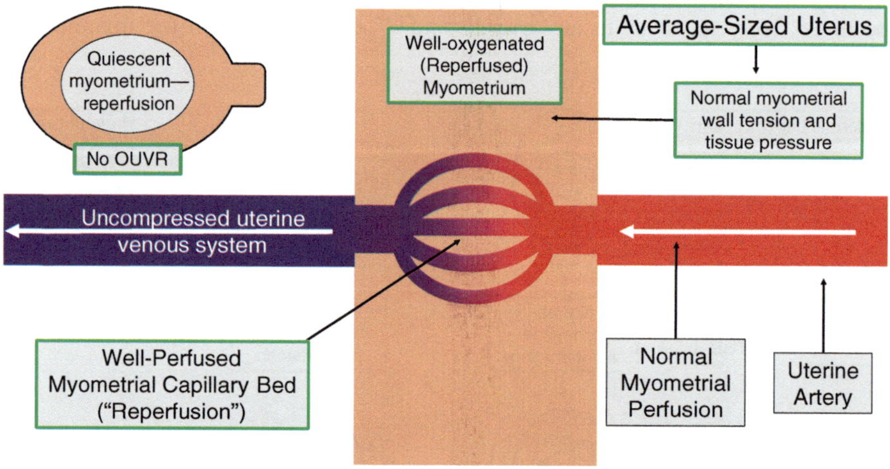

Fig. 7.18 Normal myometrial perfusion between episodes of obstruction of uterine venous return—the "reperfusion" phase. If uterine venous return is unobstructed, perfusion of the myometrium is brisk and the myometrial capillary beds are well oxygenated. If obstruction of uterine venous return does occur from time to time, the state of perfusion shown in this figure would correspond to the "reperfusion" phase within the paradigm of "ischemia and reperfusion injury." The preceding figure and this one show the postulated cyclical process of ischemia and reperfusion which might produce sterile myometrial inflammation and trigger preterm labor. *OUVR* obstruction of uterine venous return

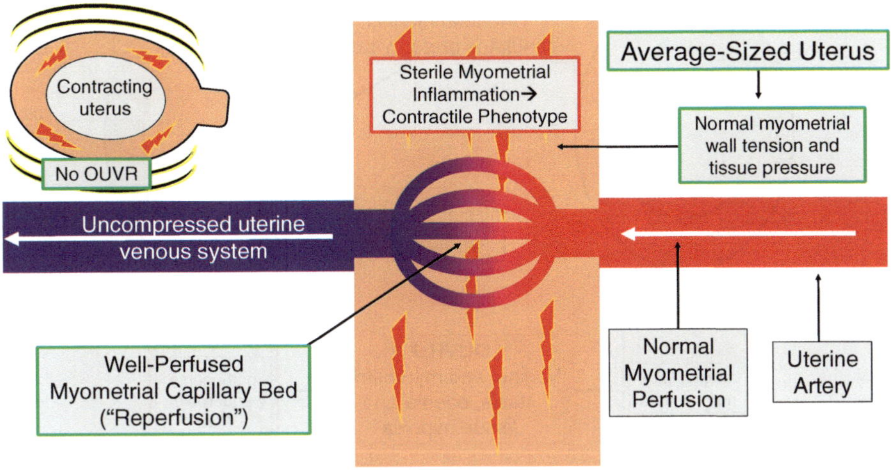

Fig. 7.19 Sterile inflammation due to myometrial ischemia and reperfusion injury has converted the myometrium to the "contractile phenotype". Normal term labor is associated with myometrial inflammation, and it is possible that ischemia and reperfusion can create a type of inflammation which prematurely activates or "takes over" the inflammatory "machinery" which normally becomes active only at term. *OUVR* obstruction of uterine venous return

already has a higher demand for oxygen combined with a more precarious oxygen supply. This would explain the higher incidence of preterm labor in "overdistended" uteruses.

Vaginal Microbiome Changes and Infectious Chorioamnionitis

Vaginal edema, stasis, and tissue hypoxia could contribute to changes in the vaginal biome which result in ascending infection and chorioamnionitis, as suggested in Fig. 7.20. The normal vaginal flora in pregnancy exist in an acidic and aerobic environment in which lactobacilli produce hydrogen peroxide, an oxidant [29, 30]. Bacterial vaginosis, which is associated with preterm labor, is associated with an abundance of anaerobic organisms [29, 30], and lower extremity edema, vulvar itching, and vaginal infections are common during pregnancy [31]. Obstruction of the inferior vena cava by the gravid uterus, together with the normal reduction of serum albumin in pregnancy, is thought to play a role in the formation of dependent edema, and maternal rest in the left lateral position is often prescribed to alleviate lower extremity edema. It is a speculation, but a biologically plausible one, that obstruction of uterine venous return might cause vaginal edema, circulatory stasis, and tissue hypoxia during pregnancy which would favor a vaginal biome dominated by anaerobic organisms which would promote ascending infection, chorioamnionitis, and preterm labor and birth. The Integrative Human Biome Project is investigating the role of the vaginal microbiome in causing preterm birth with an extensive

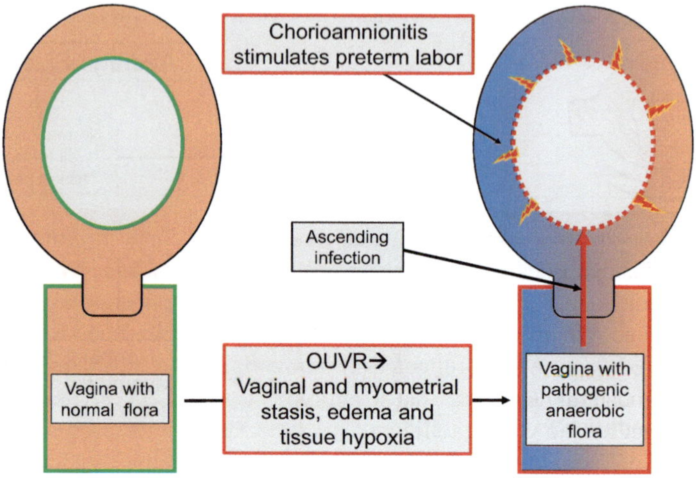

Fig. 7.20 Change in the vaginal biome and chorioamnionitis as causes of preterm labor and birth. Chorioamnionitis is a known and common cause of preterm birth, especially very early in gestation. Chorioamnionitis is associated with changes in the vaginal biome to mixed anaerobic flora, and this figure presents the theory that obstruction of uterine venous return might create venous congestion, edema, and tissue hypoxia in the vagina which could allow an unfavorable change in the vaginal biome to occur. Leg edema, vaginal infections, and vulvar itching are common in pregnancy, and the occurrence of these disorders is consistent with this theory of vaginal biome change. *OUVR* obstruction of uterine venous return

program of genomic, transcriptomic, and proteomic testing [29], but it would be unfortunate to overlook the possible role in some cases of preterm birth of a simple and correctable process such as obstruction of uterine venous return. It is possible that many of the changes in DNA transcription and translation seen in preterm birth are the *results* of such venous obstruction, rather than being the fundamental cause of preterm birth.

Summary

1. Known and suspected risk factors for preterm birth include: obesity, maternal short stature, uterine "overdistention" (a large uterus), placental abruption (decidual hemorrhage), hypoxic stress-induced activation of the fetal hypothalamic-pituitary-adrenal axis, sterile myometrial inflammation, vaginal microbiome changes, infectious chorioamnionitis, and ethnicity.
2. Maternal short stature and obesity predispose to obstruction of uterine venous return, which may increase the risk of preterm birth by exacerbating fetal, placental, myometrial, and vaginal hypoxia and by increasing abdominal venous pressures. In a woman with a tense pregnant abdomen, this physiology might resemble an incipient abdominal compartment syndrome.

3. Uterine "overdistention" (a large uterus) may predispose to preterm birth because of Laplace's law, which describes how myometrial wall tension and tissue pressure will be greater in a large uterus than in a small one. Increased wall tension and tissue pressure will tend to reduce perfusion of both myometrium and placenta.
4. Recurrent episodes of myometrial ischemia and reperfusion due to intermittent obstruction of uterine venous return might create sterile myometrial inflammation which converts the quiescent myometrial phenotype to the contractile phenotype, thus provoking preterm labor.
5. Increased decidual venous pressure caused by obstruction of uterine venous return may promote decidual hemorrhage, thrombin formation, and myometrial contraction.
6. Vaginal edema and hypoxia caused by obstruction of uterine venous return might promote a change in the vaginal microbiome, which might promote ascending infectious chorioamnionitis and preterm labor and birth.

References

1. Derraik JG, Lundgren M, Cutfield WS, Ahlsson F. Maternal height and preterm birth: a study on 192,432 Swedish women. PLoS One. 2016;11(4):e0154304. https://doi.org/10.1371/journal.pone.0154304. PMID: 27100080; PMCID: PMC4839587.
2. Kozuki N, Katz J, Lee AC, Vogel JP, Silveira MF, Sania A, Stevens GA, Cousens S, Caulfield LE, Christian P, Huybregts L, Roberfroid D, Schmiegelow C, Adair LS, Barros FC, Cowan M, Fawzi W, Kolsteren P, Merialdi M, Mongkolchati A, Saville N, Victora CG, Bhutta ZA, Blencowe H, Ezzati M, Lawn JE, Black RE, Child Health Epidemiology Reference Group Small-for-Gestational-Age/Preterm Birth Working Group. Short maternal stature increases risk of small-for-gestational-age and preterm births in low- and middle-income countries: individual participant data meta-analysis and population attributable fraction. J Nutr. 2015;145(11):2542–50. https://doi.org/10.3945/jn.115.216374. Epub 2015 Sep 30. PMID: 26423738; PMCID: PMC6457093.
3. Chan BC, Lao TT. Maternal height and length of gestation: does this impact on preterm labour in Asian women? Aust N Z J Obstet Gynaecol. 2009;49(4):388–92. https://doi.org/10.1111/j.1479-828X.2009.01006.x. PMID: 19694693.
4. Zhang G, Bacelis J, Lengyel C, Teramo K, Hallman M, Helgeland Ø, Johansson S, Myhre R, Sengpiel V, Njølstad PR, Jacobsson B, Muglia L. Assessing the causal relationship of maternal height on birth size and gestational age at birth: a Mendelian randomization analysis. PLoS Med. 2015;12(8):e1001865. https://doi.org/10.1371/journal.pmed.1001865. PMID: 26284790; PMCID: PMC4540580.
5. Cnattingius S, Villamor E, Johansson S, Edstedt Bonamy AK, Persson M, Wikström AK, Granath F. Maternal obesity and risk of preterm delivery. JAMA. 2013;309(22):2362–70. https://doi.org/10.1001/jama.2013.6295. PMID: 23757084.
6. Johansson S, Villamor E, Altman M, Bonamy AK, Granath F, Cnattingius S. Maternal overweight and obesity in early pregnancy and risk of infant mortality: a population based cohort study in Sweden. BMJ. 2014;349:g6572. https://doi.org/10.1136/bmj.g6572. PMID: 25467170; PMCID: PMC4252825.
7. Johansson S, Sandström A, Cnattingius S. Maternal overweight and obesity increase the risk of fetal acidosis during labor. J Perinatol. 2018;38(9):1144–50. https://doi.org/10.1038/s41372-018-0144-5. Epub 2018 Jun 19. PMID: 29915374.

8. https://www.uptodate.com/contents/spontaneous-preterm-birth-pathogenesis?source=mostViewed_widget. Accessed 30 July 2023.
9. Sawchuck DJ, Wittmann BK. Pre-eclampsia renamed and reframed: intra-abdominal hypertension in pregnancy. Med Hypotheses. 2014;83(5):619–32. https://doi.org/10.1016/j.mehy.2014.08.001. Epub 2014 Aug 12. PMID: 25189485.
10. Chun R, Baghirzada L, Tiruta C, Kirkpatrick AW. Measurement of intra-abdominal pressure in term pregnancy: a pilot study. Int J Obstet Anesth. 2012;21(2):135–9. https://doi.org/10.1016/j.ijoa.2011.10.010. Epub 2012 Feb 11. PMID: 22326198.
11. Gyselaers W, Lozada MJ, Pacheco LD, Tayebi S, Malbrain MLNG. Intra-abdominal pressure as an ignored parameter in the pathophysiology of preeclampsia. Acta Obstet Gynecol Scand. 2020;99(8):963–5. https://doi.org/10.1111/aogs.13898. PMID: 32683680.
12. Petrenko AP, Castelo-Branco C, Marshalov DV, Kuligin AV, Mysovskaya YS, Shifman EM, Abdulaev AMR. Physiology of intra-abdominal volume during pregnancy. J Obstet Gynaecol. 2021;41(7):1016–22. https://doi.org/10.1080/01443615.2020.1820470. Epub 2020 Nov 29. PMID: 33251897.
13. Chun R, Kirkpatrick AW. Intra-abdominal pressure, intra-abdominal hypertension, and pregnancy: a review. Ann Intensive Care. 2012;2(1):5. https://doi.org/10.1186/2110-5820-2-S1-S5. Epub 2012 Jul 5. PMID: 22873421; PMCID: PMC3390298.
14. Lozada MJ, Goyal V, Levin D, Walden RL, Osmundson SS, Pacheco LD, Malbrain MLNG. Management of peripartum intra-abdominal hypertension and abdominal compartment syndrome. Acta Obstet Gynecol Scand. 2019;98(11):1386–97. https://doi.org/10.1111/aogs.13638. Epub 2019 Jun 18. PMID: 31070780; PMCID: PMC7313226.
15. Garg D, Tyagi A, Kumar M. Intraabdominal pressure and its relation with organ dysfunction in patients scheduled for elective cesarean section: effect of supine vs left lateral tilt position. Acta Obstet Gynecol Scand. 2021;100(1):101–8. https://doi.org/10.1111/aogs.13965. Epub 2020 Aug 19. PMID: 32726457.
16. https://www.uptodate.com/contents/spontaneous-preterm-birth-pathogenesis?source=mostViewed_widget. Accessed September 16 2023.
17. https://www.cdc.gov/nchs/data/databriefs/db387-H.pdf. Accessed September 16 2023.
18. Salafia CM, López-Zeno JA, Sherer DM, Whittington SS, Minior VK, Vintzileos AM. Histologic evidence of old intrauterine bleeding is more frequent in prematurity. Am J Obstet Gynecol. 1995;173(4):1065–70. https://doi.org/10.1016/0002-9378(95)91327-0. PMID: 7485294.
19. Nishimura F, Mogami H, Moriuchi K, Chigusa Y, Mandai M, Kondoh E. Mechanisms of thrombin-Induced myometrial contractions: potential targets of progesterone. PLoS One. 2020;15(5):e0231944. https://doi.org/10.1371/journal.pone.0231944. PMID: 32365105; PMCID: PMC7197857.
20. Buhimschi CS, Schatz F, Krikun G, Buhimschi IA, Lockwood CJ. Novel insights into molecular mechanisms of abruption-induced preterm birth. Expert Rev Mol Med. 2010;12:e35. https://doi.org/10.1017/S1462399410001675. PMID: 21040617; PMCID: PMC4792258.
21. Elovitz MA, Baron J, Phillippe M. The role of thrombin in preterm parturition. Am J Obstet Gynecol. 2001;185(5):1059–63. https://doi.org/10.1067/mob.2001.117638. PMID: 11717633.
22. Vidaeff AC, Monga M, Ramin SM, Saade G, Sangi-Haghpeykar H. Is thrombin activation predictive of subsequent preterm delivery? Am J Obstet Gynecol. 2013;208(4):306.e1–7. https://doi.org/10.1016/j.ajog.2013.01.037. PMID: 23531327.
23. Elovitz MA, Saunders T, Ascher-Landsberg J, Phillippe M. Effects of thrombin on myometrial contractions in vitro and in vivo. Am J Obstet Gynecol. 2000;183(4):799–804. https://doi.org/10.1067/mob.2000.108897. PMID: 11035316.
24. Katz VL, Hansen AR. Complications in the emergency transport of pregnant women. South Med J. 1990;83(1):7–10. https://doi.org/10.1097/00007611-199001000-00004.
25. https://www.uptodate.com/contents/acute-placental-abruption-pathophysiology-clinical-features-diagnosis-and-consequences?search=abruption%20placenta&source=search_result&selectedTitle=1~150&usage_type=default&display_rank=1.
26. Chahal HS, Gelaye B, Mostofsky E, Sanchez SE, Mittleman MA, Maclure M, Pacora P, Torres JA, Romero R, Ananth CV, Williams MA. Physical exertion immediately prior to

placental abruption: a case-crossover study. Am J Epidemiol. 2018;187(10):2073–9. https://doi.org/10.1093/aje/kwy138. PMID: 29992226; PMCID: PMC6194205.
27. Phung J, Wang CA, Reeders J, Chan EC, Riveros C, Zakar T, Paul JW, Pennell CE, Smith R. Preterm labor is a distinct process from term labor following computational analysis of human myometrium. Am J Obstet Gynecol. 2022;226(1):106.e1–106.e16. https://doi.org/10.1016/j.ajog.2021.07.002. Epub 2021 Jul 7. PMID: 34245680.
28. Phung J, Wang C, Reeders J, Zakar T, Paul JW, Tyagi S, Pennell CE, Smith R. Preterm labor with and without chorioamnionitis is associated with activation of myometrial inflammatory networks: a comprehensive transcriptomic analysis. Am J Obstet Gynecol. 2023;228(3):330.e1–330.e18. https://doi.org/10.1016/j.ajog.2022.08.036. Epub 2022 Aug 21. PMID: 36002050.
29. Integrative HMP (iHMP) Research Network Consortium. The integrative human microbiome project. Nature. 2019;569(7758):641–8. https://doi.org/10.1038/s41586-019-1238-8. Epub 2019 May 29. PMID: 31142853; PMCID: PMC6784865.
30. Bagga R, Arora P. Genital micro-organisms in pregnancy. Front Public Health. 2020;8:225. https://doi.org/10.3389/fpubh.2020.00225. PMID: 32612969; PMCID: PMC7308476.
31. Ertmann RK, Nicolaisdottir DR, Kragstrup J, Overbeck G, Kriegbaum M, Siersma V. The predictive value of common symptoms in early pregnancy for complications later in pregnancy and at birth. Acta Obstet Gynecol Scand. 2023;102(1):33–42. https://doi.org/10.1111/aogs.14474. Epub 2022 Oct 27. PMID: 36300886; PMCID: PMC9780714.
32. Jansen CHJR, Kastelein AW, Kleinrouweler CE, Van Leeuwen E, De Jong KH, Pajkrt E, Van Noorden CJF. Development of placental abnormalities in location and anatomy. Acta Obstet Gynecol Scand. 2020;99(8):983–93. https://doi.org/10.1111/aogs.13834. Epub 2020 Mar 18. PMID: 32108320; PMCID: PMC7496588.

Electrical Cardiometry for Trending Maternal Cardiac Output

8

Personal Note
As we began working with electrical cardiometry in 2009, we became enthusiastic about our newly acquired ability to see changes in cardiac output and systemic vascular resistance in patients. Blood pressure is the product of cardiac output and systemic vascular resistance and—as anesthesiologists and critical care physicians—we regularly discussed those components of blood pressure in our clinical care and teaching sessions. All of us had measured cardiac output using pulmonary artery catheters or transesophageal echocardiography, but occasions requiring those highly invasive and cumbersome technologies were rare outside of critical care and cardiac anesthesia, and we never used those techniques in obstetric patients. So, in our day-to-day clinical care, cardiac output almost seemed like an heroic or mythical concept, or an eagerly sought but distant goal that was easy to discuss but difficult to see, touch, or use. But as we began to use electrical cardiometry frequently in obstetric patients we began to imagine that the measurement—or at least the *trending*—of cardiac output might become a routine part of patient care, since the technology was non-invasive, continuous, hands-free, easy to learn and apply and approved for use by the United States Food and Drug Administration (FDA). With the new technology, we saw changes in cardiac output and systemic vascular resistance as they occurred within individual pregnant patients after the administration of neuraxial anesthesia and other vasoactive medications such as oxytocin, magnesium sulfate, hydralazine, labetalol, and indigo carmine [1–3].

We were able to publish case reports and a small series [3] about some of these medication-induced hemodynamic changes, but some of our studies were rejected with the simple statement that "impedance cardiography has not been validated in pregnancy." Our growing experience was that the hemodynamic changes we saw were in the direction we expected—based on our knowledge of physiology and pharmacology—but the absolute values for stroke volume and cardiac output seemed too high. We asked ourselves, "Does electrical cardiometry really have to be *accurate* in order to be useful as a *trend indicator?*"

T. L. Archer, *Threats to Fetal, Placental and Myometrial Oxygenation*,
https://doi.org/10.1007/978-3-031-60364-8_8

Validation Studies Are Different from Trending Studies

One purpose of this chapter is to discuss the difference between "*validation studies*" and "*trending studies.*" Both types of studies compare the results obtained from a new technology with those from a reference standard, but validation studies take pairs of one-time measurements from many different people and compare the absolute values between the two technologies to see how well they agree. Trending studies, however, examine whether the values obtained by the two techniques change in the same direction within one individual over time. Electrical cardiometry appears to be very useful for identifying *trends* in cardiac output within individual pregnant women over time [1–7], but its absolute accuracy as determined by validations studies in pregnant patients is still in question, with one study favorable [4] and another not favorable [8], based on the commonly accepted 30% mean percentage error maximum for a technology to be considered "useful" [9].

Validation Studies, Bland–Altman Analysis, Standard Deviation of the Bias, and Mean Percentage Error

Figure 8.1 shows how validation studies are often structured, using cardiac output as an example of the variable being measured: many different people have cardiac output measured on one occasion with two different technologies, and the results are plotted on a graph to see whether the two technologies agree to a useful degree. In the example of Fig. 8.1, we see a "perfect validation study" (using fictitious "data"). The 31 data points—from 31 different people—lie on the line of identity, so that the "New and Perfect Technology" gives exactly the same results as the reference standard, which in this example is transthoracic echocardiography. Ideally, we would like a new technology to give the same correct absolute values as the reference standard, as shown in Fig. 8.1. Of course, this never happens in the real world, and the differences between the two technologies are most commonly analyzed using the following statistical parameters together with Bland–Altman analysis: the Pearson correlation coefficient "*r*" with its level of statistical significance, the mean bias (or average difference between the values from the new technology and those from the reference standard), the standard deviation of that mean bias, and the mean percentage error, calculated as 1.96 times the standard deviation of the mean bias divided by either the mean value from the reference standard or the mean value from the reference standard and the new technology. Figures 8.2, 8.3, 8.4, 8.5, and 8.6 use fictional data to give the reader a visual reference and a "feel" for how these various parameters are used and interact with one another, using cardiac output as the example of the quantity being measured. The figures and their captions give more detailed explanations, but the principles which I am trying to convey in these figures are the following:

1. The Pearson correlation coefficient "*r*" is valuable for many purposes but is useless for deciding whether the absolute values usefully agree between a new technology and a reference standard, unless it is derived from data which covers the

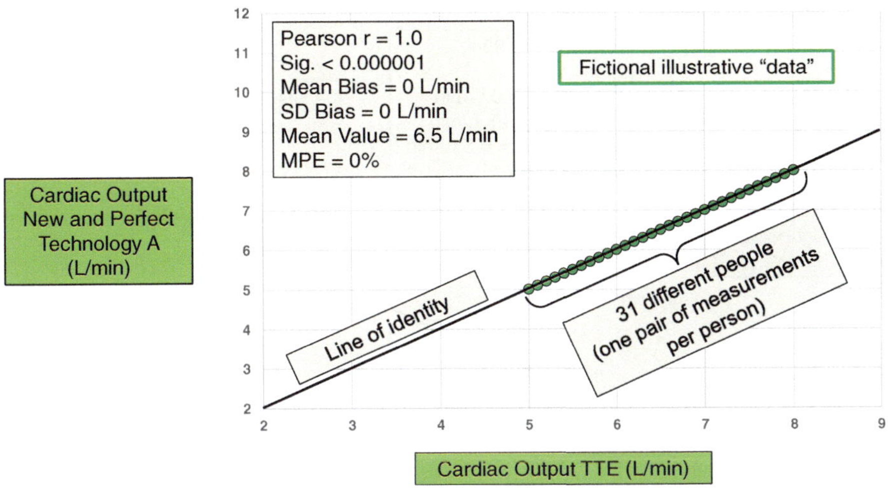

Fig. 8.1 A *validation study* for a *perfect new Technology "A,"* compared to a reference standard. Pearson correlation coefficient r = 1.0, mean bias = 0, standard deviation of the bias = 0, and mean percentage error = 0%. Validation studies commonly involve many people (31, in this fictitious example) with one pair of measurements being taken at one point in time from each person. The simultaneous measurements are performed with a reference standard technology and the new technology being evaluated. Validation studies evaluate whether the mean percentage error (defined as 1.96 times the standard deviation of the bias, divided by the average of the values obtained with the two technologies) is low enough to be "useful," with the upper limit of acceptability usually being set at 30%. Validation studies are meant to answer the question, "Does the new technology give values that are close enough to those of the reference standard—in absolute terms—to be useful?" For example, a scale that agreed with the reference standard to within one pound would probably be considered "good enough for general use" for weighing adults who weigh more than 100 pounds. Shown here is an example of a perfect technology—Technology A—which agrees perfectly with the reference standard of transthoracic echocardiography. The Pearson correlation coefficient $r = 1.0$, there is no bias (difference) between any of the values obtained with the two technologies, and therefore the mean bias is zero. Since all of the bias values are also 0, the standard deviation of the bias is 0. The average value of cardiac output with both techniques is the same—6.5 L/min. So the mean percentage error of Technology A with respect to the reference standard is (1.96 × 0)/6.5, or 0%. *L* liter, *min* minute, *MPE* mean percentage error, Pearson *r* the Pearson correlation coefficient "*r*", *SD* standard deviation, *Sig.* level of statistical significance, *TTE* transthoracic echocardiography

full range of clinically relevant values. For example, a Pearson correlation coefficient for multiple cardiac output determinations between 5.0 L/min to 5.1 L/min in an adult would not be meaningful since the clinically relevant range for cardiac output is much wider—perhaps from 2.0 to 10.0 L/min, and the lack of a statistically valid correlation between values which are almost identical on a practical and clinical level has no practical or clinical importance—despite its lack of statistical validity. In other words, do not either praise or condemn the "accuracy" of a new technology based on the Pearson correlation coefficient "*r*" from paired data points covering a narrow and clinically unimportant range of data.

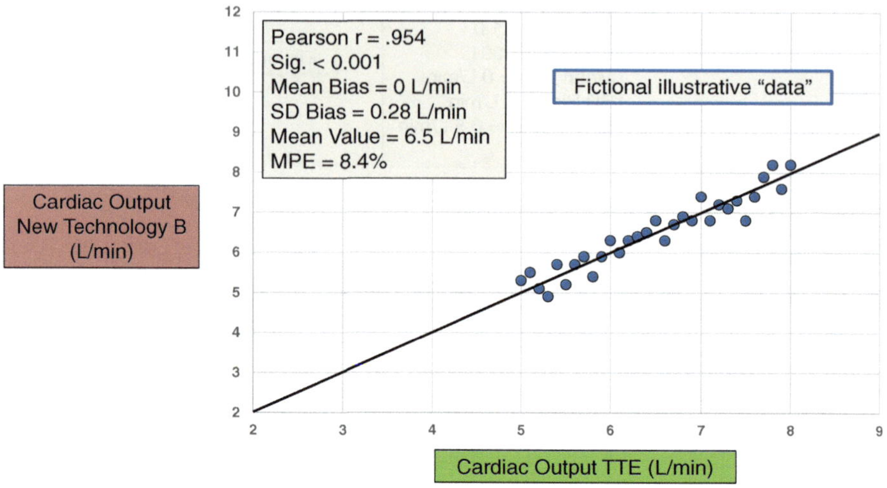

Fig. 8.2 Technology B has an excellent mean percentage error of 8.4%. This fictional example of a validation study shows what a 8.4% mean percentage error might look like graphically. The Pearson correlation coefficient *r* is very high (0.954) and highly significant. The mean bias is zero, meaning that the average of all of the biases (or differences between the new technology and the reference standard) is zero. But the biases are not all equal to zero and hence they have a standard deviation greater than zero (0.28 L/min), which means that they are scattered along both sides of the line of identity but are relatively close to that line. The mean percentage error calculation is as follows: (1.96 × 0.28 L/min)/6.5 L/min, which works out to 8.4%. *MPE* mean percentage error, *SD* standard deviation, *Sig.* statistical significance, *TTE* transthoracic echocardiography

2. The standard deviation of the bias is a key indicator of absolute accuracy or agreement, when it is compared with the mean value of the cardiac output. Strangely, perhaps, *the mean bias is in many ways less important (but much easier to understand) than the standard deviations of the bias*. The mean bias and the standard deviation of the bias play very different roles in deciding whether a new technology is useful and in how the data is interpreted.
3. The mean bias is easy to understand and compensate for. It represents a systematic and constant "inaccuracy" between the new technology and the reference standard. An informal way of explaining the significance of the mean bias would be the example of two scales for measuring weight, in which Scale B always gives a reading that is reliably and invariably 4 pounds too high in comparison to the "correct" reference standard Scale A. The key insight with respect to the mean bias is that it *reliably creates inaccuracy, but it is an inaccuracy which is easy to fix—because the inaccuracy is constant and reliable!*
4. The role of the standard deviation of the bias is much more subtle than that of the mean bias, and it describes how "inaccurate" or "untrustworthy" is the "constant" mean bias. In other words, the standard deviation of the bias shows how much variation there is *within the constant inaccuracy of the mean bias. The*

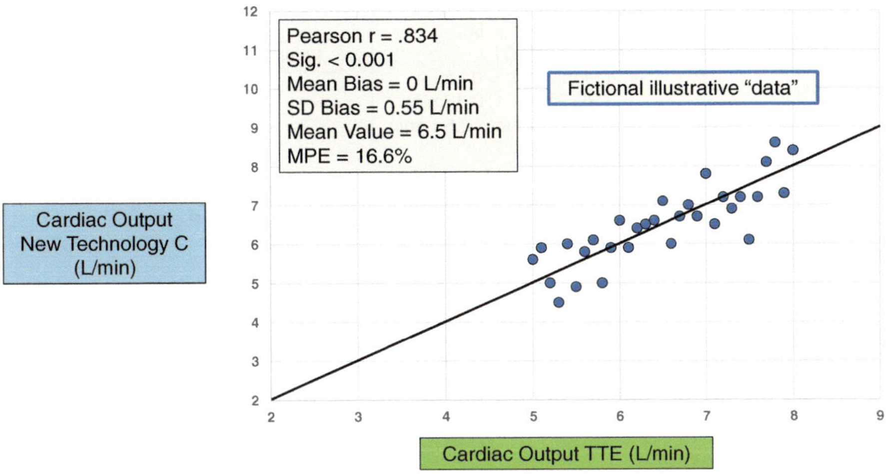

Fig. 8.3 Technology C has a good mean percentage error of 16.6%. This fictional example of a validation study shows what a 16.6% mean percentage error might look like graphically. The Pearson correlation coefficient *r* is very high (0.834) and highly significant. The mean bias is zero, meaning that the average of all of the biases (or differences between the new technology and the reference standard) is zero. But the biases are not all equal to zero and hence they have a standard deviation greater than zero (0.55 L/min), which means that they are scattered along both sides of the line of identity but are still close to that line. The mean percentage error calculation is as follows: (1.96 × 0.55 L/min)/6.5 L/min, which works out to 16.6%. *MPE* mean percentage error, *SD* standard deviation, *Sig.* statistical significance, *TTE* transthoracic echocardiography

ultimate "accuracy" or "usefulness" of a measuring technology depends on the standard deviation of the bias, and not on the mean bias, and this is a subtle point which was difficult for me to grasp.

5. To judge the importance or impact of the standard deviation of the bias, its size has to be compared to the overall size of what we are measuring. This comparison is made by calculating the *mean percentage error* of the technique. For example, on a percentage basis, a standard deviation of the bias of one pound is much more important in measuring the weight of a 5 pound cat than it would be for measuring the weight of an 800 pound gorilla.
6. Normally, the standard deviation of the bias is multiplied by 1.96 so that 95% of the values as measured by the new technology will be within the mean percentage error which results from the calculation. For example, if the mean percentage error is 16.6%, it means that 95% of values as measured by the new technology will fall within 16.6% of the "correct" value as determined by the reference standard.
7. Here is an example of a mean percentage error calculation using the (fictitious) "data" in Fig. 8.3: Mean percentage error = (1.96 × 0.55 L/min)/6.5 L/min = 16.6%. In this example, the standard deviation of the bias is 0.55 L/min and the

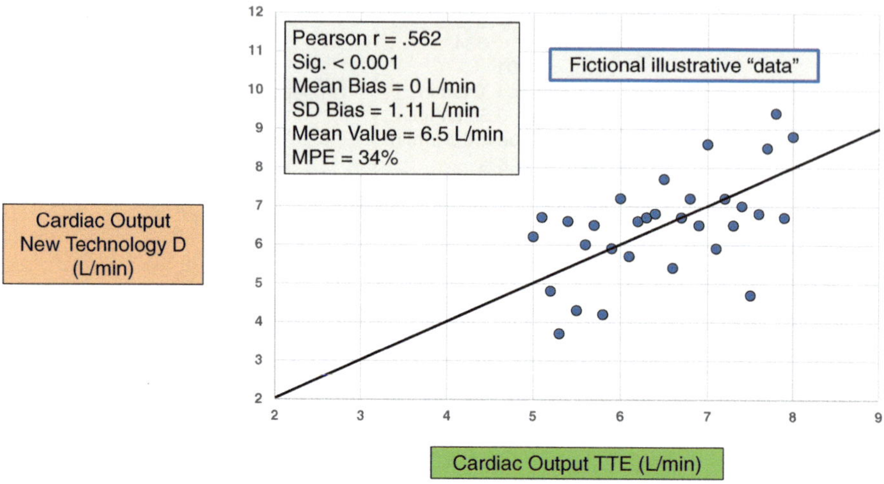

Fig. 8.4 Technology D has an "unacceptable" mean percentage error of 34%. This fictional example of a validation study shows what a 34% mean percentage error might look like graphically. The Pearson correlation coefficient *r* is high (0.562) and still highly significant (as is the case in Fig. 8.7). The mean bias is zero, meaning that the average of all of the biases (or differences between the new technology and the reference standard) is zero. But the biases are not all equal to zero and hence they have a standard deviation greater than zero (1.11 L/min), which means that they are scattered along both sides of the line of identity, but much farther from that line. The mean percentage error calculation is as follows: (1.96 × 1.11 L/min)/6.5 L/min, which works out to 34%. Please note that the mean percentage error of this example exceeds the arbitrary, but widely accepted, 30% threshold for "usefulness" of a new technology. At this point, when the technology might be deemed "not useful" or "not acceptable" in a validation study, the Pearson correlation coefficient between the two sets of measurements is still moderately high and highly significant. This fact demonstrates that mean percentage error may be a more stringent criterion for usefulness of a new technology than the Pearson correlation coefficient r, or its level of significance. But a further corollary of this observation is that—at least in the example of Fig. 8.7—the Pearson correlation coefficient *r* together with its high significance do indicate that there is probably a meaningful relationship of some sort between the parameters, even if the absolute values of the technology being evaluated are so incorrect as to be "not useful." For example, the new technology might be useful for *trending* the value of interest, even though the absolute values are deemed "not useful." *MPE* mean percentage error, *SD* standard deviation, *Sig.* statistical significance, *TTE* transthoracic echocardiography

mean value of what we are measuring (by both the new technology and the reference standard in this contrived example) is 6.5 L/min. The 16.6% means that 95% of the cardiac output values which we obtain using New Technology C will fall within 16.6% of the reference value. A mean percentage error of 30% is often (and arbitrarily) accepted as the highest "acceptable" value for mean percentage error, in order for a new technology to be considered useful. Obviously, hidden within all of this apparent mathematical certitude, there is a lot of judgment and guesswork!

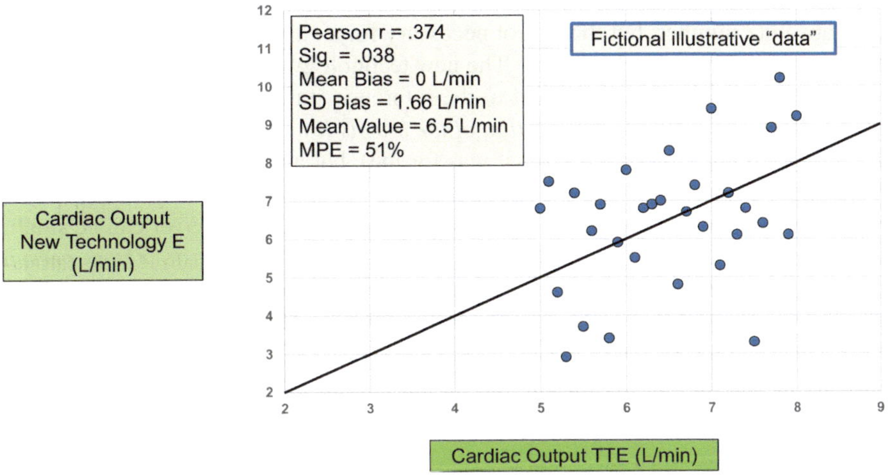

Fig. 8.5 Technology E has a terrible mean percentage error of 50.1%. This fictional example of a validation study shows what a 50.1% mean percentage error might look like graphically. The Pearson correlation coefficient *r* is 0.374 and is still significant, with sig. = 0.038. The mean bias is still zero, meaning that the average of all of the biases is zero. But the biases are not all equal to zero and have a large standard deviation (1.66 L/min) compared to the average value of the data (6.5 L/min), which means that they are very widely scattered along both sides of the line of identity. The mean percentage error calculation is as follows: (1.96 × 1.66 L/min)/6.5 L/min, which works out to 50.1%. Please note that the mean percentage error of this example far exceeds the arbitrary, but widely accepted, 30% threshold for "usefulness" of a new technology in a validation study. At this point, when the technology might be deemed "worthless" in a validation study, the Pearson correlation coefficient between the two sets of measurements is still positive at 0.374 and is significant at sig. = 0.038, and this can be seen in the upward slope of the data points going from left to right in the graph. *Another key message of this exercise is that a high mean percentage error does not mean that a technology is worthless or cannot detect hemodynamic trends. It merely means that the absolute values of the new technology are not reliable in comparison to the reference standard. As we will see, EC appears to be very useful for trending purposes but has a variable mean percentage error which probably depends on the sample of people studied* [4, 8]. *MPE* mean percentage error, *SD* standard deviation, *Sig.* statistical significance, *TTE* transthoracic echocardiography

Mean Bias: Easy to Understand But Not Important for the "Accuracy" of a Validation Study

The title of this section is meant to sound surprising or paradoxical. How can a big and consistent difference between the absolute values of two data sets not affect the "usefulness" of the new technology that is being evaluated? If the new technology consistently gives a much smaller or greater value than the reference standard, doesn't that fact automatically make the new technology "wrong," "unreliable," and "not useful?" The answer is, *"No! A large mean bias by itself is not very important because it is easy to fix."*

We would like the absolute values produced by the two technologies to be the same absolute number, but that is not necessary for a validation study to be considered favorable to a new technology. The new technology can have a (desirable) low mean percentage error with respect to the reference standard despite a large mean bias, *as long as the standard deviation of the bias is low*, as shown in Fig. 8.6. This is a difficult point to grasp (at least it was for me), but an important one, and a further explanation is given in the caption to Fig. 8.6. Another way of expressing this truth is that the mean bias can be large and the mean percentage error can be small, as long as the *mean bias itself—large or small—is relatively constant from person to person. What is important is that the bias does not change very much from one person to another.* If this is the case, then the standard deviation of the bias will be small, even though the mean bias may be large.

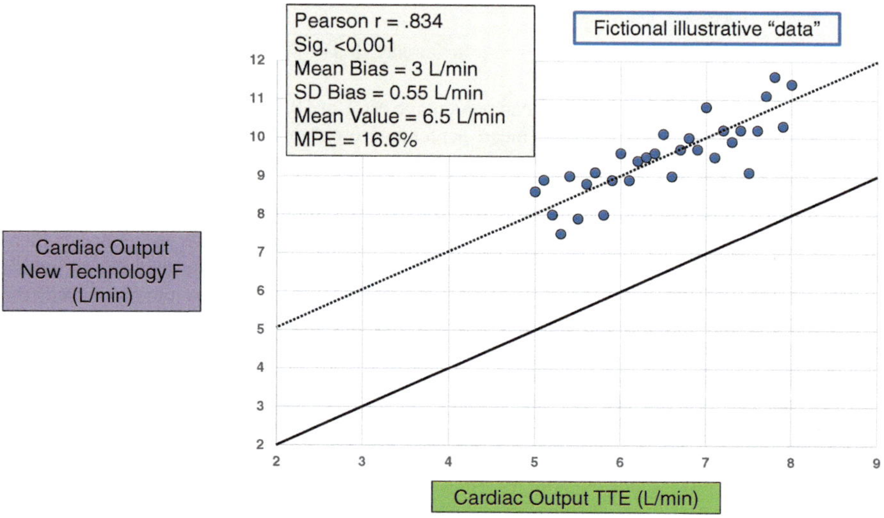

Fig. 8.6 Technology F has a good mean percentage error of 16.6%, but also a mean bias of 3 L/min. This example illustrates the important principle that *in a validation study the mean bias is much less important than the standard deviation of the bias*. The reason for this is that a mean bias can be simply compensated for, by subtracting the mean bias from the values obtained with the new technology in order to get the values that would have been obtained using the reference standard. A non-zero mean bias with a low standard deviation of the bias suggests that there is something intrinsic to the new method which systematically and uniformly increases or decreases the measurement from what would be obtained from the reference standard itself. In a sense, a high mean bias—by itself—means very little, since it can be corrected for, by using simple addition or subtraction. In the example of this figure, each fictitious data point from the new technology has a value 3 L/min higher than the corresponding data point in Fig. 8.3. Therefore, the mean bias is 3 L/min, rather than zero, but everything else is the same, including the mean percentage error. In a sense, the New Technology F shown in this figure is just as good as the New Technology C shown in Fig. 8.3, even though the absolute values obtained with New Technology F are systematically 3 L/min higher than those obtained with New Technology C. *We could even say—in a sense—that New Technology F is "just as accurate" as New Technology C, since the standard deviation of the bias is the same with both technologies! MPE* mean percentage error, *SD* standard deviation, *Sig.* statistical significance, *TTE* transthoracic echocardiography

Figure 8.7 shows real data from a validation study of electrical cardiometry for the measurement of cardiac output in pregnant women, using transthoracic echocardiography as the reference standard [8]. This validation study had "good news" and "bad news:" across the full clinically relevant range of values, the Pearson correlation coefficient between the stroke volume values obtained by electrical cardiometry and transthoracic echocardiography was 0.458 with sig.= 0.002, but the mean percentage error was 43.7%—more than enough to prevent electrical cardiometry from being considered "useful" for the measurement of absolute values of stroke volume and cardiac output. Also, the mean bias of the stroke volume determination was 15.6 mL. So, this validation study of electrical cardiometry showed two

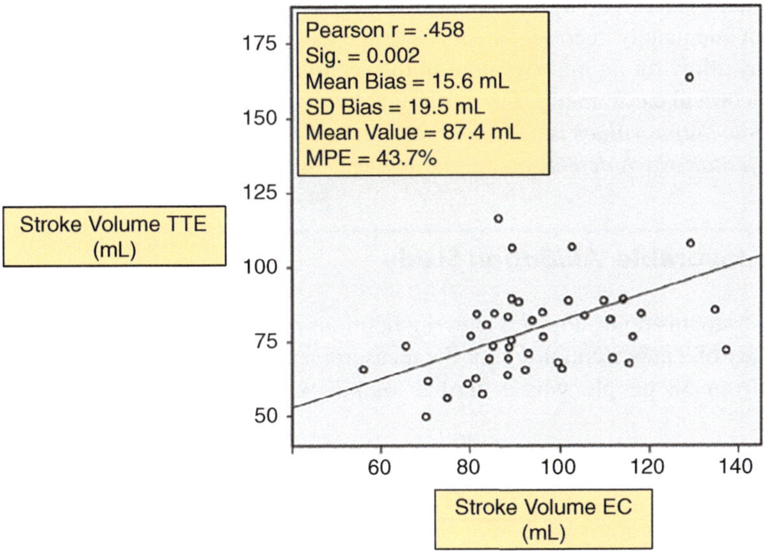

Fig. 8.7 A real validation study of electrical cardiometry for the measurement of stroke volume, using transthoracic echocardiography as the reference standard. Good and highly significant correlation but bad mean percentage error. These are the actual results for stroke volume (not cardiac output) for our validation study of electrical cardiometry using transthoracic echocardiography as the reference standard [8]. Our study showed a mean percentage error of 43.7%, putting the technology in the "not useful" category for the determination of absolute values of stroke volume and cardiac output in comparison to transthoracic echocardiography. Qualitatively, the real data in this figure resemble the data in Fig. 8.5, which has a mean percentage error of 50.1%. From our clinical impressions, we felt that electrical cardiometry trended stroke volume well within single patients over time, but were dismayed that this validation study in a group of people showed such a modest correlation (although with high significance) and such a high bias and mean percentage error. We asked ourselves, "Why doesn't electrical cardiometry do a better job of getting the absolute values right?" Our study proposed one modification of the EC algorithm to improve its absolute accuracy, and this chapter will present another approach to improving it, *but the lesson I want you to take away from this chapter is that a technology for the "measurement" of cardiac output can fail in a validation study and yet be a useful tool for the trending of cardiac output, despite the fact that the absolute values obtained from EC are far from correct. EC* electrical cardiometry, *MPE* mean percentage error, *SD* standard deviation, *Sig.* statistical significance, *TTE* transthoracic echocardiography

problems with the technology—a large mean percentage error (which is a serious problem) and a large mean bias (which is not a serious problem, as we have just explained). In contrast to that study, a more recent validation study of electrical cardiometry for the measurement of cardiac output in pregnant women using trans-thoracic echocardiography as the reference standard [4] showed a much lower mean percentage error of approximately 23%, based on my calculations from the data given in the paper.

The explanation for the difference between the two studies may be that the more recent study involved participants with much lower mean weights—*and with a much lower standard deviation of their weights*—than was the case in the earlier study [8]. Variations in patient weight appear to affect the estimate of cardiac output in pregnant patients in a systematic way that the electrical cardiometry algorithm may not adequately account for, and—as we will see later on in this chapter—this fact may allow for an improvement in the accuracy of the absolute values obtained from electrical cardiometry. *But again, I want to emphasize that absolute accuracy of cardiac output values is not required for a new technology to be useful as a trending indicator which detects positional changes in maternal cardiac output.*

An Unfavorable *Validation* Study

To illustrate this point, Fig. 8.8 shows a fictitious example of an unfavorable validation study of a new technology for the measurement of cardiac output. The fictitious data—from 38 people whose cardiac output was measured once with the two

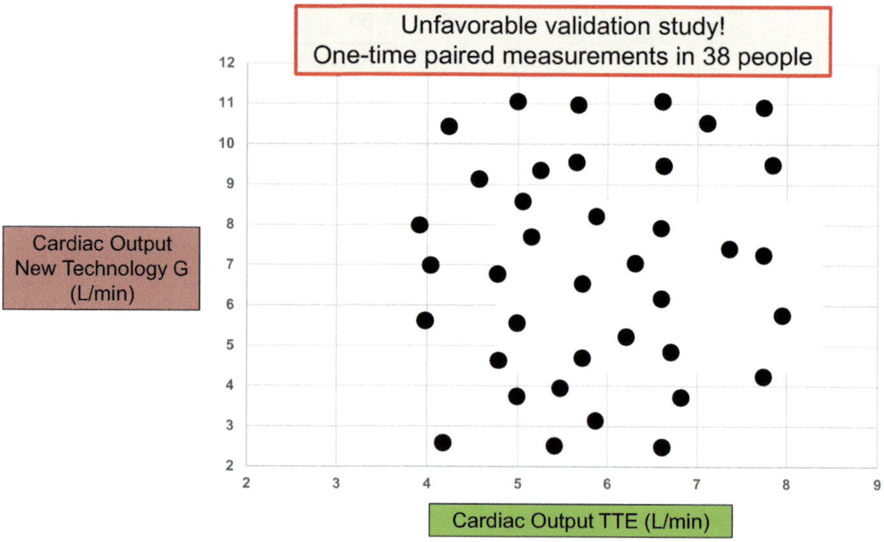

Fig. 8.8 An unfavorable validation study. These are results from a fictitious study comparing a new technology to a reference standard, with 38 one-time measurements of cardiac output from 38 different people. The correlation coefficient will not be significant and the mean percentage error will be very high. The new technology will be judged to be worthless for measuring the absolute values of cardiac output. *TTE* transthoracic echocardiography

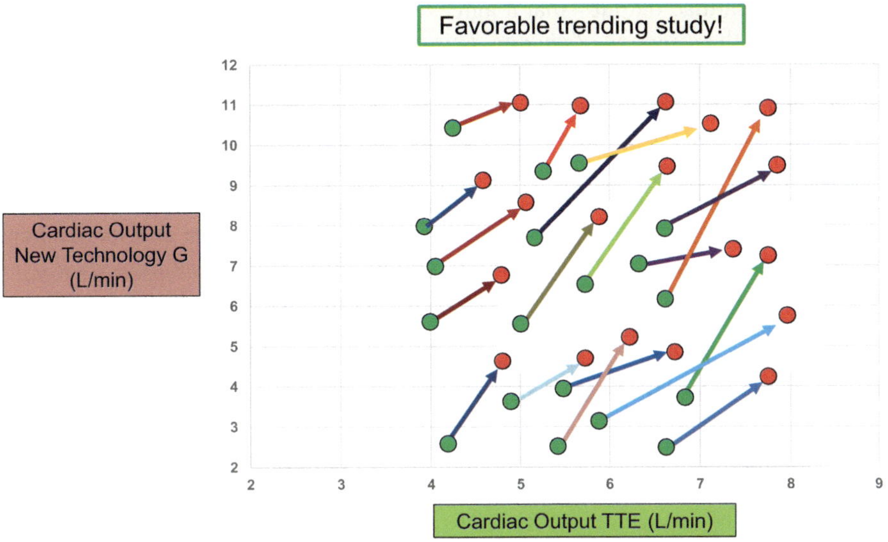

Fig. 8.9 A favorable trending study. These fictional data points are the same as those shown in Fig. 8.8, but the imaginary "experimental conditions" were different: In this imaginary experiment, 19 individuals had their cardiac outputs measured with the two technologies before and immediately after exercise. Each green dot represents the cardiac output of one person before exercise and a colored line connects each green dot with the cardiac output in that same individual after exercise, recorded as a red dot. The reference standard shows that cardiac output increases after exercise in each of the 19 people studied, and the new technology agrees with the reference standard in every case. This could be described as an "individual" trending study with 19 participants. Concordance analysis (one method of evaluating trending studies) would show a concordance rate of 100%—meaning that the direction of change was correctly identified by the new technology in all 19 cases. *TTE* transthoracic echocardiography

technologies—looks like a swarm of bees and there is no recognizable correlation between the values produced by the two technologies. If confronted with this "validation study" I am sure that we would agree that the new technology was worthless. But now look at Fig. 8.9.

But a Favorable *Trending* Study

Figure 8.9 shows the same fictitious data points shown in Fig. 8.8, but the fictitious experiment which produced these data points was different. Figure 8.9 shows *pairs* of data points from 19 different people, with a different colored line connecting the two data points for each person. The green data points represent an individual's cardiac output measurement before exercise, whereas the red data points represent that same individual's cardiac output after exercise. *For each of the 19 fictitious individuals whose "data" is shown in* Fig. 8.9*, the reference standard and the new technology agree in showing an increase in cardiac output after exercise—even though the absolute values do not agree at all between the two technologies!* This is how I am defining the successful "trending ability" of a new technology for "measuring" cardiac output—that it agrees with the reference standard technology in identifying the *direction of change. This ability to know whether the cardiac output is increasing or decreasing within a single person over time should be sufficient for the detection and correction of obstruction of uterine venous return—using electrical cardiometry or any other cardiac output trending technology.* For this limited but important purpose, the results of validation studies of new technology are irrelevant. This may seem like a strong statement, but I believe it is true. What is needed for the detection of obstruction of uterine venous return and its resultant decreases in cardiac output is *reliable trending ability within one individual over time*—not correct one-time absolute values of cardiac output.

Another Unfavorable Validation Study

Figure 8.10 shows more fictional data (obtained using a reference standard and a new technology) from a fictional validation study consisting of 21 one-time paired measurements of cardiac output from 21 pregnant patients resting in the left lateral decubitus position. Looking at these data points we see another "swarm of bees" and can say with confidence that—as a validation study—this data shows the new technology to be worthless for obtaining correct absolute values of cardiac output.

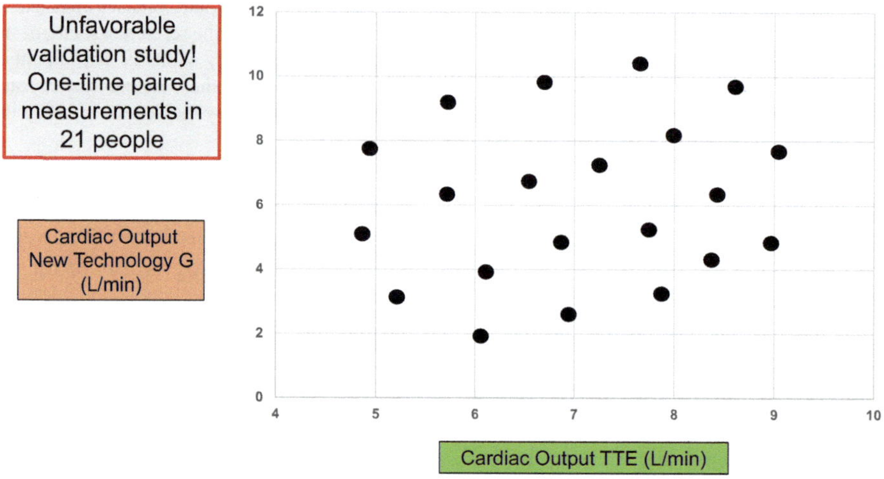

Fig. 8.10 Another unfavorable validation study. This figure shows fictional data (obtained using a reference standard and a new technology) from an imaginary validation study consisting of 21 one-time paired measurements of cardiac output from 21 pregnant patients resting in the left lateral decubitus position. Looking at the data points we see what looks like another "swarm of bees" and can say with confidence that—as a validation study—this data shows the new technology to be worthless for obtaining correct absolute values of cardiac output. *L/min* liters per minute, *TTE* transthoracic echocardiography

Another Favorable Trending Study

Figure 8.11 shows the same fictional data points as in Fig. 8.10, but the circumstances of the data collection were very different from those in the validation study of Fig. 8.10. In Fig. 8.11, we now see a collection of data points from four different patients over the course of a 20 min "loading dose" of magnesium sulfate. This fictitious data (in which the mean percentage error differences between "patients" are grossly exaggerated for illustrative purposes) presents two theories which I believe to be true about electrical cardiometry, based on our published and unpublished work: (1) Electrical cardiometry reliably shows increasing trends of cardiac output over time in patients receiving a loading dose of magnesium sulfate (even though the absolute values are probably incorrect) and (2) lower body mass index and weight are associated with a systematic increase in the electrical cardiometry-derived estimate of cardiac output for a given "true" cardiac output as measured by the reference standard. In statistical terms, this theorized relationship can be re-stated as follows: decreasing BMI or weight is associated with an increasing mean bias of the cardiac output determination by electrical cardiometry. Or even more concisely, one could say that "when one is using electrical cardiometry, thinner patients will appear to have higher cardiac outputs." *But it is probable that, despite the increasing mean bias with decreasing body mass index—as shown in* Fig. 8.11*—the mean percentage error for a given patient with a given body mass index will be acceptably low.*

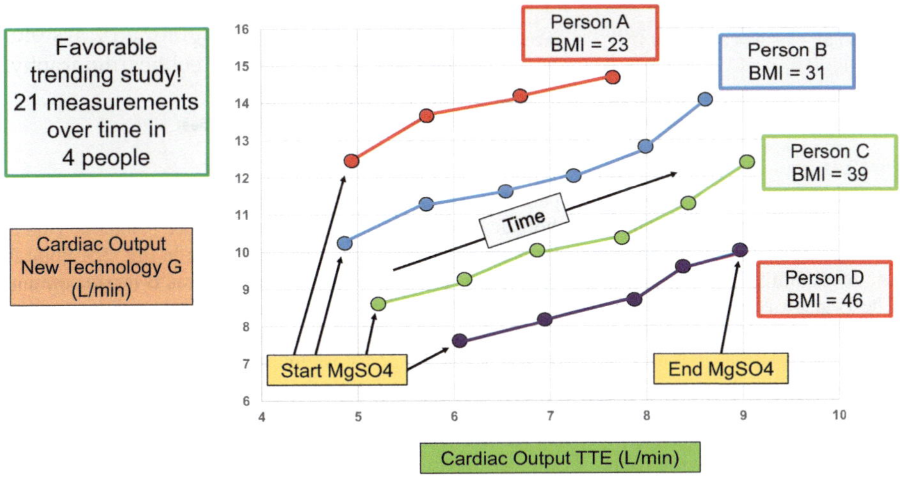

Fig. 8.11 Another favorable trending study. This figure shows the same data points as in Fig. 8.10, but the imaginary circumstances of the data collection have changed from those of the "validation study" shown in Fig. 8.10. In what is now a fictional "trending study," we see a collection of data points from four different patients over the course of a 20 min "loading dose" of magnesium sulfate. This fictitious data makes two points which I believe to be true about electrical cardiometry (based on our published and unpublished work): (1) electrical cardiometry reliably demonstrates a truly increasing trend of cardiac output over time, such as that which occurs with magnesium sulfate or oxytocin administration and (2) lower body mass index is associated with a systematic increase in the electrical cardiometry-derived cardiac output reading corresponding to a given "true" cardiac output as measured with the reference standard. *L/min* liters per minute, *$MgSO_4$* magnesium sulfate, *TTE* transthoracic echocardiography

Electrical Cardiometry Reliably Trends Cardiac Output Within Individuals Over Time, Despite Incorrect Absolute Values

Figure 8.12 shows a real (non-fictional) example of such trending, in which electrical cardiometry follows changes in stroke volume as demonstrated by transthoracic echocardiography [5, 10]. The Pearson correlation coefficient "r" between the

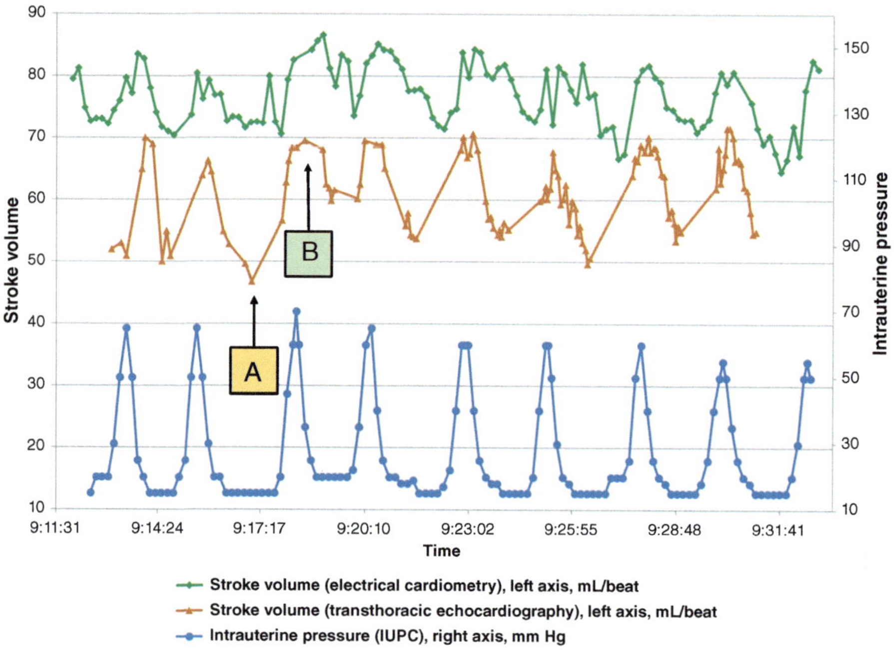

Fig. 8.12 Autotransfusion during pain-free labor: electrical cardiometry correctly identifies trends in stroke volume, using transthoracic echocardiography as the reference standard. This is stroke volume data from the same patient whose cardiac output data is shown in Fig. 2.5. Point A is a minimum value for stroke volume during an autotransfusion cycle, whereas B is a maximum. The Pearson correlation coefficient r between the stroke volumes by electrical cardiometry and transthoracic echocardiography in the data shown was 0.549, sig. <0.001, but it should be noted that the correlation coefficient might have been higher if not for the specific data recording methods used. A recorded stroke volume measurement from transthoracic echocardiography comes from a single heartbeat, whereas each recorded measurement from electrical cardiometry is the average of the values for the preceding ten heartbeats, and measurements are recorded every ten seconds. Additionally, the timing of the two measurements was not exactly simultaneous, since each transthoracic echocardiography measurement was paired with the electrical cardiometry measurement which most closely followed it in time, with up to a 20 s delay being allowed. Because of this averaging of the electrical cardiometry data and the lack of precise simultaneity of measurement, changes recorded by electrical cardiometry tended to lag those from transthoracic echocardiography and are also damped or "smoothed" in magnitude in comparison to the transthoracic echocardiography readings. This lagging and smoothing effect is also seen in Fig. 8.17 for the ICON parameter from electrical cardiometry in comparison to the Vmean parameter from transthoracic echocardiography. Because of the differences in recording techniques, the calculated correlation coefficient between electrical cardiometry and transthoracic echocardiography data may be lowered when a patient's hemodynamics are changing rapidly, as in the data shown. *IUPC* intrauterine pressure catheter [10]

stroke volumes as measured by electrical cardiometry and transthoracic echocardiography was 0.549, sig. <0.001, and it should be noted that the correlation coefficient might have been higher if not for the specific data recording methods used, as explained in the caption of Fig. 8.12. When the Bland–Altman technique is applied to this single-patient stroke volume data (which changes over time), the mean percentage error is 14.5% and the mean bias is 19.4 mL. For cardiac output [10], the mean percentage error is 14.8% and the mean bias is 1.64 L/min, and from these four values we can see that stroke volume and cardiac output fit the model displayed in Fig. 8.6—namely, that the mean percentage errors are low, but the mean bias values are high. As explained in Fig. 8.6, this picture suggests that electrical cardiometry may be useful for trending stroke volume and cardiac output, but that the absolute values will be very questionable. This lack of agreement of absolute values for stroke volume and cardiac output between the two technologies is probably due to the fact that the ICON parameter from electrical cardiometry gives a poor implicit absolute estimate of Vmean. That said, it appears that electrical cardiometry does a better job of estimating the absolute duration of systole since left ventricular ejection time from electrical cardiometry appears to agree well with envelope time from transthoracic echocardiography both within individuals over time [5] and between individuals [8]. In one validation study [8], mean envelope time from transthoracic echocardiography was 279 ms (SD = 23) and mean left ventricular ejection time (LVET) from electrical cardiometry was 274 ms (SD = 22). The mean bias between the two techniques for the duration of systole was −4.9 ms, and the mean percentage error was 12.7%. This is a reassuring absolute agreement between the two technologies, which is similar to that shown in Fig. 8.3, in which the absolute values of the two technologies agree quite well.

Figure 8.13 shows *simulated and schematic* graphical and numerical data from transthoracic echocardiography corresponding to the two points of minimum and maximum stroke volume in an autotransfusion cycle, marked as “A” and “B” in Figs. 8.12 and 8.13. Figure 8.12 contains real patient data, whereas the data in Fig. 8.13 is *simulated* data produced for illustrative purposes.

The graphical data example shown in Fig. 8.13 is included to give the reader a better understanding of how transthoracic echocardiography derives the mean systolic blood flow velocity in the left ventricular outflow tract, along with the duration of systole, from the area of the “velocity–time integral,” which is, in fact, the “stroke distance.” The stroke distance is then multiplied by the left ventricular outflow tract area to arrive at the stroke volume, as shown geometrically and algebraically in Figs. 8.18 and 8.21, respectively. It should be noted that Vmean is not derived directly but rather is calculated by dividing the VTI (also called the “stroke distance”) by the duration of systole (also called the “envelope time”).

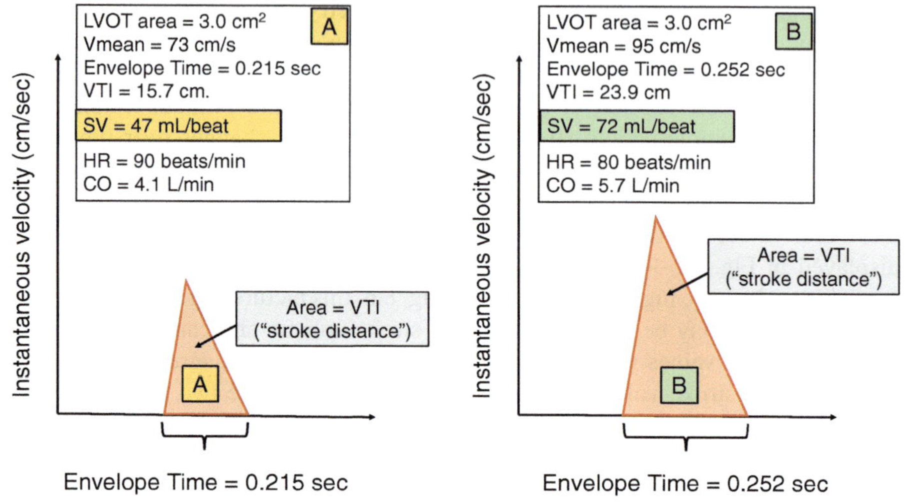

Fig. 8.13 Velocity–time integrals from transthoracic echocardiography allow calculation of envelope time, stroke distance, and Vmean (*simulated data*). The difficult part of measuring cardiac output with transthoracic echocardiography is obtaining the velocity–time integral (VTI) or stroke distance, which is calculated graphically by tracing the area under the velocity–time curve (or "envelope") for a single heartbeat. Obtaining the proper echocardiographic view for this measurement requires considerable skill and training, *and this measurement must be repeated every time a new cardiac output is desired, which requires the continuing presence of a highly trained technician or physician.* To obtain the stroke volume, the stroke distance is multiplied by the left ventricular outflow tract area, which is calculated from the measurement of left ventricular outflow tract diameter. The measurement of the left ventricular outflow tract diameter is the easy part of obtaining the stroke volume with transthoracic echocardiography, since it only needs to be performed once for each patient and is obtained from a transthoracic echocardiography view (the left parasternal long axis view) that is relatively easy to acquire. The data shown in this figure is simulated and the difference between the graphical sizes of the velocity–time integral envelopes is exaggerated for illustrative purposes, but relevant real patient data has been reported elsewhere [5]. Note that there is roughly a 40% difference between the minimum and maximum stroke volume over the autotransfusion cycle shown (between points "A" and "B" in Fig. 8.12 and in this figure), and this information regarding the "volume responsiveness" of the heart (and its position on the Starling curve) might prove useful in evaluating the "volume status" and cardiac function of pain-free laboring patients. (Pain increases the heart rate, which tends to decrease the stroke volume, making the increase in stroke volume during autotransfusion less predictable during painful labor than during pain-free labor.) *CO* cardiac output, Envelope time the duration of systolic blood flow from transthoracic echocardiography, *HR* heart rate, *LVOT* area left ventricular outflow tract area, obtained from measured left ventricular outflow tract diameter as $\pi \times$ (left ventricular outflow tract diameter/2)^2, Vmean mean systolic blood flow velocity in the left ventricular outflow tract as determined by transthoracic echocardiography, *VTI* velocity–time integral (or "stroke distance"), the distance that blood travels forward in the ascending aorta during one heartbeat, derived graphically as the area of the VTI

How Electrical Cardiometry Works

As shown in Fig. 8.14 [12], electrical cardiometry works by passing an insensible alternating current of fixed maximum amplitude through the thorax and analyzing the associated voltage changes specific to the cardiac cycle. The ratio of the voltage to the fixed maximum amplitude current is the *magnitude* of the *impedance*, which is the equivalent for alternating current of *resistance* for direct current. The sine wave of the voltage is shifted out of phase with that of the alternating current, and changes in the degree of that phase shift during the cardiac cycle are utilized in another impedance cardiography technology called "bioreactance."

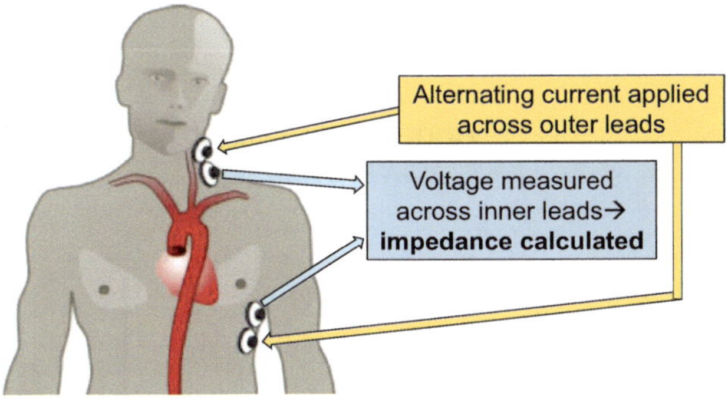

Fig. 8.14 How electrical cardiometry works. Electrical cardiometry works by passing an insensible alternating current of fixed maximum amplitude between the outer thoracic electrode patches and analyzing the voltage changes specific to the cardiac cycle which are produced between the inner electrode patches. The ratio of the voltage to the fixed maximum amplitude alternating current is the *magnitude of the impedance*, which is the equivalent for alternating current of *resistance* for direct current. Modified from [11] with permission

Blood Acceleration Decreases the Magnitude of Thoracic Impedance

In the model of electrical velocimetry (upon which electrical cardiometry is based), the decrease in thoracic impedance during systole is due to the alignment of red blood cells caused by blood acceleration, as shown in Fig. 8.15 [11]. This alignment facilitates the passage of electrical current, reducing the magnitude of the impedance. This alignment of accelerating red blood cells is not an all-or-none process. The greater the blood acceleration during systole, the greater the degree of red blood cell alignment—and the greater and more rapid will be the decrease in thoracic impedance during systole. *The maximum rate of decrease in thoracic impedance during systole is termed ICON, as shown in* Fig. 8.16 [12], *and ICON is a key parameter within the system of electrical cardiometry which I will now explain in greater detail.*

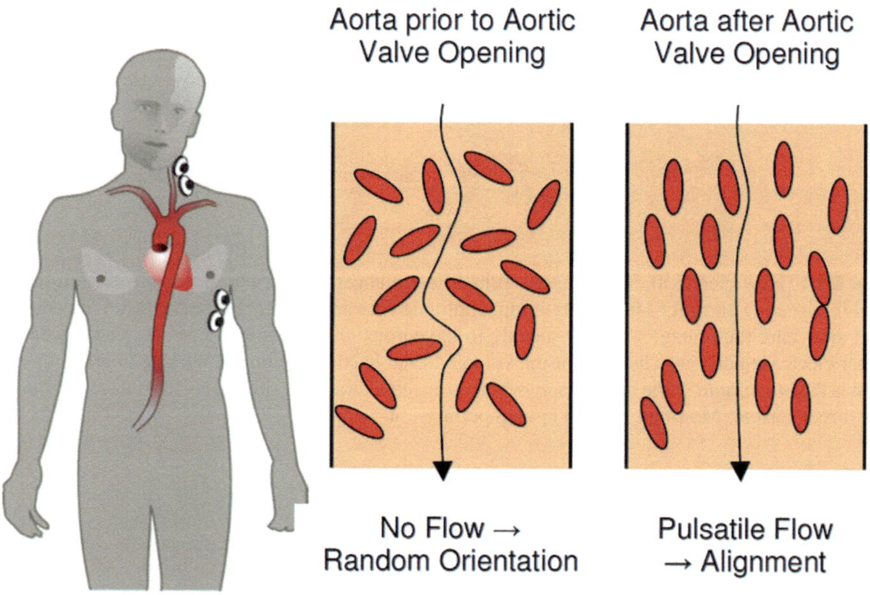

Fig. 8.15 Systolic blood acceleration causes red blood cell alignment, reduces thoracic impedance, and creates the ICON parameter. In the model of electrical velocimetry (upon which electrical cardiometry is based), the decrease in thoracic impedance during systole is due to the alignment of red blood cells *caused by blood acceleration.* This alignment facilitates the passage of electrical current, reducing the magnitude of the impedance. This alignment of accelerating red blood cells is not an all-or-none process. The greater the blood acceleration during systole, the greater the degree of red blood cell alignment—and the greater and more rapid will be the reduction in thoracic impedance during systole. *The maximum rate of decrease in thoracic impedance during systole is termed ICON and is shown graphically in* Fig. 8.16. From [11] with permission

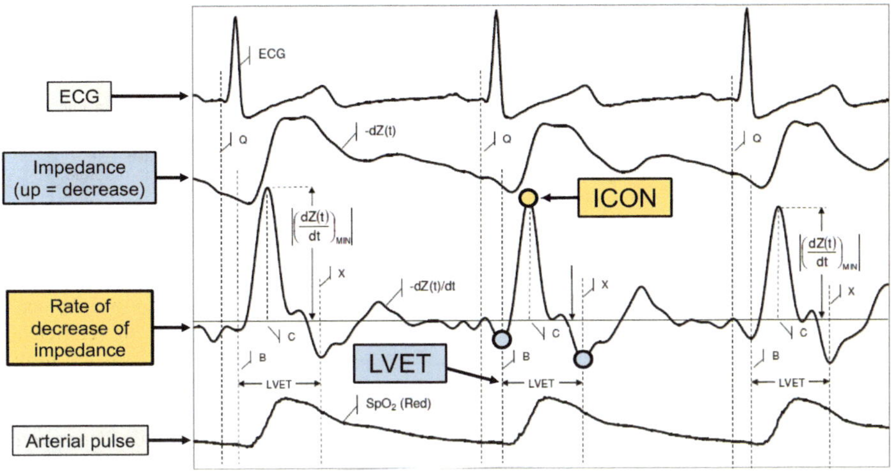

Fig. 8.16 Three data streams obtained from electrical cardiometry. The top three data streams (electrocardiogram, magnitude of thoracic impedance, and rate of decrease in impedance during systole) are obtained with electrical cardiometry. The bottom tracing is an arterial pulse waveform for comparison. Note that the tracing for magnitude of thoracic impedance has its y-axis reversed, with an upward deflection representing a *decrease* in impedance—which is done to make the impedance tracing resemble an arterial pressure waveform. The tracing for the rate of decrease in impedance during systole supplies two key parameters for the calculation of stroke volume: ICON (which correlates with Vmean from transthoracic echocardiography *only within a single individual,* as shown in Fig. 8.17) and the left ventricular ejection time (LVET), which correlates closely with the envelope time from transthoracic echocardiography *both within and between individuals* [5, 8]. The product of ICON and LVET constitutes an electrical cardiometry analog of the velocity–time integral, or stroke distance, obtained from transthoracic echocardiography. I think that this is a valuable insight which should be investigated further, since the stroke distance in a given person is always directly proportional to the true stroke volume, since the area of the left ventricular outflow tract in one person is fixed, and stroke volume is the product of the stroke distance and that fixed area. *ECG* electrocardiogram, *ICON* maximum rate of decrease in thoracic impedance during systole (the name stands for "index of contractility" and correlates with the maximum systolic blood acceleration in the ascending aorta within a single individual over time), *LVET* left ventricular ejection time. Modified from [11] with permission

ICON (or "Index of Contractility")

ICON is thought to correlate with the degree of systolic blood acceleration within the ascending aorta during systole and is used to derive an "index of mean blood velocity" during systole. This apparent transformation of a *degree of acceleration* into a *mean velocity* seems like a "leap of faith," but—*within individual patients over time*—ICON does appear to track mean systolic blood velocity ("Vmean") in the left ventricular outflow tract as measured by transthoracic echocardiography [5]. This tracking relationship is shown in Fig. 8.17, and the caption to that figure explains the apparent time lag between changes in Vmean and ICON.

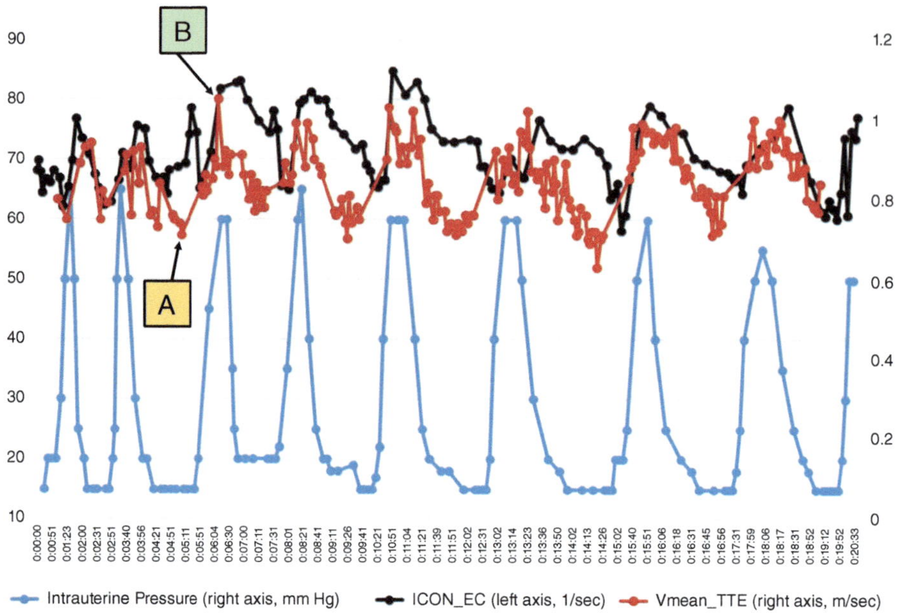

Fig. 8.17 ICON from electrical cardiometry correlates with Vmean from transthoracic echocardiography within one laboring patient. This figure shows Vmean and ICON during the same time period and circumstances as are shown in Fig. 8.12. Vmean is the mean systolic blood flow velocity in the left ventricular outflow tract as measured by transthoracic echocardiography. The ICON parameter from electrical cardiometry tracks Vmean well within this laboring patient, as stroke volume and cardiac output increase and decrease due to uterine contractions and autotransfusion. But the changes in ICON appear delayed at times and damped in amplitude compared to the changes in Vmean, probably due to the electrical cardiometry recording settings used [5] (Fig. 8.12). Points A and B correspond to the similarly labeled data points in Figs. 8.12 and 8.13. The correlation coefficient between ICON and Vmean for this data was $r = 0.51$, sig. = 0.000. *ICON_EC* index of contractility from electrical cardiometry, *Vmean_TTE* mean systolic blood velocity in the left ventricular outflow tract from transthoracic echocardiography

The key to the absolute accuracy—or inaccuracy—of electrical cardiometry for the determination of stroke volume is the following: the ICON parameter from electrical cardiometry can be used to calculate an estimate of Vmean, which then gives an estimate of stroke distance when it is multiplied by the duration of systole, the absolute values of which appear to be given accurately by electrical cardiometry [5, 8]. For measuring the absolute duration of systole, left ventricular ejection time from electrical cardiometry appears to agree well with envelope time from transthoracic echocardiography both within individuals over time [5] and between individuals [8]. In one validation study [8], mean envelope time from transthoracic echocardiography was 279 ms (SD = 23) and mean left ventricular ejection time (LVET) from electrical cardiometry was 274 ms (SD = 22). The mean bias between the two techniques for the duration of systole was −4.9 ms, and the mean percentage error was 12.7%.

This is a reassuring absolute agreement between the two technologies, which is similar to that shown in Fig. 8.3, in which the absolute values of the two technologies agree quite well. This stroke distance equivalent—obtained entirely from electrical cardiometry data—can then be multiplied by the area of the left ventricular outflow tract—or an estimate based on patient height—to obtain an estimate of the absolute stroke volume.

This is the logical progression of the attempt of this chapter to make electrical cardiometry "look like" transthoracic echocardiography, both conceptually and mathematically. In the current electrical cardiometry algorithm, the stroke distance equivalent is multiplied (or "scaled") by a proprietary "patient constant" which is predominantly based on patient weight (according to the manufacturer). This particular use of the weight parameter seems highly questionable if the purpose is to convert or "scale" the stroke distance into a volume, as shown in Fig. 8.18, in which the "proper" factor for scaling the stroke distance to become a volume is seen to be the area of the left ventricular outflow tract, rather than the patient's weight.

Another problem with the current electrical cardiometry algorithm appears to be that the specific relationship between ICON and Vmean appears to be different from person to person, depending on weight, body mass index, breast size, and age, as suggested in Fig. 8.19.

In other words, blood acceleration determines both Vmean and ICON, but other factors—which vary between individuals and have nothing to do with blood acceleration—appear to affect ICON as well. Each person appears to have her own relationship between Vmean and ICON, based not only on Vmean but also on other inter-individual variables (such as weight) which have nothing to do with blood acceleration, as shown schematically in Fig. 8.19.

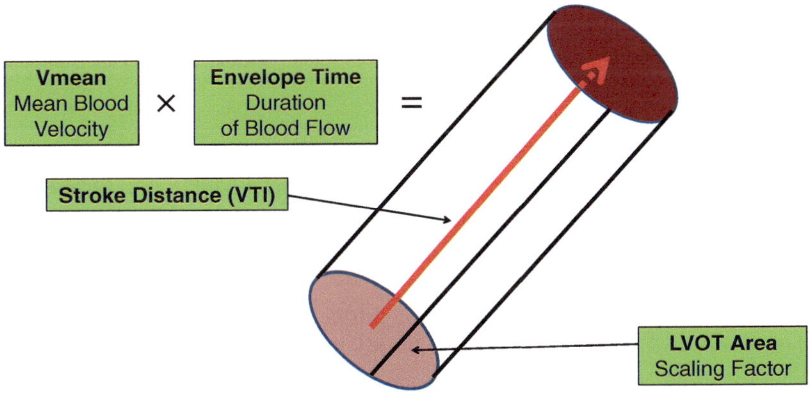

Fig. 8.18 Stroke volume conceptualized as the volume of a cylinder. This figure shows the same calculation as shown in Fig. 8.21, but here it is visualized as computing the volume of a cylinder. This is a very useful way of visualizing the process and it corresponds well to what is actually being measured in transthoracic echocardiography: velocity, time, and area (derived from diameter). *LVOT* left ventricular outflow tract, *Vmean* mean systolic blood flow velocity in the left ventricular outflow tract from transthoracic echocardiography, *VTI* velocity–time integral (or "stroke distance")

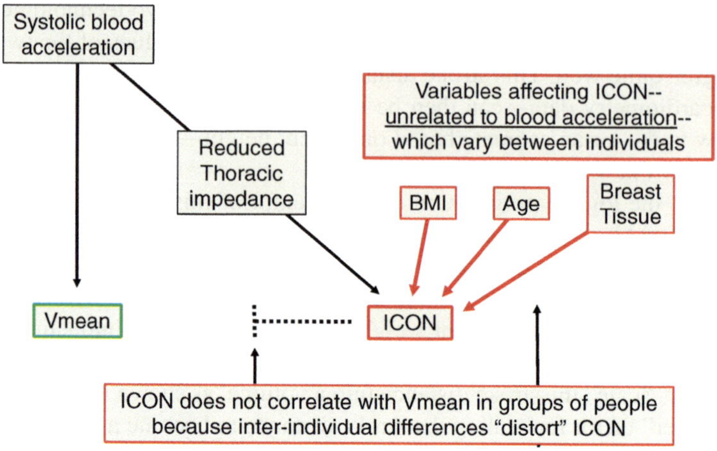

Fig. 8.19 One-time paired measurements in multiple individuals: why a validation study fails for electrical cardiometry. ICON does not correlate with Vmean in groups of people because inter-individual differences "distort" ICON in different ways. It would be very convenient if the only factor affecting the ICON measurement were blood acceleration and the reduction in thoracic impedance which that acceleration causes. But many other factors—which are extraneous to blood acceleration and stroke volume measurement, such as weight, body mass index (BMI), breast size or age—affect ICON as well, as suggested in this figure. Within a single individual, these extraneous factors still have their effect, *but that effect on ICON is constant over time*. Therefore, within a single individual, the effect of changing blood acceleration on ICON over time can be appreciated against a constant "background" (see Figs. 8.17 and 8.20). In groups of people, however, the blood acceleration which produces ICON still exists, of course, but from person to person the variation in the extraneous factors affecting ICON "overwhelms" the effect of blood acceleration, and ICON varies widely for a given true Vmean, depending on the specific weight, body mass index, breast size, and age of each individual participating in a group study, as suggested in this figure. *BMI* body mass index, *ICON* maximum rate of decrease in thoracic impedance during systole, *Vmean* mean systolic blood flow velocity in the left ventricular outflow tract from transthoracic echocardiography

When inter-individual factors (such as variations in weight) do not obscure the sought-for individual relationship of ICON to Vmean, ICON does trend reliably with Vmean within a single person over time—as shown in a laboring patient in Fig. 8.17 and schematically in Fig. 8.20.

The ability to usefully trend changes in cardiac output, without necessarily having the correct absolute values, is well accepted in modern fluid management [13, 14] and it would almost certainly be adequate in the management of pregnant patients when the primary goal is to avoid obstruction of uterine venous return by detecting a positional decrease in cardiac output.

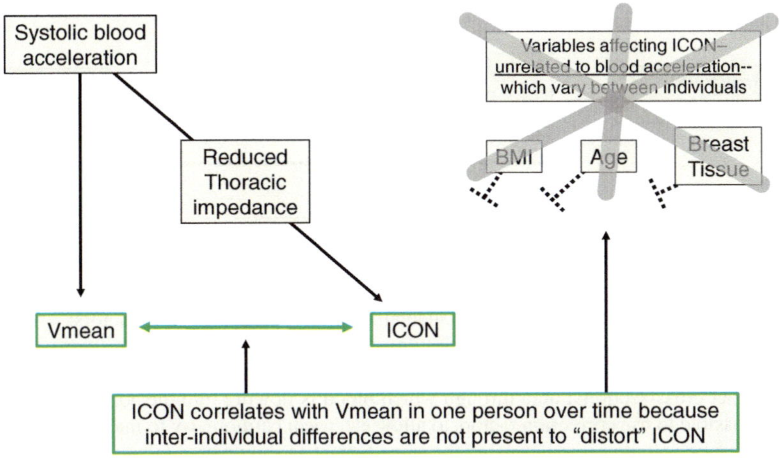

Fig. 8.20 Multiple paired measurements in a single individual over time: why a trending study succeeds for electrical cardiometry. ICON correlates with Vmean within one person over time because inter-individual differences are not present to "distort" ICON. Within a single individual, weight, body mass index, breast size, or age do not change over time. Within a single individual, these extraneous factors still have their effect, *but that effect on ICON is constant over time*. Therefore the effects of changing blood acceleration on both ICON and Vmean can be appreciated against a constant "background"—and ICON and Vmean trend together. *BMI* body mass index, *ICON* maximum rate of decrease in thoracic impedance during systole, *Vmean* mean systolic blood flow velocity in the left ventricular outflow tract from transthoracic echocardiography

Improving the Absolute Accuracy of Electrical Cardiometry

Although it is not needed for the purpose of detecting obstruction of uterine venous return within individual patients, Ballas et al. [12] and Anyikam et al. [15] have proposed methods for improving the absolute accuracy of electrical cardiometry in pregnant patients. These proposed modifications of the electrical cardiometry algorithm would make it correspond better with transthoracic echocardiography, both conceptually and mathematically. Figure 8.21 shows how stroke volume is calculated using transthoracic echocardiography, and Fig. 8.18 shows how this calculation can be conceptualized as the calculation of the volume of a cylinder. In our validation study with 44 pregnant non-laboring women, ICON from electrical cardiometry did not correlate significantly with Vmean from transthoracic echocardiography [8], as shown in Fig. 8.22, but Ballas et al. have developed a formula

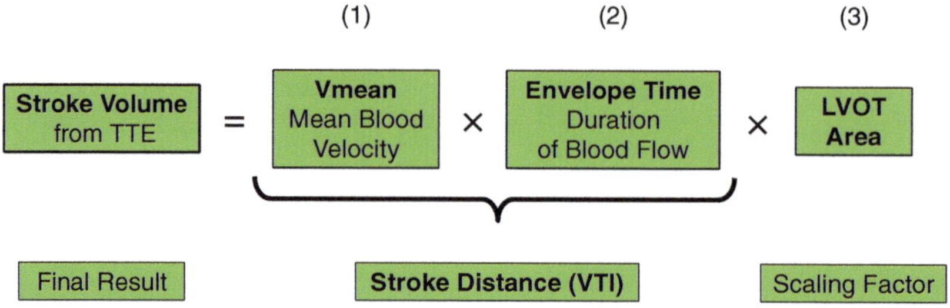

Fig. 8.21 Calculation of stroke volume from transthoracic echocardiography. In transthoracic echocardiography, the stroke volume is calculated as the product of three factors: Vmean (mean blood flow velocity in the left ventricular outflow tract during systole), envelope time (the duration of systolic blood flow in the left ventricular outflow tract during systole), and the left ventricular outflow tract cross-sectional area through which blood is flowing into the aorta during systole. It may be possible to use correction factors to allow electrical cardiometry to make usefully accurate *absolute* stroke volume estimates using the same format as shown here (also see Fig. 8.23). *LVOT* left ventricular outflow tract, *TTE* transthoracic echocardiography, *Vmean* mean systolic blood flow velocity in the left ventricular outflow tract from transthoracic echocardiography, *VTI* velocity–time integral (or stroke distance)

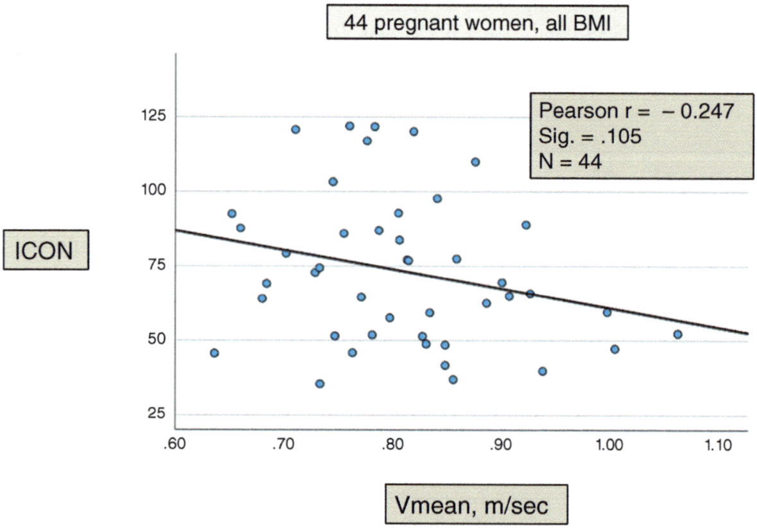

Fig. 8.22 In a multiple person validation study ICON has no correlation with Vmean—because of inter-individual variations in BMI and other factors. Unlike the situation within a single individual over time, there is no correlation between ICON and Vmean in a group of individuals. This may be due to "interference" in the "visibility" of the relationship due to inter-individual variations in BMI, weight, breast size, and age, as suggested in Fig. 8.19. *BMI* body mass index, *ICON* index of contractility (from electrical cardiometry), *Vmean* mean velocity of blood flow in the left ventricular outflow tract during systole (from transthoracic echocardiography)

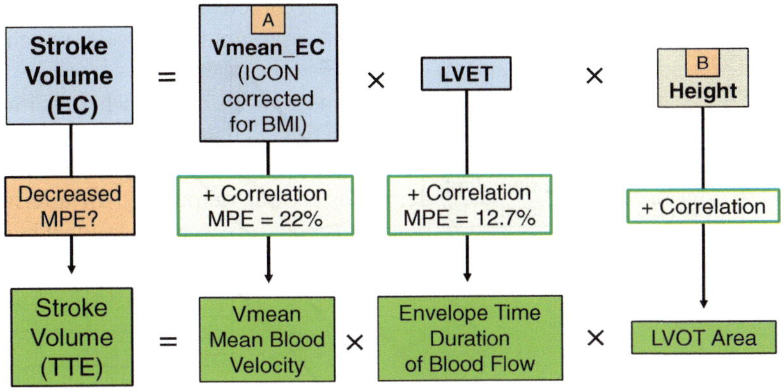

Fig. 8.23 Electrical cardiometry can be made to "look like" transthoracic echocardiography. With the modifications to ICON based on body mass index proposed by Ballas et al. [12] and the use of patient height to estimate left ventricular outflow tract area as proposed by Anyikam et al. [15], electrical cardiometry stroke volume values might attain better absolute agreement with transthoracic echocardiography values, as suggested in this figure. Left ventricular ejection time from electrical cardiometry has been shown in at least two studies [5, 8] to agree with envelope time from transthoracic echocardiography with a low mean percentage error. The modification of ICON using body mass index proposed by Ballas et al. results in a 22% mean percentage error for the estimation of Vmean from electrical cardiometry data alone. This estimate of Vmean using ICON and body mass index is shown in the figure as "Vmean_EC" and is labeled with an "A." Finally, the use of height to estimate left ventricular outflow tract area (shown as modification "B" in the figure) would eliminate the need to independently measure left ventricular outflow tract diameter using hand-held transthoracic echocardiography. Thus, with these two modifications—"A" and "B"—perhaps electrical cardiometry would give absolute estimates of stroke volume in better agreement with those obtained from transthoracic echocardiography in pregnant patients. *BMI* body mass index, *EC* electrical cardiometry, *ICON* "index of contractility" defined as maximum rate of decrease in thoracic impedance during systole, which correlates with Vmean within individual people over time, *LVET* left ventricular ejection time, *LVOT* left ventricular outflow tract, *MPE* mean percentage error, *TTE* transthoracic echocardiography, *Vmean_EC* a prediction of Vmean (separately obtained from TTE) using only ICON and body mass index (BMI)

which corrects the measured ICON value for the body mass index and thereby predicts Vmean (as would be measured by transthoracic echocardiography) with a 22% mean percentage error in pregnant patients [12]. Also, Anyikam et al. have proposed using patient height (which is correlated with left ventricular outflow tract area, unlike patient weight) as a "scaling factor" for the electrical cardiometry equivalent of stroke distance [15], and the Ballas and Anyikam proposals are shown together schematically in Figs. 8.23 and 8.24.

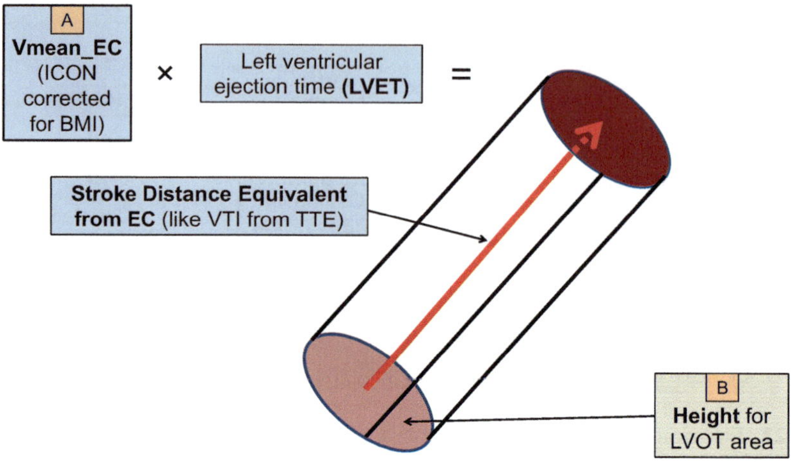

Fig. 8.24 The proposed revision of the electrical cardiometry algorithm, visualized as the calculation of the volume of a cylinder. This figure is meant to be analogous to Fig. 8.18. In this analogy, the "stroke distance equivalent" (from electrical cardiometry data only) is the product of "Vmean_EC" as proposed by Ballas et al. [12] and the left ventricular ejection time. This "stroke distance equivalent" is then "scaled" by an estimate of left ventricular outflow tract area based on patient height [15]. *Using those two modifications, it may be possible to obtain absolute stroke volume estimates based only on electrical cardiometry data alone, which have an acceptably low mean percentage error in comparison to transthoracic echocardiography. If this were possible, it might mean that electrical cardiometry could not only be a highly useful tool for trending cardiac output in pregnant patients but also a valuable tool for measuring its absolute value with "useful" accuracy! BMI* body mass index, *EC* electrical cardiometry, ICON "index of contractility" defined as maximum rate of decrease in thoracic impedance during systole, which correlates with Vmean within individual people over time, *LVET* left ventricular ejection time, *LVOT* left ventricular outflow tract, *MPE* mean percentage error, *TTE* transthoracic echocardiography, *Vmean_EC* a prediction of Vmean (separately obtained from TTE) using only ICON and body mass index, *VTI* velocity–time integral

With these two modifications of electrical cardiometry, it may be possible to use electrical cardiometry data alone—namely ICON, left ventricular ejection time, weight or BMI, and height—to obtain more accurate absolute estimates of Vmean, envelope time, and left ventricular outflow tract area which can then be used to calculate stroke volume and cardiac output. This improvement in the absolute accuracy of electrical cardiometry might make it less frequently necessary to use the much more cumbersome and labor-intensive procedure of transthoracic echocardiography when a usefully accurate absolute estimate of cardiac output is required. In this modification process, electrical cardiometry would be improved in two ways: (1) it would come to resemble transthoracic echocardiography more closely than it does at present, both conceptually and mathematically, and (2) the absolute value results for stroke volume and cardiac output in pregnant patients might have a much lower mean percentage error in comparison to transthoracic echocardiography than they have at present—meaning, in short, that they would be "more accurate" in comparison to an accepted reference standard.

An Example of Correcting ICON for BMI to Arrive at an Estimate of Vmean

Although it is not necessary to follow the argument of this book, I am providing in this chapter an example of how one might correct ICON for BMI in order to arrive at a more accurate absolute estimate of Vmean, which is derived from transthoracic echocardiography. Note that this process derives an estimate of a value normally acquired using the labor-intensive technique of transthoracic echocardiography but uses only electrical cardiometry data (ICON and BMI), which is very easy to acquire in a continuous and hands-free manner. This example is based on the data set from [8], which is an expanded version of the data acquired and used by Ballas et al. and Anyikam in [10, 12, 15]. This example is not meant to be definitive in any way but is included here as an example of the statistical methods which can be used to clarify the relationship between two variables (such as Vmean and ICON) when a third variable (such as BMI) has a strong influence on one of the first two variables considered (ICON, in this case).

The example is presented in Figs. 8.25, 8.26, 8.27, 8.28, and 8.29 and their captions, but this example is included only for interested readers, since it is quite "technical" and reviewing it is not necessary in order to follow the main argument of this book. The data used for this example were obtained during the studies which are described in [8], but much of this data was not published in those references. I received permission to use this previously unpublished data from Dr. Ruth Waterman, Professor and Chair of the Department of Anesthesiology of the University of California San Diego, and from UC San Diego Services and Support.

Correlations

		BMI	Vmean	ICON	ICON_div_Vmean
BMI	Pearson Correlation	1	.625**	−.645**	−.752**
	Sig. (2-tailed)		<.001	<.001	<.001
	N	39	39	39	39
Vmean	Pearson Correlation	.625**	1	−.254	−.505**
	Sig. (2-tailed)	<.001		.119	.001
	N	39	39	39	39
ICON	Pearson Correlation	−.645**	−.254	1	.957**
	Sig. (2-tailed)	<.001	.119		<.001
	N	39	39	39	39
ICON_div_Vmean	Pearson Correlation	−.752**	−.505**	.957**	1
	Sig. (2-tailed)	<.001	.001	<.001	
	N	39	39	39	39

**. Correlation is significant at the 0.01 level (2-tailed).

Fig. 8.25 Correlation matrix used to correct ICON for BMI in order to obtain an improved absolute estimate of Vmean based solely on electrical cardiometry data

Review of basic concepts and goals of this exercise: "Vmean" is a value and concept derived from transthoracic echocardiography. It is the mean velocity of blood flow in the left ventricular outflow tract during systole and is multiplied by the envelope time (or duration of systole, also obtained from transthoracic echocardiography) to obtain the velocity–time integral, also known as the "VTI" or the "stroke distance." This stroke distance is then multiplied by the area of the left ventricular outflow tract in order to calculate the stroke volume, as shown in Figs. 8.18 and 8.21. The mean systolic blood flow velocity (measured by transthoracic echocardiography as "Vmean") appears to be the "weak link" in obtaining an accurate absolute estimate of stroke volume from electrical cardiometry, because the implicit blood velocity assumptions used within the current version of electrical cardiometry do not appear to give good results in pregnant women. Unlike Vmean, the duration of systole ***can*** be estimated with a low mean percentage error from the electrical cardiometry parameter "left ventricular ejection time."

Therefore, improving the estimate of Vmean (which would be obtained using transthoracic echocardiography) based on electrical cardiometry information alone would greatly improve the absolute accuracy of the stroke volume estimate obtained from electrical cardiometry. *We have called this estimate or prediction of the transthoracic echocardiography parameter Vmean, based on EC information alone, "Vmean_EC."*

Correlation matrix for BMI, Vmean, ICON, and ICON/Vmean for 39 pregnant women with BMI ≤40. This example begins with the correlation matrix shown in this figure from 39 pregnant women whose BMI ≤40. This matrix shows that (1) Vmean does not correlate significantly with ICON in this group of pregnant women (see also Fig. 8.26), (2) BMI correlates very well (positively and with a high Pearson correlation coefficient and high significance) with Vmean (see also Fig. 8.27), which is consistent with the basic physiological concept that heavier pregnant women require a higher cardiac output than lighter women, and that a higher Vmean may be part of the maternal cardiovascular system's solution to that need, and (3) BMI correlates very well (negatively and with a high Pearson correlation coefficient and high significance) with ICON (see also Fig. 8.28), which is consistent with the idea that adipose tissue lowers ICON in some systematic way that has nothing to do with the observed positive correlation between Vmean and ICON which is found within individuals over time, and (4) BMI correlates very well (negatively and with a high Pearson correlation coefficient and high significance) with ICON/Vmean (see also Fig. 8.29), which suggests that for a given true Vmean (1.0 m/s, for example), the ICON value which corresponds to that velocity will decrease as the person's BMI increases. *BMI* body mass index, ICON index of contractility (from electrical cardiometry), ICON_div_Vmean the quantity ICON divided by the quantity Vmean, Vmean mean velocity of blood flow in the left ventricular outflow tract during systole (from transthoracic echocardiography)

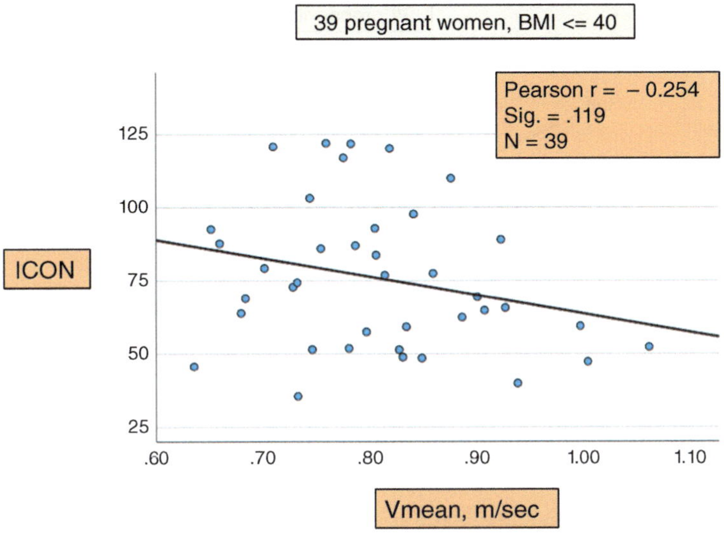

Fig. 8.26 ICON from electrical cardiometry completely fails to estimate Vmean from transthoracic echocardiography in a validation study of 39 pregnant women with BMI ≤40. Compare this figure (which contains real data) [8] with the fictitious example shown in Fig. 8.8 (in which cardiac output is the variable being measured). Within one individual over time, ICON tracks Vmean usefully, but in this real validation study it fails completely to estimate Vmean—probably due to interference from factors (such as BMI, breast size, or age) which vary from person to person. *BMI* body mass index, *ICON* index of contractility, from electrical cardiometry, *Vmean* mean velocity of blood flow in the left ventricular outflow tract during systole, from transthoracic echocardiography

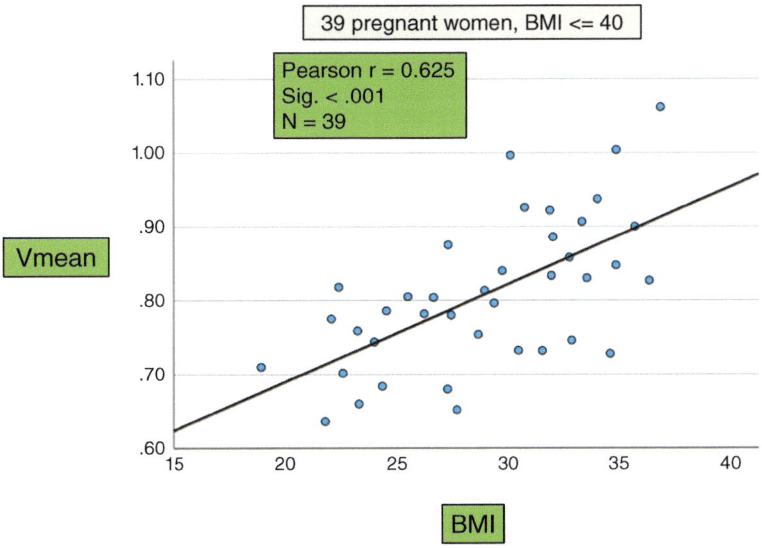

Fig. 8.27 Vmean from transthoracic echocardiography increases with increasing BMI in a validation study of 39 pregnant women with BMI ≤40 [8]. This finding is consistent with the fact that heavy pregnant women will need a higher cardiac output than lighter women, and that an increased Vmean—an additional stress on the maternal cardiovascular system—is part of the solution to that need. *BMI* body mass index

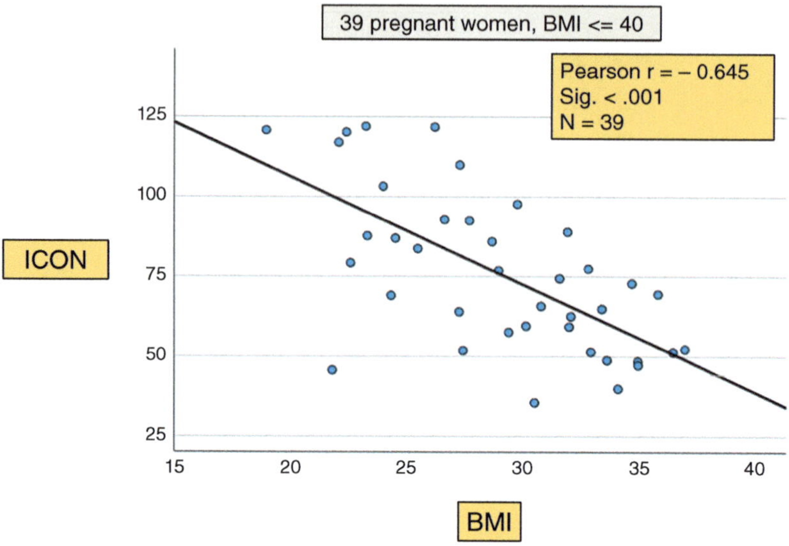

Fig. 8.28 ICON from electrical cardiometry decreases with increasing BMI in a validation study of 39 pregnant women with BMI ≤40 [8]. This data shows a profound "disconnect" between ICON and Vmean when multiple individuals are studies together. Within an individual, ICON tracks Vmean over time, but in a group of healthy pregnant women with differing body mass indices, increasing BMI systematically decreases the ICON parameter. This "interference" in the relationship between Vmean and ICON by factors having nothing to do with blood acceleration or velocity is shown schematically in Fig. 8.19

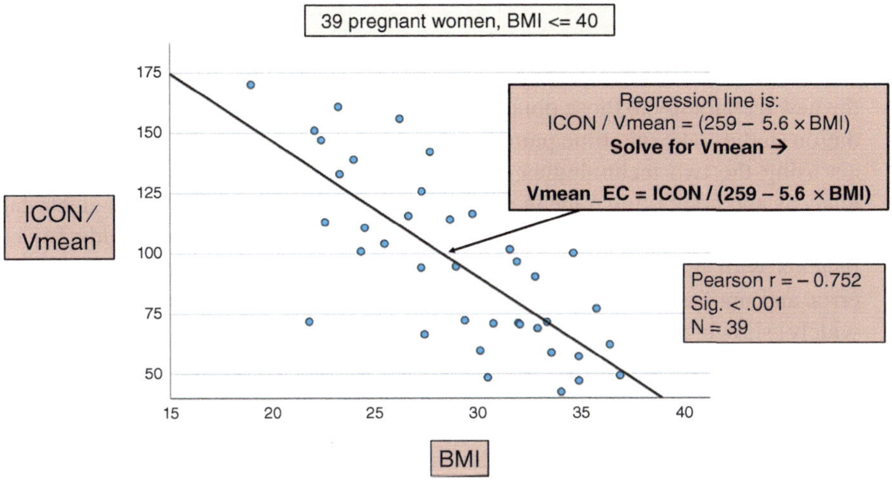

Fig. 8.29 The ratio of ICON to Vmean decreases with increasing BMI in a validation study of 39 pregnant women with BMI ≤40. This is the key figure for the process of trying to "correct" ICON for BMI in order to enable electrical cardiometry to produce useful absolute estimates (or "predictions") of the Vmean parameter using electrical cardiometry data alone. If this were possible in current practice, it would save large amounts of time and effort by making labor-intensive transthoracic echocardiography unnecessary in many clinical situations, even when absolute values for cardiac output are desired, rather than just trends. The process is as follows: the ratio of ICON to Vmean is plotted against the BMI and a regression equation is determined which describes the relationship between that ratio (ICON/Vmean) and BMI. The regression equation for the data shown in the figure is: ICON/Vmean = (259 – 5.6 × BMI). This equation is then solved for Vmean, which becomes "Vmean_EC" since it is an estimate of a transthoracic echocardiography parameter utilizing only electrical cardiometry data (ICON). This equivalent equation is: Vmean_EC = ICON/(259 – 5.6 × BMI). It can be seen from this equation that for a given true Vmean (1.0 m/s, for example), an increase in BMI will produce a decrease in ICON, which is what is observed in the graphical figures. Summary and discussion of this example: This example demonstrates a method of deriving an absolute estimate of Vmean which would be obtained from transthoracic echocardiography, utilizing only the ICON parameter from electrical cardiometry. This estimate of Vmean is called "Vmean_EC." *The example shown does not represent the identical process used in* [5, 8, 10, 12], *and the results of this example (while based on similar real data) will differ from the results presented in those references.* This example is presented as an educational exercise only and is meant to stimulate further research

Absolute Accuracy of Cardiac Output "Measurements" Not Needed for Detecting and Preventing Obstruction of Uterine Venous Return

Finally, it needs to be reiterated that absolute accuracy of cardiac output measurements would almost certainly not be necessary for the detection and prevention of obstruction of uterine venous return. Furthermore, it should be emphasized that other techniques may be developed which are superior to electrical cardiometry for trending maternal cardiac output during pregnancy and thereby preventing obstruction of uterine venous return.

Chapter Summary

1. Validation studies of new technology compare the absolute values obtained from the new technology to those obtained using a reference standard. Generally, validation studies take one-time paired measurements from many different individuals using the two technologies, and compare the results using Bland–Altman analysis and computing a mean percentage error. Validation studies of electrical cardiometry in pregnant patients have been equivocal—with one study [4] in patients with little variation in body weight showing a low mean percentage error and another study (in which the weights of the participants varied more widely) showing a much higher mean percentage error [8].
2. Trending studies evaluate whether a new technology agrees with a reference standard in identifying *the direction of change of cardiac output within one individual over time.* Electrical cardiometry appears to successfully identify trends in cardiac output within individuals over time, and this should be sufficient to use it (or any other successful trending technology) for cardiac output-guided maternal positioning to avoid obstruction of uterine venous return.
3. Within individual patients over time—but not between one-time paired measurements from multiple individuals—the ICON parameter from electrical cardiometry correlates with Vmean, which is the mean systolic blood velocity in the left ventricular outflow tract as measured by transthoracic echocardiography. But ICON is also affected by weight, body mass index, breast size and age, and these inter-individual differences—which have nothing to do with blood acceleration or velocity—probably prevent electrical cardiometry from giving acceptably accurate absolute values for cardiac output in pregnant patients. What this means is that each person probably has her own relationship between ICON and Vmean, depending on several individual factors.
4. The absolute accuracy of the stroke volume and cardiac output estimates from electrical cardiometry in pregnant patients may be able to be improved using correction factors involving patient BMI or weight, and height and the ICON parameter from electrical cardiometry. With respect to the duration of systole, electrical cardiometry seems to agree well with transthoracic echocardiography, both within single patients over time and between patients.

References

1. Archer TL, Conrad BE. Electrical velocimetry follows the hemodynamics of drug therapy and aortocaval compression in preeclampsia. Int J Obstet Anesth. 2011;20(1):91–2. https://doi.org/10.1016/j.ijoa.2010.08.001. Epub 2010 Dec 3. PMID: 21126865.
2. Archer TL. Electrical velocimetry elucidates the hemodynamics of hypertension caused by indigo carmine. J Clin Anesth. 2011;23(2):166–8. https://doi.org/10.1016/j.jclinane.2010.02.013. PMID: 21377084.
3. Archer TL, Conrad BE, Suresh P, Tarsa M. Electrical velocimetry demonstrates the increase in cardiac output and decrease in systemic vascular resistance accompanying cesarean delivery

and oxytocin administration. J Clin Anesth. 2012;24(1):79–82. https://doi.org/10.1016/j.jclinane.2011.02.014. PMID: 22284326.
4. Yoshida A, Kaji T, Yamada H, Yonetani N, Sogawa E, Yamao M, Maeda K, Sata M, Irahara M. Measurement of hemodynamics immediately after vaginal delivery in healthy pregnant women by electrical cardiometry. J Med Invest. 2019;66(1):75–80. https://doi.org/10.2152/jmi.66.75. PMID: 31064959.
5. Archer TL. Transthoracic echocardiography and electrical cardiometry elucidate the hemodynamics of autotransfusion during labor under epidural analgesia. Int J Obstet Anesth. 2017;31:113–5. https://doi.org/10.1016/j.ijoa.2017.03.010. Epub 2017 Mar 24. PMID: 28676402.
6. Feng SM, Liu J. Electrical velocimetry has limited accuracy and precision and moderate trending ability compared with transthoracic echocardiography for cardiac output measurement during cesarean delivery: a prospective observational study. Medicine. 2020;99(34):e21914. https://doi.org/10.1097/MD.0000000000021914.
7. Liu Y, Pian-Smith MC, Leffert LR, Minehart RD, Torri A, Coté C, Kacmarek RM, Jiang Y. Continuous measurement of cardiac output with the electrical velocimetry method in patients under spinal anesthesia for cesarean delivery. J Clin Monit Comput. 2015;29(5):627–34. https://doi.org/10.1007/s10877-014-9645-8. Epub 2014 Dec 16. PMID: 25510959.
8. Martin E, Anyikam A, Ballas J, Buono K, Mantell K, Huynh-Covey T, Archer T. A validation study of electrical cardiometry in pregnant patients using transthoracic echocardiography as the reference standard. J Clin Monit Comput. 2016;30(5):679–86. https://doi.org/10.1007/s10877-015-9771-y. Epub 2015 Sep 24. PMID: 26403606.
9. Critchley LA, Lee A, Ho AM. A critical review of the ability of continuous cardiac output monitors to measure trends in cardiac output. Anesth Analg. 2010;111(5):1180–92. https://doi.org/10.1213/ANE.0b013e3181f08a5b. Epub 2010 Aug 24. PMID: 20736431.
10. Ballas J, et al. Abstract/Poster # 733: Electrical cardiometry provides a continuous, non-invasive method of trending cardiac output in labor. Am J Obstet Gynecol. 2014;210(1):S359. Accessed at: https://www.ajog.org/article/S0002-9378(13)01831-0/fulltext.
11. https://osypka-asia.com/pdf/technique.pdf. Accessed 21 September 2023.
12. Ballas J, et al. Abstract/Poster # 734: Electrical cardiometry, when controlled for body mass index, accurately predicts the velocity-time integral utilized by transthoracic echocardiography to measure maternal cardiac output in pregnancy. Am J Obstet Gynecol. 2014;210(1):S359–60. Accessed at: https://www.ajog.org/article/S0002-9378(13)01832-2/fulltext.
13. Monnet X, Marik PE, Teboul JL. Prediction of fluid responsiveness: an update. Ann Intensive Care. 2016;6(1):111. https://doi.org/10.1186/s13613-016-0216-7. Epub 2016 Nov 17. PMID: 27858374; PMCID: PMC5114218.
14. Shi R, Monnet X, Teboul JL. Parameters of fluid responsiveness. Curr Opin Crit Care. 2020;26(3):319–26. https://doi.org/10.1097/MCC.0000000000000723. PMID: 32332283.
15. Anyikam A, et al. Abstract/Poster #467: Predicting left ventricular outflow tract area to improve thoracic impedance cardiography estimation of cardiac output among antepartum patients. Am J Obstet Gynecol. 2015;212(1):S238. Accessed at: https://www.ajog.org/article/S0002-9378(14)01568-3/fulltext.

Parallels Between Myometrium and Myocardium

9

Personal Note
In anesthesiology training, discussions of the determinants of *myocardial* oxygen supply and demand are frequent and detailed, since a solid knowledge of the subject is required to take care of patients. In order to maximize the heart's supply of oxygen and minimize its demand, anesthesiologists, cardiologists, and other critical care physicians routinely adjust a patient's heart rate, heart volume (preload), and systolic and diastolic blood pressures. For the long-term health of the heart, cardiologists use medications such as beta-blockers and antagonists of the renin–angiotensin–aldosterone system to prevent or at least slow the harmful remodeling of cardiac muscle which occurs in response to stress.

Despite the fact that the heart and the uterus are both hollow and contractile muscular organs which need oxygen to do their essential jobs, little research has been performed on the determinants of *myometrial* oxygen supply and demand. Susan Wray and others have emphasized the dangers of myometrial hypoxia [1] and have suggested that myometrial hypoxia may play a role in dysfunctional labor [2]. Wiberg-Itzel et al. have studied amniotic fluid lactic acid as an indicator of dysfunctional labor [3], and I have suggested that obstruction of uterine venous return may play a role in dysfunctional labor [4], but compared to the amount of research performed on the oxygenation of cardiac muscle, the myometrium has received little attention.

Myometrial and Myocardial Oxygen Supply and Demand

On 24 June 2023, I entered search terms regarding myometrial and myocardial oxygenation into the PubMed online search engine and obtained the results shown in Table 9.1. The immense difference between the number of publications about the oxygenation of the heart and the uterus supports my contention that the short- and long-term oxygenation of the myometrium have not received sufficient attention.

T. L. Archer, *Threats to Fetal, Placental and Myometrial Oxygenation*,
https://doi.org/10.1007/978-3-031-60364-8_9

Table 9.1 PubMed references for search terms found on 24 June 2023

Search term	Number of references
Myometrial oxygen demand	0
Myocardial oxygen demand	3093
Myometrial oxygen supply	22
Myocardial oxygen supply	4920
Myometrial oxygen supply and demand	0
Myocardial oxygen supply and demand	1374
Myometrial perfusion	119
Myocardial perfusion	54,751
Myometrial hypoxia	95
Myocardial hypoxia	14,009
Myometrial oxygenation	107
Myocardial oxygenation	40,374

The current treatment for a failing myometrium during labor is oxytocin, not oxygen, not more oxygen supplied by improved perfusion, and I have never heard obstetricians discussing how to increase myometrial oxygen supply or decrease myometrial oxygen demand—although it may be a common part of obstetrics training of which I am simply unaware. Also, I am not aware of any attempts to resuscitate a hypoxic myometrium inside the mother, although it has been proposed [5].

Applying Cardiac Physiology to the Uterus

In this book, I have tried to apply to the uterus the same biomechanical and physiological principles that have been applied to the heart, involving Laplace's law, tissue pressure, perfusion pressure, and tissue oxygenation. What can we learn from work on the *myocardium* that might be applicable to the *myometrium*?

One lesson is that cardiologists have regarded increased myocardial tissue pressure as an impediment to myocardial perfusion, oxygenation, and function. Figure 9.1 and its caption present the role of tissue pressure in limiting tissue perfusion when tissue pressure exceeds venous pressure. One term for this type of perfusion limited by external tissue pressure (or alveolar gas pressure within the lung) is "sluice flow." Sluice flow may occur in chorionic villi when increased intervillous space pressure literally "squeezes" fetal perfusion out of the chorionic villi, until umbilical artery pressure is high enough to overcome the increased tissue pressure within the chorionic villi (see Fig. 4.8).

One surrogate measurement cardiologists use to track myocardial tissue pressure is the left ventricular end-diastolic pressure (LVEDP). This pressure compresses the *myocardium* from the *inside* of the cardiac chamber and reduces perfusion of the subendocardium, much as an obese abdominal wall might compress an area of *myometrium* from the *outside* of the uterus and thereby limit myometrial or placental perfusion.

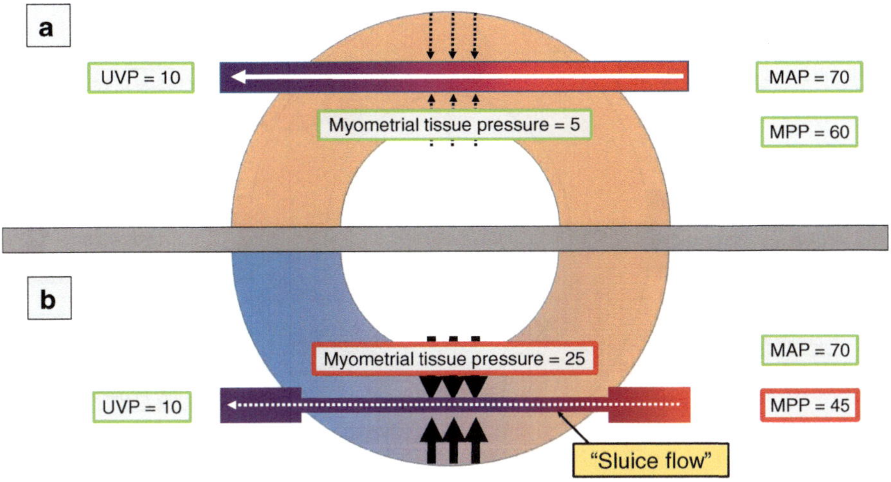

Fig. 9.1 What is the perfusion pressure of a tissue? What is "sluice flow"? Perfusion pressure is usually defined simply as the arterial inflow pressure minus the venous outflow pressure. In panel (**a**), the myometrial perfusion pressure is the mean arterial pressure (70 mmHg) minus the uterine venous pressure (10 mmHg), or 60 mmHg. But what happens if the tissue being perfused is edematous or under tension or external pressure, and the tissue pressure is higher than the venous pressure? In this case, perfusion pressure is defined as mean arterial pressure minus tissue pressure, as shown in panel (**b**), in which the myometrial perfusion pressure is the mean arterial pressure (70 mmHg) minus the myometrial tissue pressure (25 mmHg), or 45 mmHg. This is an example of the reduced pressure differential driving "sluice flow" within the myometrium. But "sluice flow" occurs within the chorionic villi as well—and wherever tissue pressure exceeds venous pressure. Obstruction of uterine venous return increases intervillous space pressure, which will compress the chorionic villi, raising their own tissue pressure and opposing fetoplacental perfusion (see also Fig. 4.8). This is one of the key concepts presented in this book: that increased intervillous space pressure will decrease chorionic villus perfusion, in the phenomenon which has been named "sluice flow." *Please note: Pressures (shown in mmHg) are only approximate and meant for illustrative purposes only*. *MAP* mean arterial pressure, *MPP* myometrial perfusion pressure, *UVP* uterine venous pressure

Elevations of left ventricular end-diastolic pressure are associated with myocardial ischemia, infarction, and heart failure [6, 7], leading to the theory that elevated left ventricular end-diastolic pressure increases myocardial tissue pressure and decreases myocardial perfusion and oxygenation, and some cardiac therapies do intentionally reduce left ventricular end-diastolic pressure, such as the use of nitrates in angina or diuretics in heart failure. Figure 9.2 shows the favorable myocardial perfusion associated with low tissue pressure as quantified by a low left ventricular end-diastolic pressure, and Fig. 9.3 shows how the oxygenation of the myocardium may deteriorate when the left ventricular end-diastolic pressure is elevated, in another example of "sluice flow."

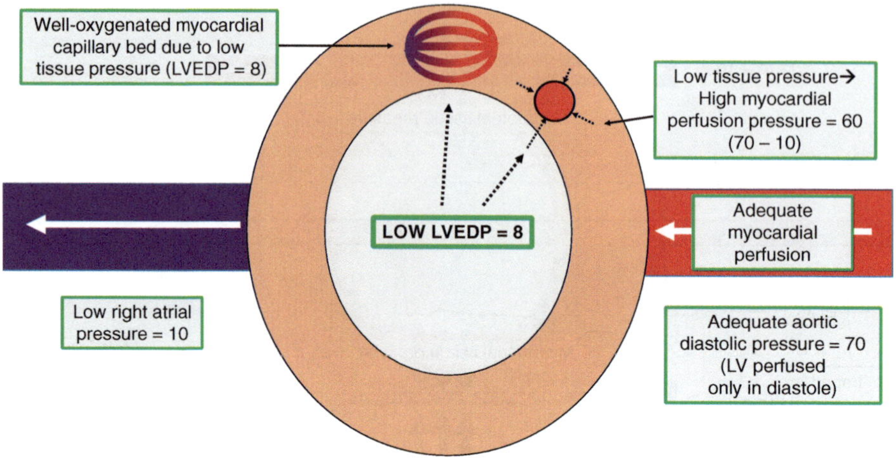

Fig. 9.2 Low tissue pressure and high perfusion pressure in the healthy heart. In this healthy heart (which could also be a healthy uterus!), the low tissue pressure in the wall of the left ventricle (8 mmHg) means that the perfusion pressure of the ventricle is the diastolic blood pressure in the aortic root minus the right atrial pressure, since the left ventricle is only perfused during diastole and the coronary circulation drains into the right atrium. In this example, the perfusion pressure of the left ventricle is 60 mmHg (or 70–10) and the myocardium is well oxygenated. *Please note: Pressures (shown in mmHg) are only approximate and meant for illustrative purposes only. LV* left ventricle, *LVEDP* left ventricular end-diastolic pressure

Elevated myometrial tissue pressure may have a similar effect within the uterus, reducing perfusion of *both the myometrium and the placenta*. The causes of increased myometrial tissue pressure may be increased uterine size (via Laplace's law) or the external myometrial compression produced by obesity or short stature. For both myocardium and myometrium, the causes of decreased oxygen supply are shown in Fig. 9.4, and the causes of increased oxygen demand are shown in Fig. 9.5.

Many of these stresses are unavoidable, of course, but we should do what we can—both during labor and earlier in gestation—to optimize fetal, placental, and myometrial oxygenation. It would seem appropriate to investigate whether "position therapy" might reduce dangerous levels of myometrial tissue pressure in some patients, as well as decrease uterine venous pressure. We should do what we can to improve perfusion of the myometrium and placenta, even if some of the impediments to perfusion cannot be eliminated.

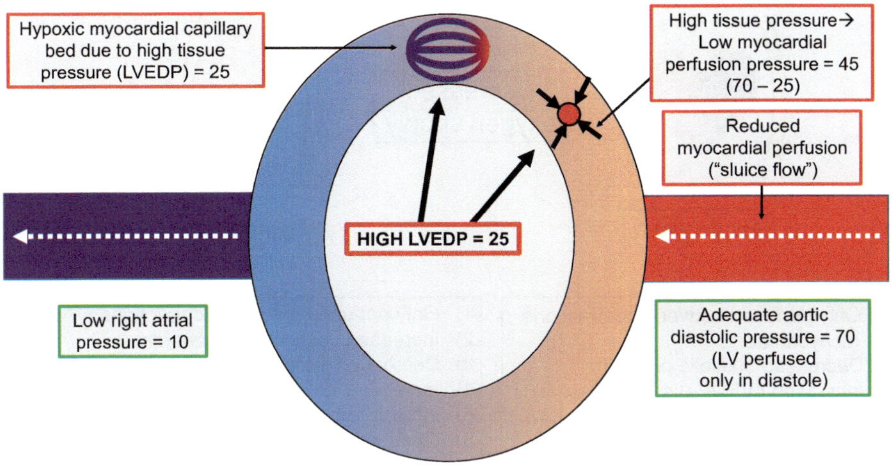

Fig. 9.3 High tissue pressure and low perfusion pressure in the ischemic and failing heart. In this ischemic and failing heart (which could also be the uterus of a short and obese woman lying in the supine position during labor), the high tissue pressure in the wall of the left ventricle (25 mmHg) means that the perfusion pressure of the ventricle is the diastolic blood pressure in the aortic root minus the elevated tissue pressure (25 mmHg). In this example, the perfusion pressure of the left ventricle is 45 mmHg (or 70–25) and the myocardium is ischemic, which will cause it to contract poorly and continue to fail. The treatment in this cardiac patient might involve decreasing myocardial oxygen requirements by diuresing the patient to reduce heart size or by opening up blocked coronary arteries. Analogous treatment in a uterus that was ischemic due to increased tissue pressure might be for the patient to avoid the supine position, which would reduce the pressure of the obese abdominal wall on the myometrium, as well as decrease uterine venous pressure. *Please note: Pressures (shown in mmHg) are only approximate and meant for illustrative purposes only. LV* left ventricle, *LVEDP* left ventricular end-diastolic pressure

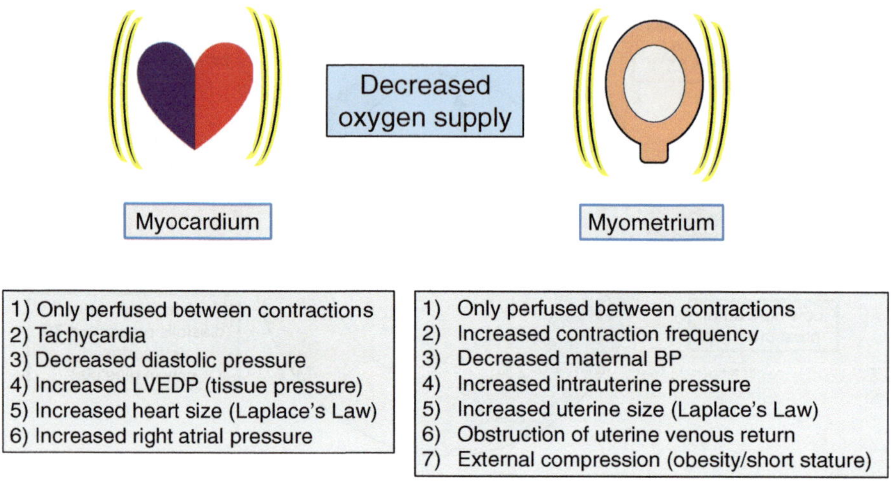

Fig. 9.4 The causes of decreased myocardial and myometrial oxygen supply. For both the heart and the myometrium, frequent contractions increase oxygen demand and limit oxygen supply. This is the most important message regarding oxygen supply and demand for both organs. But perfusion pressure, or the arterial inflow pressure minus the venous outflow pressure (or the tissue pressure, when it exceeds venous pressure), plays a major role in the oxygen supply of both organs as well. For example, each of the following three scenarios will reduce myometrial oxygen supply: (1) a reduction in maternal blood pressure, perhaps caused by neuraxial anesthesia or obstetric hemorrhage, (2) an increase in uterine venous pressure, perhaps caused by obstructed uterine venous return, or (3) an increase in tissue pressure, perhaps caused by obesity, short maternal stature, or a large uterus (via Laplace's law). Please note the particularly bad effect that uterine enlargement has on myometrial wall tension, and hence on both myometrial oxygen demand and supply: an enlarged uterus at a given intracavitary pressure has a higher wall tension than a normal-sized uterus with the same intracavitary pressure. This is Laplace's law. But in the real world, the physical size limitations of the abdominal cavity will probably increase overall intra-abdominal pressure, which will be at least partially transmitted to the amniotic fluid. Hence, an enlarged uterus will almost certainly have increased intrauterine pressure and (by Laplace's law) will have a greatly increased myometrial wall tension and tissue pressure. Therefore, in an enlarged uterus, oxygen demand is *increased* because wall tension is increased and there is an increased total amount of myometrial tissue which requires oxygen. Furthermore, oxygen supply is *decreased* because myometrial tissue pressure is increased, which decreases myometrial perfusion pressure through the mechanism of "sluice flow." On top of these disadvantages, the large uterus, by its very size, has an increased probability of obstructing its own venous return, compared to a smaller uterus! *The final result is that uterine "overdistention" (a large uterus) can be expected to cause multiple problems in obstetrics, and that obstructed uterine venous return—if present—can only be expected to make those problems worse*. *BP* arterial blood pressure, *LVEDP* left ventricular end-diastolic pressure

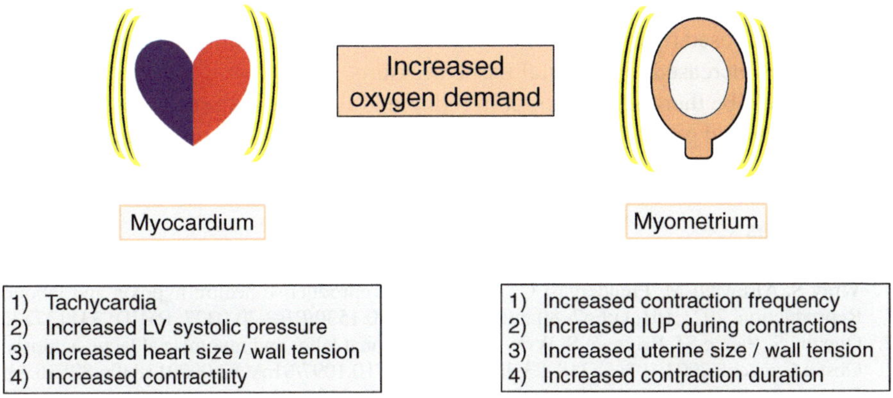

Fig. 9.5 The causes of increased myocardial and myometrial oxygen demand. Both the heart and the uterus are muscular organs which require oxygen in order to contract, and the more frequently they contract, the more oxygen they require. Furthermore, both organs receive oxygenated blood only between contractions—and not during them. In other words, the more frequently both muscular chambers contract, the more oxygen they require and the less they get! Laplace's law applies to both organs as well, which means that for a given intracavitary pressure, the larger the chamber, the greater the wall tension and the greater the oxygen consumption. So, in summary, a large uterus which contracts frequently will need much more oxygen than a small uterus which contracts less often. *IUP* intrauterine pressure, *LV* left ventricular

Summary

1. Unlike the heart, the myometrium's supply and demand for oxygen—independent of the oxygen requirements of the fetus—have received very little attention. During labor, the focus is on the fetus and there appears to be little interest in the myometrium's independent oxygen needs during both labor and earlier in gestation.
2. The same analytic approach can be used for the myometrium as for the heart, focusing on the following facts:
3. Laplace's law applies to both organs. Both a large heart and a large ("overdistended") myometrium have oxygen supplies that are precarious in comparison to those of smaller organs, because of increased oxygen demand and decreased oxygen supply when the organs are larger.
4. Both organs are perfused only between contractions.
5. For both organs, increased frequency of contractions increases oxygen demand and reduces oxygen supply.
6. Myocardial tissue pressure can be estimated from the left ventricular end-diastolic pressure, and elevations of left ventricular end-diastolic pressure are associated with myocardial infarction and heart failure. Elevations of myometrial tissue pressure could be caused by a large uterus (from Laplace's law) or

from external pressure from an obese abdominal wall or from the other constraints imposed by maternal short stature. Lateral positioning may reduce some causes of increased myometrial tissue pressure.

7. There may be therapeutic benefit in reducing myometrial tissue pressure during both labor and gestation to protect both the fetus and the myometrium.

References

1. Wray S, Alruwaili M, Prendergast C. Hypoxia and reproductive health: hypoxia and labour. Reproduction. 2021;161(1):F67–80. https://doi.org/10.1530/REP-20-0327. PMID: 33112773.
2. Quenby S, Pierce SJ, Brigham S, Wray S. Dysfunctional labor and myometrial lactic acidosis. Obstet Gynecol. 2004;103(4):718–23. https://doi.org/10.1097/01.AOG.0000118306.82556.43. Erratum in: Obstet Gynecol. 2004;103(6):1344. PMID: 15051564.
3. Wiberg-Itzel E. Amniotic fluid lactate (AFL): a new predictor of labor outcome in dystocic deliveries. J Matern Fetal Neonatal Med. 2022;35(25):7306–11. https://doi.org/10.1080/14767058.2021.1946790. Epub 2021 Nov 10. PMID: 34758684.
4. Archer TL. Obstructed uterine venous return: a preventable cause of dysfunctional labor? Reproduction. 2021;161(4):V15–7. https://doi.org/10.1530/REP-21-0002. PMID: 33617462.
5. Archer TL. Obstetric anesthesia: a case-based and visual approach. Chapter 32. Archer TL ed. Springer Nature Switzerland AG.
6. Li YY, Bush CA, Orsini A, Mi Z, Leier CV. Predictors of inpatient outcomes in hospitalized patients after left heart catheterization. Am J Cardiol. 2009;103(4):486–90. https://doi.org/10.1016/j.amjcard.2008.10.012. Epub 2008 Dec 25. PMID: 19195507.
7. Salem R, Denault AY, Couture P, Bélisle S, Fortier A, Guertin MC, Carrier M, Martineau R. Left ventricular end-diastolic pressure is a predictor of mortality in cardiac surgery independently of left ventricular ejection fraction. Br J Anaesth. 2006;97(3):292–7. https://doi.org/10.1093/bja/ael140. Epub 2006 Jul 11. PMID: 16835254.

Discussion and Suggestions for Research 10

A Well-Known Problem Hiding in Plain Sight

On the one hand, the main idea of this book may appear strange and even simplistic—that obstruction of uterine venous return by the gravid uterus might play an important role in many of the most serious and well-known disorders of pregnancy—preeclampsia, fetal growth restriction, preterm birth, dysfunctional labor, and postpartum uterine atony and infection. On the other hand, it is well-known and well-accepted that positional obstruction of uterine venous return does occur and that it can cause acute problems during the second half of gestation and—especially—late in pregnancy. The need to avoid aortocaval compression and the supine hypotensive syndrome of pregnancy when caring for pregnant patients is such a well-accepted principle of general medical care that one might say it is *a well-known problem hiding in plain sight* during the second half of gestation. It seems plausible that such a well-known anatomical problem could harm the fetus, placenta, myometrium, and vagina in the second half of pregnancy in a slow and insidious manner that was much less dramatic—and much harder to recognize—than the maternal hypotension, loss of consciousness, and acute fetal distress which are commonly associated with acute aortocaval compression and the supine hypotensive syndrome of pregnancy.

The validity of this theory—and the possible value of investigating it—does not depend on any specific technology or method for detecting obstruction of uterine venous return. The purpose of this book is to point out that such obstruction probably occurs with some frequency during the second half of gestation, that it might harm the fetus, placenta, myometrium, and vagina in a subtle and unrecognized way, and that it deserves further investigation. How it is investigated is an open question, but we have proposed that positional reductions in maternal cardiac output can be used as an objective indicator of positional obstruction of uterine venous return at the inferior vena cava.

T. L. Archer, *Threats to Fetal, Placental and Myometrial Oxygenation*,
https://doi.org/10.1007/978-3-031-60364-8_10

The Special Danger from *Venous* Obstruction to Uteroplacental Perfusion and Cardiac Output

Figures 1.11 and 1.12 show four locations at which placental perfusion might be limited within the maternal and uterine circulations: (1) at the spiral arteries of the placenta, (2) by maternal cardiovascular disease which limits cardiac output, (3) by obstruction of the inferior vena cava with decreased cardiac output and increased uterine venous pressure, and (4) by increased myometrial tissue pressure which increases the resistance of the placental and myometrial vessels which pass through it.

Figure 1.16 shows how a limitation of maternal cardiac output which is imposed from the venous side of the circulation may constitute a particularly dangerous situation for both the mother and the fetus, since uterine and lower body venous obstruction at the inferior vena cava not only decreases cardiac output into the arterial side of the circulation but also increases uterine venous pressure as well, which can directly cause placental dysfunction.

Which Is More Dangerous to the Fetus: Decreased Cardiac Output or Increased Uterine Venous Pressure?

Increased uterine venous pressure from obstruction of uterine venous return may be more of a problem than the reduction in overall maternal cardiac output caused by that obstruction. Another way of saying this is that decreased cardiac output may very well serve as a *signal* or *marker* of obstruction of uterine venous return, *without being the primary cause of the injury due to that obstruction.* Maternal cardiac disease causing a reduction in cardiac output is associated with an increased incidence of both preeclampsia and fetal growth restriction, *but in the case of obstruction of uterine venous return accompanied by a decrease in maternal cardiac output, it may be difficult to know what proportion of the resulting injury comes from the reduction in cardiac output per se and what proportion is due to the increase in uterine venous pressure, which may compress chorionic villi and reduce fetoplacental perfusion in what has been termed "sluice flow* [1]." But one might theorize that both the *flow* and the *pressure* effects of obstruction of uterine venous return can be harmful and that they both should be prevented, if possible.

Uterine Venous Pressure

A key assumption of this book is that when obstruction of uterine venous return occurs, uterine venous pressure increases. On the one hand, this effect would seem obvious, but its potential significance is so great that the fact should be established beyond the shadow of a doubt, and its effect should be understood quantitatively. When I have discussed aortocaval compression with other health care professionals, they immediately focus on its effect on maternal cardiac output and blood pressure, *but almost no one seems to consider what might be happening on the venous side of the uterine circulation* [2]. Even authors who have emphasized the importance of the venous system in pregnancy may not have paid sufficient attention to the possible importance of obstruction of uterine venous return in the pathogenesis of pregnancy-related diseases.

An increase in uterine venous pressure may be more harmful overall than a modest decrease in cardiac output or blood pressure. Not only would increased uterine venous pressure decrease uteroplacental perfusion (thereby decreasing the pO_2 in the intervillous space) but it would also increase the hydrostatic pressure within the intervillous space. This increased hydrostatic pressure might reduce fetoplacental perfusion since the chorionic villi have been shown to be compressible. This situation in which chorionic villus tissue pressure exceeds extra-placental umbilical venous pressure—and therefore functions as the limiting factor on chorionic villus perfusion—has been termed "sluice flow [1]". One can therefore imagine that increased uterine venous pressure may be a *double threat* to fetal, placental, and myometrial oxygenation—from the maternal side but also from the fetal side of the placenta's double circulation. For these reasons, the possible deleterious effects of increased uterine venous pressure on the fetus and myometrium should be a focus of research.

Separate and Differing Oxygen Needs for the Fetus, Placenta, and Myometrium

A common implicit assumption—at least regarding labor—appears to be that if the fetus is doing well, then the entire uterus is doing well. This assumption probably arises for at least two reasons: (a) besides the mother, the fetus is the major focus of pregnancy—emotionally, morally, legally, and financially and (b) the almost universal utilization of external fetal heart rate monitoring throughout pregnancy has perhaps distracted attention from a possible need to independently evaluate the well-being of the placenta and the myometrium—apart from that of the fetus. *If it could be accomplished, this independent assessment of the well-being of the placenta and myometrium might provide an opportunity to prevent hypoxic injury to the placenta, fetus, and myometrium—rather than merely detecting its results and timing delivery accordingly!*

The Importance of Myometrial Tissue Pressure for Uteroplacental Perfusion

The myometrium—by means of its wall tension and tissue pressure—has the power to restrict and even eliminate both fetal and myometrial oxygenation! To use a somewhat violent (but accurate) metaphor, the myometrium has a "stranglehold" on the placenta's and its own (myometrial) perfusion and oxygenation. By the time dysfunction or injury of the placenta or myometrium affects the fetal heart rate or myometrial contractility, it may be too late. Hypoxic or ischemic damage to the placenta or myometrium may have already occurred. In other words, changes in fetal heart rate or myometrial performance may be the *end results* of pre-existing and long-standing oxygenation problems for the placenta and myometrium—*which we might have been able to detect and prevent much earlier in gestation or labor.*

Methods for Predicting and Preventing Placental and Myometrial Injury in the Second Half of Pregnancy

No methods exist for evaluating the well-being of the placenta or the myometrium in real time. There is a fetal heart rate monitor for evaluating the well-being of the fetus in real time, but there is no "placental well-being monitor" and there is no "myometrial well-being monitor." Of course, obstetricians frequently measure intrauterine pressure to assess the adequacy of uterine contraction strength, but intrauterine pressure is almost certainly the *result* of the myometrium's well-being (or lack of it), and not the *cause*. *The hemodynamic approach proposed in this book attempts to detect hemodynamic conditions in real time which may be in the process of injuring the placenta or myometrium.* The idea behind the approach I propose is to intervene in the hemodynamics of the second half of pregnancy so as to avoid problems by optimizing fetal, placental, myometrial, and vaginal oxygenation at all times.

Rigorous intervention to optimize oxygenation may be unnecessary in many healthy pregnancies which do not face other health challenges, but it might make an important difference in pregnancies threatened by health problems such as obesity, short stature, diabetes, chronic hypertension, or a genetic predisposition to pre-eclampsia. This is a re-statement of the idea shown in Fig. 1.24 where only the 20% of pregnancies (a hypothetical percentage) affected by a "first hit" vulnerability might be significantly benefited by the prevention of a "second hit" caused by obstruction of uterine venous return. Our emerging capacity to quickly, safely, and easily detect obstruction of uterine venous return would make it viable to screen large numbers of pregnant women during gestation in order to estimate the number of women who might be affected by this problem. Such a screening program should be an early part of future research.

Prevention of Preterm Labor and Birth

There is circumstantial evidence to suggest that maximization of maternal cardiac output and minimization of uterine venous pressure during gestation might prevent or delay preterm birth. Both obesity and short maternal stature are associated with preterm birth and this fact suggests that the cause of preterm birth might have something to do with increased intra-abdominal pressure. Both obesity and short stature will tend to compress the uterine venous system—either at the inferior vena cava or by direct compression of myometrial tissue—and the alternating impairment and restoration of adequate uterine perfusion could trigger preterm birth by the ischemia and reperfusion mechanism or by the fetal hypoxic stress mechanism as discussed in Chap. 7. Changes in the vaginal microbiome conducive to infectious chorioamnionitis are also possible results of obstruction of lower body venous return at the inferior vena cava, much as lower body edema is a known and common occurrence in pregnancy.

If there is a positional component to this impaired perfusion, then perhaps cardiac output-guided maternal positioning could help delay delivery and allow more time for intrauterine fetal development. Avoidance of obstruction of uterine venous return using cardiac output-guided maternal positioning might be effective only if used before the onset of premature labor or—in the case of non-infectious causes of preterm labor—it might be used to stop preterm labor even after it has started.

Preterm Birth: Research Suggestions

Exploratory research might compare the degree of positional variation of cardiac output in patients admitted to the hospital because of preterm labor, with the variation seen in patients who do not experience preterm labor. Alternatively, a randomized therapeutic trial could be performed on patients admitted to the hospital because of preterm labor, with one group receiving standard care while the other group received standard care plus cardiac output-guided maternal positioning.

Prevention of Dysfunctional Labor and Uterine Atony

A study of the use of cardiac output-guided maternal positioning for the prevention or treatment of dysfunctional labor would give results quickly since the endpoints—cesarean or vaginal delivery—would be clear-cut and immediate. As in the case of preterm labor, the "position therapy" could be initiated in two ways: (1) only if dysfunctional labor develops, in an attempt to restore myometrial function via "intramaternal resuscitation of the uterus" or (2) it could be administered to all patients at the onset of labor, in an attempt to prevent dysfunctional labor by providing maximum myometrial perfusion and oxygenation throughout the entire course of labor. If cardiac output-guided maternal positioning were found to decrease the incidence of dysfunctional labor, such management might bring the "best of both worlds" to labor—a pain-free labor (with an epidural) and the possible optimal uteroplacental perfusion benefits of the high maternal mobility encouraged by midwives.

Prevention of Preeclampsia and Fetal Growth Restriction

Both preeclampsia and fetal growth restriction appear to develop over the course of weeks or even months, and any hemodynamic intervention to prevent, delay, or reduce the injury from these disorders would probably have to be maintained for a relatively long period of time. Spinapolice et al. [3] showed a reduction in the incidence of preeclampsia in women who spent four hours per day resting in the left lateral position, but to the best of my knowledge this study has not been repeated. Furthermore, the study as performed seems to have had the limitation *that it was implicitly assumed that resting in the left lateral position relieved obstruction of uterine venous return and that patients who did not rest in that position for four hours per day did experience obstruction of uterine venous return.* A similar study should be performed now, but this time utilizing the objective determination of the positional uterine hemodynamics of each patient, rather than making assumptions about uterine perfusion based solely on patient position.

The therapeutic intervention possibly required—that of avoiding those maternal positions associated with a reduced cardiac output—might or might not be inconvenient for the patient, but we do not have any knowledge of the dimensions of the potential problem of obstruction of uterine venous return earlier in gestation. Suffice it to say that if it were shown that prevention of obstruction of uterine venous return using cardiac output-guided maternal positioning reduced the incidence or severity of preeclampsia or fetal growth restriction, this would be a powerful inducement to a pregnant woman to cooperate with the daily "position therapy" required. If proven to be effective, *such "position therapy" would hopefully be seen—by the mother herself, her care-givers, and by society at large—as a beneficial part of routine prenatal care* which would increase the probability that babies would be born in the best possible condition for achieving their full potential during the rest of their lives. The inconvenience involved in prenatal "position therapy" would hopefully be perceived as more than justified by the fact that such treatment would reduce the future burden of disability on individuals, families, and society.

Choice of Cardiac Output Trending Technology for Future Research

At least three technologies have been widely used for the measurement and trending of maternal cardiac output during pregnancy: transthoracic echocardiography, the USCOM Doppler monitor [4], and impedance cardiography (with electrical cardiometry as an example of that technology). MRI scanning has begun to be used for research purposes but is time-consuming and costly and appears to be impractical for widespread clinical use at this time.

Transthoracic Echocardiography May Not Be the Best Reference Standard for Studies of Positional changes of Maternal Cardiac Output During Pregnancy

"Formal" transthoracic echocardiography, which acquires cardiac images and velocity-time integrals through echocardiographic "windows" in the chest wall, may not be suitable for measuring cardiac output in all relevant maternal positions, since the transthoracic echocardiography view required for measurement of the velocity–time integral (VTI) is usually acquired most easily from the left lateral position and may be unobtainable from the supine or right lateral positions.

The USCOM Doppler Hemodynamic Monitor

Unlike "formal" transthoracic echocardiography, the USCOM Doppler monitor obtains the velocity–time integral from the ascending aorta through the sternal notch echocardiographic window at the base of the neck, and this sternal notch window for obtaining the velocity–time integral will probably work well in all maternal positions. Much valuable hemodynamic research in pregnancy has been performed using both the USCOM monitor and formal transthoracic echocardiography, but both of these technologies require the presence and intervention of a trained operator whenever hemodynamic measurements are required, since the technique is not hands-free. If electrical cardiometry—or any other continuous and hands-free technology (such as bioreactance or optical plethysmography)—is found to trend satisfactorily with USCOM, that other technology might be a more convenient and ultimately more useful alternative to USCOM for the detection of obstruction of uterine venous return. This replacement of USCOM by an easier-to-use, continuous, and hands-free technology might be another fruitful area for research. Other even simpler surrogate techniques for trending maternal cardiac output might also be developed, such as optical plethysmography or even heart rate and its variation.

Closing Appeal for More Research

At present, we have very little systematic knowledge about the incidence—let alone the impact—of obstruction of uterine venous return during pregnancy. The potential benefit of this research is great, and I hope that someone reading this book decides to investigate further. I hope that you have enjoyed reading this book and that some of the ideas presented in it will be of use to you in your clinical care and future research.

References

1. Power GG, Longo LD. Sluice flow in placenta: maternal vascular pressure effects on fetal circulation. Am J Phys. 1973;225(6):1490–6. https://doi.org/10.1152/ajplegacy.1973.225.6.1490. PMID: 4202497.
2. Gyselaers W. Origins of abnormal placentation: why maternal veins must not be forgotten. Am J Obstet Gynecol. 2023;228(6):613–21. https://doi.org/10.1016/j.ajog.2022.12.014. Epub 2022 Dec 17. PMID: 36539026.
3. Spinapolice RX, Feld S, Harrigan JT. Effective prevention of gestational hypertension in nulliparous women at high risk as identified by the rollover test. Am J Obstet Gynecol. 1983;146(2):166–8. https://doi.org/10.1016/0002-9378(83)91047-5. PMID: 6846433.
4. Information from the manufacturer about the USCOM Doppler hemodynamic monitor can be found at: https://www.uscom.com.au/products/uscom1a/overview/.

Index

T. L. Archer, *Threats to Fetal, Placental and Myometrial Oxygenation*,
https://doi.org/10.1007/978-3-031-60364-8

E

F

H

I

L

M

N

O

GPSR Compliance

The European Union's (EU) General Product Safety Regulation (GPSR) is a set of rules that requires consumer products to be safe and our obligations to ensure this.

If you have any concerns about our products, you can contact us on ProductSafety@springernature.com

In case Publisher is established outside the EU, the EU authorized representative is:

Springer Nature Customer Service Center GmbH
Europaplatz 3
69115 Heidelberg, Germany

Batch number: 10732090

Printed by Printforce, the Netherlands